Preoperative Assessment and Perioperative Management

Edited by

Mark Radford
Divisional Director of Nursing (Surgery) University Hospitals
Coventry and Warwickshire NHS Trust, UK
Visiting Professor at Birmingham City University, UK

Alastair Williamson
Consultant Anaesthetist
Good Hope Hospital, Heart of England Foundation Trust, UK

Clare Evans
Consultant Nurse (Perioperative care) Bristol Royal Infirmary,
United Bristol Healthcare NHS Trust, UK

Preoperative Assessment and Perioperative Management
Mark Radford
Claire Evans
Alastair Williamson

ISBN: 978-1-905539-02-4

First published 2011

Illustrations by Mary Blood except figures 6.6 and 6.7 reproduced from David Lynes (ed.), *The Management of COPD in Primary and Secondary Care* (M&K Publishing, 2007)

Photographs copyright © The Contributors, 2011.

British Library Cataloguing in Publication Data

A catalogue record for this book is available from the British Library

Notice

Clinical practice and medical knowledge constantly evolve. Standard safety precautions must be followed, but, as knowledge is broadened by research, changes in practice, treatment and drug therapy may become necessary or appropriate. Readers must check the most current product information provided by the manufacturer of each drug to be administered and verify the dosages and correct administration, as well as contraindications. It is the responsibility of the practitioner, utilising the experience and knowledge of the patient, to determine dosages and the best treatment for each individual patient. Any brands mentioned in this book are as examples only and are not endorsed by the publisher. Neither the publisher nor the authors assume any liability for any injury and/or damage to persons or property arising from this publication.

To contact M&K Publishing write to:

M&K Update Ltd · The Old Bakery · St. John's Street

Keswick · Cumbria CA12 5AS

Tel: 01768 773030 · Fax: 01768 781099

publishing@mkupdate.co.uk

www.mkupdate.co.uk

Designed by Mary Blood

Typeset in 10pt Univers Light

Printed in England by Reeds Printers, Penrith

Contents

PREFACE

Preoperative assessment of the surgical patient is a key part of the perioperative process. However, it is one that cannot be separated from the other aspects of perioperative management, both clinical and administrative, that ensure the safe and effective treatment of surgical patients. There are a number of books on the market that examine perioperative management, anaesthesia and surgical nursing that are only able to touch on the preoperative assessment process. *Preoperative Assessment and Perioperative Management* sets out to be different, by bridging the gap between these texts and the evolving and developing area of practice that preoperative assessment has become in modern healthcare.

In order to achieve this, *Preoperative Assessment and Perioperative Management* aims to deliver the core clinical aspects of practice, linked to the education and service development needs of a perioperative service. The challenge for such a book is to integrate this knowledge effectively, using the best evidence base, for use in everyday practice. The brief to the contributors was to help define preoperative assessment using their expertise to highlight best practice. They have achieved this, ensuring that the reader has access to the thoughts of some of the leading experts in international perioperative practice. The contributors have done this in an open and accessible style that will guide readers through some complex and demanding subjects to enable them to deliver better frontline care to surgical patients.

Preoperative Assessment and Perioperative Management is also a helpful text for a range of professionals who wish to understand more about the management of patients undergoing surgery.

Preoperative Assessment and Perioperative Management covers three main aspects:

- the core clinical skills and knowledge to assess patients prior to surgery
- specialist areas of preoperative practice
- service development and management of the perioperative systems.

We hope that you enjoy reading this book, as much as we enjoyed editing it.

Mark Radford
Alastair Williamson
Clare Evans

Acknowledgements

MR

I would like to thank (once again!) Sam, Ellie and Isobel for putting up with me doing another publishing idea on top of an already busy life. To Alastair, Clare, Mike and Ken (MandK) for persevering with this project that seems to have gone on for a lifetime, and next time I shall take your advice. Finally, to all the perioperative staff at Good Hope Hospital, who have in their own small way contributed to this book over the years of working with you all.

CE

I would like to thank my family and friends for their support and encouragement – yet again. To all the staff I have worked with in Oxford, London and Bristol who have brought rich experiences to my working life, making this journey an adventure. Lastly, thanks to Mark, for the invitation to share this experience – please learn to take no as a final answer!

Professor Mark Radford BSc (Hons), RGN, PGDip (ANP), MA (Med. Ed.), ENB 183

Mark Radford is currently Divisonal Director of Nursing for Surgery at University Hospitals Coventry and Warwickshire and a Visiting Professsor of Nursing at Birmingham City University. He was previously a Consultant Nurse in Perioperative Emergency Care at Good Hope Hospital, part of Heart of England Foundation Trust. His clinical work has focused on the management of emergency surgery and trauma patients. As a nurse he has previously worked in anaesthetics, preoperative assessment, critical care and AandE in the UK and Europe. He has also worked as an adviser to the Department of Health, NCEPOD, MHRA and NICE on a range of areas including perioperative hypothermia, emergency management and nurse prescribing. He has published widely on advanced practice nursing and perioperative care. His research focuses on clinical decision-making, expertise and sociological issues in healthcare.

Dr Alastair Williamson MB ChB (Cantab), FRCA

Dr Alastair Williamson is a Consultant Anaesthetist at Good Hope Hospital, part of Heart of England Foundation Trust. Since his appointment in 1999, he has been actively involved in the support and development of Preoperative Assessment Services at the hospital, and in particular the development of the role of the Perioperative Emergency Care Team. He was involved locally and nationally as an Anaesthetic Clinical Lead in the NHS Modernisation Agency's National Theatre and Preoperative Assessment Programme. He has presented at national and international conferences on the role of preoperative assessment in modern surgical services. Based on this work, he has developed a keen interest in process re-design and the use of Lean Six Sigma methodologies in clinical re-design both in emergency and elective clinical pathways. Clinically he has a keen interest in total intravenous anaesthesia (TIVA), both for major colorectal surgery and day case surgery.

Clare Evans RGN, BSc (Hons), MSc (ANP)

Clare Evans is currently a Consultant Nurse, Perioperative Care, at University Hospitals Bristol Foundation Trust. Her clinical work is focused on improving quality and safety of care for surgical patients, supporting the preoperative assessment and optimisation of elective surgical patients and developing a day of surgery admission unit. She has previously worked as a Consultant Nurse at Chelsea and Westminster Healthcare NHS Trust and as Nurse Practitioner, Neurosurgery, in Oxford. Her interests lie in developing nursing practice and hospital processes to offer quality patient care.

Contributors

Dr John Andrzejowski MB ChB, FRCA
Consultant Neurosurgical Anaesthetist
Royal Hallamshire Hospital, Sheffield

Dr Andrew Blann PhD, FRCPath
Consultant Clinical Scientist and Senior Lecturer
University Department of Medicine, City Hospital, Birmingham, UK

Dr John Carlisle BSc, MB ChB, MRCP, FRCA
Consultant Anaesthetist
South Devon Healthcare NHS Foundation Trust

Mrs Clare Hammond RGN, BA (Hons)
Day Case Unit Nurse Manager
University Hospital of North Staffordshire, Stafford, UK

Dr Munirul Haque MBBS, MRCP (UK)
Consultant Physician (Acute Medicine)
Good Hope Hospital, Heart of England Foundation Trust

Ms Christine Hughes RGN, DipN, Cert Ed, BSc (Hons), CAS
Perioperative Specialist Practitioner
East Cheshire NHS Trust

Mr Ciaran Hurley RN, MA, BMedSci, PGDipEd
Senior Lecturer
University of Sheffield, Sheffield, UK

Dr David Kennedy BSc, PhD, CSci, FRCPath
Consultant Clinical Scientist (Biochemistry)
Good Hope Hospital, Heart of England Foundation Trust

Mrs Liz Kenny RGN, BSc (Hons)
Staff Nurse
Calderdale Royal Hospital, Halifax, West Yorkshire, UK

Dr Ross Kerridge MB BS, FRCA, FANZCA
Director of Perioperative Services
John Hunter Hospital, New South Wales, Australia

Dr Stefan Jankowski MB ChB, FRCA
Consultant Neurosurgical Anaesthetist
Royal Hallamshire Hospital, Sheffield

Liz Lees RGN, Dip N, BSc (Hons), Dip HSM, Msc
Consultant Nurse (Acute Medicine)
Birmingham Heartlands Hospital
Heart of England Foundation Trust, Birmingham, UK

Dr David Lynes PhD, BSc (Hons), Dpsn, EGN, RGN Head of Education
Respiratory Education UK
University Hospital Aintree, UK

Dr Simon Moore MB, ChB, FRCA
Consultant Anaesthetist
Good Hope Hospital, Heart of England Foundation Trust, UK

Dr Cheng Ong FRCA
Consultant Anaesthetist
Guy's and St Thomas' Hospital, London, UK

Dr Adrian Pearce FRCA
Consultant Anaesthetist
Guy's and St Thomas' Hospital, London, UK

Mrs Helen Pickard RGN, BSc, MSc (ANP), PGCert (Med. Ed.)
Consultant Nurse (Acute Medicine)
Good Hope Hospital, Heart of England Foundation Trust

Dr Sudarshan Ramachandran BSc, MRCS, LRCP, PhD, FRCPath
Consultant Chemical Pathologist
Good Hope Hospital, Heart of England Foundation Trust

Dr Ian Smith Bsc, MB BS, MD, FRCA
Consultant Anaesthetist and Senior Lecturer
University Hospital of North Staffordshire, Stafford, UK

Dr Jonathan Thompson BSc (Hons), MB, ChB, MD, FRCA
Senior Lecturer and Honorary Consultant,
University of Leicester and University Hospital Leicester NHS Trust, UK

Mrs Hilary Walsgrove RGN, DPSN, BSc, MSc
Senior Lecturer
Bournemouth University, UK

Dr Simon P. Young MB ChB, MD, FRCA
Specialist Registrar and Honorary Lecturer,
University of Leicester and University Hospital Leicester NHS Trust, UK

Chapter **1**

The evolving role of the preoperative assessment team

Liz Kenny

SUMMARY

This chapter will describe:
- the development of preoperative assessment in the UK
- the development of the preoperative assessment nurse role and benefits of nurse-led POA
- the role of the nurse in preoperative assessment
- the future role of preoperative assessment
- collaboration between POA nurses, anaesthetists and allied healthcare professionals.

INTRODUCTION

This chapter discusses the development of the preoperative assessment team (POA) by reviewing published and unpublished sources and also integrates personal experiences. It discusses studies that compare the work of dedicated preoperative assessment teams, including nurses and doctors, and the importance of a collaborative role with allied healthcare professionals.

The development of preoperative assessment and the role of the nurse

Preoperative assessment in the UK has traditionally been carried out by medical staff. In 1972, nursing staff were identified as having some involvement in POA on a general surgical ward in Cardiff; however, nurses were simply acknowledged as part of the process.[1] As the specialty of POA has evolved, the role of the nurse has been enhanced and developed.

This has been reflected in the last 15 years as many health organisations and government departments have produced policies, protocols and guidance advising on how POA services and roles should be developed (see Box 1.1). Since the 1990s, many studies and articles have been published concerning the POA specialty; the majority have the nurse in a pivotal role in the POA process. Some authors describe the nurse's role as that of a coordinator, liaising between the patient/carers and other healthcare professionals to ensure the patient's surgical journey is smooth. This is consistent with the developing role of the POA nurse.[2,3,4,5]

Box 1.1 Policies, protocols and guidance affecting the POA nurse's role

1991 New Deal for Junior Doctors (Calman-Hine Report) – NHS Management Executive. London: HMSO

1992 Scope of Professional Practice – UKCC, London

1997 The New NHS: Modern and Dependable – Department of Health. London: HMSO

1999 Making a Difference. Strengthening the Nursing, Midwifery and Health Visiting Contribution to Health and Healthcare – Department of Health. London: HMSO

2000 NHS Plan – Department of Health. London: HMSO

2001 Preoperative assessment: The role of the anaesthetist – Association of Anaesthetists of Great Britain and Ireland

2002 Improving Orthopaedic Services: A guide for clinicians, managers and commissioners. NHS Modernisation Agency

2002 Functioning as a Team? – The National Confidential Enquiry into Perioperative Deaths

2002 National good practice guidance for day surgery – NHS Modernisation Agency

2003 National good practice guidance on preoperative assessment for inpatient surgery – NHS Modernisation Agency

2003 European Working Time Directive – Council of the European Union (2003/88/EC).

2005 Nurse Practitioners: an RCN guide to the nurse practitioner role, competencies and accreditation – RCN

In the mid-1990s, the registered nurse in POA is described as a coordinator, performing general observations such as blood pressure recordings and urinalysis, giving information to the patient about their forthcoming admission, treatment and further information about any special requirements whilst the senior house officer performs the clerking of the patient and orders tests.[6] In Liverpool, Australia, authors describe nurses in the POA and Same Day Admission Unit reviewing patients who do not need medical input, although the role of the nurse was not further specified.[7] By 2000, the nurse's role is described as multifunctional, addressing many factors affecting the patient's admission to hospital, making appropriate arrangements and referrals to ensure the patient journey is smooth both in and out of hospital.[4]

The 2002 National Confidential Enquiry into Perioperative Deaths (NCEPOD)[8], highlighted the fact that the surgeon was no longer the only consultant involved or responsible for the individual patient's care, implying a shared care responsibility, which had eroded the continuity previously in place in the UK NHS. An example of fragmented and substandard multi-disciplinary care was reported in 2005 that had resulted in an untimely death. This led to recommendations that the lead clinician role should be revitalised to minimise oversights generated by a growing number of teams and to improve continuity in care.[9] Historically, at the author's hospital, the POA nurse role incorporated the task of monitoring and promoting the ongoing treatment of a caseload of patients deemed unfit for surgery, through case management. This activity ensures that a healthcare professional with medical knowledge and experience oversees the care of an unfit patient who still requires surgery by promoting communication between teams of allied health professionals (AHPs) in primary and secondary care, surgeons, anaesthetists and physicians, to achieve the goal of safe admission. Previously a surgical secretary with limited medical knowledge and limited access to medical advice undertook this aspect of care. However it is clearly more suitable for this practice to be integrated into the national role of the POA nurse.

Gradually, additional clinical focus was attached to the POA nurse role and the valuable input of health promotion was incorporated[3,6,10,11] as advised in the core principles of the NHS Plan in 2000. A 1997 paper[12] described the results of a study in which 30 surgical patients were advised by POA nurses to stop smoking preoperatively using the method routinely practised and a further 30 were given additional health promotion input. Patients described the approach used by the POA nurse and the leaflet devised for the study as most helpful. This additional input improved the rate of reducing and stopping smoking from 50% of the routine group to 80% of the treatment group. The collaborative role of health promotion in the POA clinic has also been examined in Liverpool, Australia,[13] in a study in a POA clinic in which 124 patients were randomly assigned to an experimental group and 86 patients to the routine care pathway in an attempt to improve the standard of smoking cessation information given to patients. A multifaceted intervention was developed which included the use of opinion leaders, consensus processes, computer-delivered cessation care, computer-generated prompts for care provision by clinic staff, staff training and performance feedback. POA nurses were more efficient than the anaesthetists in both groups and it was considered that this was for two reasons. Firstly, the anaesthetists did not receive any performance feedback. Secondly, the anaesthetists may have felt they were offering redundant advice that had been previously given in the POA clinic.

A natural addition to the role of the POA nurse is to act as a central point of contact for the patient, as a named nurse, and as a link between primary and secondary care for patients.[3,10] Qualified nurses remain the central figure for the patient in need, are often said to be valuable to patients, are expected to know about individual plans of care, meet needs and be an advocate even though much direct care is being performed by unqualified members of staff.[14] It has been reported that patients feel more at ease with a POA nurse than with a doctor, are more relaxed about answering medical questions and feel more able to ask medical questions, although no evidence supporting these assumptions is discussed in the paper.[15]

As discussed previously, the POA nurse role has been promoted in many NHS policies. Increasing commercial pressure in the NHS has led to the role of the POA nurse expanding to include taking on more clinical interventions and case management. At the author's hospital the POA nurse has a generalist role, preoperatively assessing in a nurse-led unit for multiple surgical specialties with the support of an Integrated Care Pathway (ICP) and local guidelines and protocols. In other areas of the world, the role of the POA nurse is dedicated to a single surgical specialism, dictated by the size of the local population, hospital or Trust or popularity of the specialism. Box 1.2 shows examples of the variety of POA specialisms although it must be noted that the list of specialties is not exhaustive.

An example of a POA nurse working away from the POA clinic is described at the Good Hope Hospital, Birmingham, where a POA service for emergency surgical patients ensures rapid access to surgery.[16] The nurse is able to coordinate the surgical care process from AandE, to the ward then into theatre. The role supports the anaesthetic, surgical and nursing teams by assisting in the prioritisation and optimisation of the patient's condition and by initiating investigations and prompting further treatment. The development of the POA nurse role in this manner proves that the knowledge and skills are highly adaptable and effective.

Nurse-led POA has been discussed since the 1990s but the lack of POA nurse education programmes leads one to assume that training must be undertaken 'in-house'.[17] A 1996 article written by a POA nurse highlighted the lack of structured training programmes when she described being trained 'in-house' for her new POA role[18] and others too have discussed 'in-house' training programmes[16,19] developed to allow a study of the appropriateness of nurse-led preoperative assessment. The development of a competency framework has been recommended, incorporating a range of strategies to evaluate the skills and performance of the POA nurse and assess by observation, witness testimony and self-assessment.[17] The use of a competency framework would ensure that consistent standards of education are met locally and nationally, to achieve safe practice in POA. Such a framework would standardise 'in-house' POA nurse training programmes but would need to follow a rigorous guideline development process by a group of POA healthcare experts. An example of such a focused preoperative competency framework can be seen in Chapter 20.

University-based POA education is now available in the UK. The POA book and CD *Preoperative Assessment: Setting a Standard through Learning*[20] and on-line 'e-learning' modules run by the University of Southampton are evidence of a need for knowledge, skills and theory-based education. A POA lead nurse developed two BSc modules in 'POA assessment and planning' and 'Health assessment and physical examination' that run at Bournemouth University.[21] Other university-based courses are currently available – for example, a module called 'Principles in pre-assessment' at De Montfort University in Leicester addresses current developments, management issues, legislative influences and the expanding role of the POA

Box 1.2 Preoperative assessment specialist areas

From The Preoperative Association First National Conference Abstract Book 2004 and The Preoperative Association Second National Conference Abstract Book 2005

Orthopaedics

Lancashire Teaching Hospitals NHS Trust

East Birmingham PCT and Birmingham Heartlands and Solihull NHS Trust

Manchester Royal Infirmary

The Robert Jones and Agnes Hunt Orthopaedic and District Hospital

Leeds Teaching Hospitals

The Conquest Hospital, St Leonards-on-Sea

York Hospital

Hillingdon Hospital, Uxbridge

Day Case Surgery

Kidderminster Hospital

Mid Yorkshire NHS Trust

Derbyshire Royal Infirmary

Urology

Hope Hospital, Salford

Paediatrics

Chelsea and Westminster Hospital, London

Radiotherapy, Plastics and Burns

St Albans City Hospital, Hertfordshire

Cardiothoracic Surgery

King's College Hospital NHS Trust

Opthalmology

North Cheshire Hospitals NHS Trust

Emergency Care

Good Hope Hospital, Sutton Coldfield

Chelsea and Westminster Hospital, London

nurse. The module also focuses on practical aspects of POA and critically explores areas such as clinical examination, history taking and anaesthetic practice. Bangor University has recently developed a POA module where students are to be taught physical assessment skills, neck and airway assessment, respiratory assessment, cardiovascular assessment, management of clinical conditions and many other preoperative assessment-related topics. Sadly, the York University 'Principles of pre-assessment' module is no longer running.

Physical examination skills, including auscultation, are being performed by POA nurses[10,22] although there is ongoing debate as to its necessity. Some POA nurses have been trained to Masters level in anatomy, physical examination and test ordering modules.[23,24] A small study to compare safety and appropriateness of POA nurses assessing patients, instead of junior doctors, found the nurses to be effective in their practice and superior in their history taking.[25] The POA nurses were given 30 hours' training in history taking and the physical examination skills of inspection, palpation, percussion and auscultation. The Southampton-based team argues that, although the nurses were trained in physical examination and the study found they were effective in their practice, further evidence pertaining to nurses performing these skills should be sought to examine if it can be safely undertaken before allowing it to become common practice. In 1996, POA nurses in the US were performing physical examination.[26] Another US paper reports Nurse Practitioners (NP) (qualified nurses educated to a degree level, employed in a NP post) assessing patients preoperatively.[27] Part of their role is to perform physical examination skills but the paper does not discuss specific POA training, education or type of documentation used to support the role. The Association of Anaesthetists of Great Britain and Ireland (AAGBI)[28] suggests the POA nurse uses a screening questionnaire to identify patients with health problems and, when these patients are identified, that they should be seen by a surgical or anaesthetic house officer who should perform the preliminary clerking and examination of the patient. In a number of studies and geographical locations, robust questionnaires are used in the nurse-led preoperative assessment process which don't incorporate physical examination skills and this has not been reported as an omission in care provision.[15,29-32] At the author's hospital, auscultation is not performed by the POA nurses as it is thought that history taking skills are effective in assessing any undiagnosed or uncontrolled abnormalities. Local anecdotal evidence supports the view that efficient history taking provides enough information to identify patients with uncontrolled or undiagnosed health conditions.

The preoperative assessment team

Preoperative assessment management involves the coordination of a range of healthcare professionals in the management of care, including medical staff, nurses, and allied healthcare professionals (AHPs). To improve the care provided to patients, POA nurses should be aware of AHPs who can assist and enhance the patient's surgical journey. In most UK NHS hospitals, POA services actively promote and incorporate interdisciplinary collaboration of AHPs in primary and secondary care, including physiotherapists, occupational therapists, clerical staff and specialist nurses such as stoma care, breast care and diabetic nurses and, predominantly, anaesthetists. In addition, the POA nurse is a member of a team with mixed skills including qualified nurses, clerical coordinators and healthcare assistants, allowing the POA nurse to dedicate their time to clinical duties instead of clerical duties.

A multi-disciplinary and multi-agency approach is essential in POA, drawing on the skills of appropriate health professionals to ensure the patient is fully prepared to undergo elective surgery.[32] Occupational therapists and physiotherapists within the multi-disciplinary team work in some POA clinics.[33] Even back in 1972 a social worker attended the POA clinic to assist with any 'difficulties regarding social or domestic commitments'.[1] Discharge planning is often mentioned in POA literature and is an integral part of the POA service, involving social services and GP referrals.[7] One POA clinic is reported as involving a theatre nurse, occupational therapists, physiotherapists, a social worker and doctors,[34] describing the clinical and educational collaboration as very effective and also as enjoyable for its participants. Discharge planning is part of the POA nurse's responsibility and should be incorporated into the POA integrated care planning approach, an example of which can be found in Chapter 15.

Pharmacists are involved in POA in some areas. For example, in Dudley, UK the POA nurses were reported to accept that collaboration with the pharmacists was vital for the patient.[35] In another POA clinic, pharmacists attended a POA clinic to review every patient. The POA nurses and doctors and the ward nurses and doctors identified the completing of discharge documentation as the most valuable service.[36]

Nurses or junior doctors in the POA specialism?

As previously stated, traditionally POA has been performed by medical staff, supported by nurses.[2,6] A number of studies have examined the quality of the POA performed by junior doctors and POA nurses and advantages identified if nurses can be viewed as equals in performing POA: the junior doctors can be freed up to participate in the outpatients department, attend theatre and gain further experience in other areas.[37,38] A team from Reading performed a prospective study in which 100 patients were preoperatively assessed by a registered nurse using a proforma and then preoperatively assessed by a junior doctor in the traditional manner.[38] The study made direct comparisons of the information collated by both professional groups excluding physical clinical examination information as it wasn't performed by the nurses. It concluded that the nurse was as accurate as the junior doctor when taking a surgical history. Comparisons of the work of nurses and junior doctors were made in a quantitative study in Southampton, UK, involving 1847 patients from four different surgical sites within the UK.[23] The results were comparable between the two groups: overall 15% in the junior doctors' group made errors possibly affecting management, compared to 13% in the nurses' group.

Further comparisons were undertaken in Epsom, UK, where the effectiveness of pre-admission clerking by both the nurse and doctor was measured.[39] The results revealed that the nurses under-ordered investigations and the doctors over-ordered investigations, which identified a need for a protocol. Both groups cancelled a similar number of patients for health reasons, although the nurses were more likely to make valid referrals for further medical opinion. As no patients seen by either the nurses or doctors had their surgery cancelled due to problems unidentified at POA, it was concluded that nurses were as effective as doctors in the pre-clerking role. In another study, at a nurse-led POA clinic at the Royal Hallamshire in Sheffield,[25] sets of medical notes were examined and the information gathered by doctors was compared to that gathered by the nurses in a nurse-led POA clinic.[31] In their opinion the nurses' documentation was of more value as it contained information regarding anaesthetic history, allergies, family history and medication. In Newcastle, a qualitative study compared the information gathered by nurses using a structured questionnaire in a nurse-led oral surgery day case clinic, to that of information gathered by clinicians in an outpatients department.[15] The review of 57 sets of medical notes highlighted gaps in the information collected by the clinicians, ultimately promoting the use of dedicated time to POA the patient and the use of the questionnaire in the nurse-led clinic. A team from Oxford undertook a quantitative study in which 2726 patients were assessed in a nurse-led POA clinic with a view to being admitted to a short stay mixed surgical ward in a hospital without integrated acute services to support them in the event of a medical emergency.[40] Using guidelines and policies drawn up in collaboration with anaesthetists and surgeons, the nurses were able to POA patients effectively. The rates for cancellation of surgery were 11% in other areas of the Trust where POA did not occur. The study noted a 3.9% cancellation rate in POA clinic and 5% on day of admission. The POA nurses in Oxford and Newcastle were also able to refer patients accordingly to both anaesthetists and surgeons if the need arose.

A growing number of POA services, nationally and internationally, are nurse-led initiatives which result in greater nurse autonomy and better relations with physicians, leading to a positive impact on multi-disciplinary teamwork.[41] They also stated that nurse-led initiatives have been identified in a number of settings and studies suggest better care and patient outcomes, commonly indicating that this may be linked to the nurses' focus on patient involvement, patient education and the ability to provide psychological support. Nurse-led POA offers a more holistic approach to preoperative screening than the traditional medically orientated approach and enhances the service by integrating other duties into the role such as health promotion and discharge planning as previously discussed in this chapter.[11] Following the introduction of nurse-led POA clinics in Grimsby, same day admissions increased from 16% to 60%, which suggests that the initiative may provide major cost benefits for the NHS whilst also enhancing overall patient care.[42]

Collaboration between POA nurses and anaesthetists

From a US perspective, an anaesthesia-based POA service is described where nurses review the medical records of patients.[26] They are also trained to perform physical assessments of patients using standardised protocols and policies and refer patients to the anaesthetists if deemed unfit for surgery. The nurses were trained specifically to assist the anaesthetists following a sharp increase in attendance at the POA centre. A Californian study reports that specially trained nurses are part of an anaesthesia care team.[43] In Utrecht, in the Netherlands, a quantitative research study was performed in which 4540 patients were preoperatively assessed on separate occasions by a specially trained nurse and then by an anaesthetist.[22] The two professional groups agreed on 87% of the patient assessments. The study proposed that nurses could act as diagnostic filters, identifying patients who need further input from the anaesthetists.

Positive results from POA collaboration were seen at the Cromer hospital in East Anglia where a high number of 'on the day' cancellations of day case patients by anaesthetists was noted.[44] A consultant anaesthetist collaborated with the POA staff and his colleagues, and reviewed and re-wrote protocols in 2002 that reduced the cancellation rate from 5% to 2.5% by 2005.

Other POA collaborations include POA nurses working with junior surgeons and anaesthetists when the patient was deemed at risk due to medical status.[37] A study from 2003 reported POA nurses referring 27% of patients to the anaesthetist and 3.1% to surgeons for further advice regarding preoperative care.[40] In 1997, some POA nurses were collecting information from patients and highlighting any potential problems to the consultant surgeon by sending a referral via the secretary.[31] In Calderdale and Huddersfield NHS Trust, the POA nurses perform an assessment which is supported by strict protocols and guidelines incorporated within an ICP. In 2006, a retrospective, unpublished audit of the POA nurse-led service provided evidence that approximately 20% of the total number of patients assessed by the POA nurses were referred to the anaesthesia clinic: 10% following the identification of potentially uncontrolled, undiagnosed or complex health problems and 10% due to the nature of the surgery required, for example, major abdominal surgery.

The future of preoperative assessment

POA has become a permanent part of the elective surgical process, performed by qualified nurses, often using a form of documentation that is integrated into the patient's paper records. However, the Electronic Patient Record (EPR) is the future, when all patients' records will be accessible on line;[45,46] therefore a single IT solution is likely to emerge in the NHS which can link to other aspects of patient care and assessment. There are a number of POA software packages available that advise when preoperative tests are indicated, following the completion of a health questionnaire.[47,48,49] This can be done using touch screen technology, used over the phone with voice recognition software or a touch tone phone, or can be completed remotely, e.g. in the patient's home or GP surgery. These data collection styles have been designed with medical input to ensure valid information is collected. In the US, a study indicated that the use of a computerised POA tool by an anaesthetist increased the number of clinical conditions identified in a set of medical notes, compared to the original process in which trained personnel reviewed medical notes.[50] Another US study indicates that the touchtone phone method was liked by patients, they found the system easy to use (similar to other services such as banking via touch tone phones) and the patients indicated that they were 'likely to be as truthful with their doctor'.[48]

One of the POA software programs generates a preoperative plan,[47] indicating when an anaesthetic assessment is required and could indicate if any additional preoperative tests could be performed before the patient attends the anaesthesia clinic, saving the patient and the hospital valuable time in extra appointments. Risk stratification programs that predict risk according to the patient's health condition[50,51] could be integrated into the program to assist in the filtering of appropriate patients to an anaesthesia clinic, potentially reducing inappropriate referrals (see Chapter 2). Computerised record-keeping data would allow allied health professionals, e.g. physiotherapists and occupational therapists, easy access to a patient's data away from the POA clinic, thus reducing the amount of time a patient spends in the POA clinic.

Computerised POA health questionnaires, designed for completion by a patient, lead one to consider the effect upon a POA service's skill mix. Selection criteria for day case patients are already part of the POA process and could be extended within the POA software package to identify patients with complex or uncontrolled health conditions to be reviewed by a POA nurse who could decide if an anaesthesia assessment is required. Otherwise, healthcare assistants (HCAs) or administration assistants could perform more tasks, such as assisting with completion of the questionnaire. For uncomplicated patients, the same staff could follow the generated preoperative plan, performing general observations, swabs for infection control and providing printed pre- and postoperative information as indicated. At Calderdale and Huddersfield NHS Trust, an HCA implements an individual preoperative plan, devised by the POA nurse at the original POA appointment, when undertaking a telephone questionnaire and making admission arrangements for inpatients. A telephone questionnaire allows the HCA to assess whether the patient is still fit for surgery. The introduction of a POA software program would initially be expensive but could change the skill mix in a POA clinic, reducing staffing costs in the long term.

Telemedicine involves the use of communications and information technologies for the delivery of clinical care.[52] These are accepted methods of reviewing patients, which are especially useful if patients live long distances from specialist care centres. Often POA is performed over the phone if a patient has dementia or a disability that would make a POA appointment distressing. Occasionally, anaesthetists use the telephone to establish if a referred patient needs to attend the anaesthesia clinic. Used in conjunction with computerised POA programs, telemedicine could reduce the volume of patients attending the POA clinics.

Conclusion

The future make-up of the preoperative assessment team is likely to go through further changes as more technological solutions are applied to patient care in the surgical journey. The whole challenge of delivering new service models is examined in more detail in Chapter 18. However, the role of the nurse in POA will continue, due in part to the patients' need to share their health story with a healthcare professional who is able to tailor their care package to their individual requirements. The POA team has the ability to identify potential problems with health and social circumstances, act independently and have advanced communication and teaching skills.[5] As we have seen from this chapter, in the 1990s the POA nurses' role was often described in the literature as a 'clerical' coordinator who ensured that the patient was reviewed by the surgeons and AHPs attending the POA clinic, but this has changed radically. In the new millennium, in some hospitals, it has developed into that of a dedicated POA nurse competently practising in an advanced role as a 'clinical' coordinator. The POA nurse completes a holistic assessment, gives preoperative information, provides a named nurse service, appropriately refers and collaborates with doctors and AHPs, manages a caseload of unfit patients, coordinating care and services in order to improve the patient's surgical journey. Where the role is performed without direct medical input, e.g. in nurse-led clinics, the POA nurse is an experienced nurse whose autonomous role is supported by policies, documentation, protocols and anaesthetic services. Unfortunately, it has been found that staff working directly with patients are less likely to know about service changes and developments that could benefit patients[53] and, as the dedicated POA nurse role has the potential to become isolated, special efforts need to be made by the POA nurses and the managers of all service types to keep up to date regarding service changes and developments. The continuing education of the POA team is necessary and the attainment of professional competencies is essential for POA nurses to further develop their role.[17]

The already advanced nature of the POA nurse's role involves increased responsibility, as they often work alone and without direct medical supervision. Some specialist nurses work in primary care areas and integrate POA in their practice.[54] Difficulties matching the role of the POA nurse to any of the Agenda for Change job profiles have been identified and the development of a template for a generic POA nurse has been proposed.[55] It is anticipated that the development of competencies could help POA nurses to meet the requirements of the Knowledge and Skills Framework.[21]

The introduction of 'computerised care' to POA removes the ideal opportunity for a patient to discuss any anxieties or concerns about pending surgery at a time when some patients feel vulnerable and powerless, whether the surgery is because of a life-threatening disease or not. Computerised care removes the opportunity for a healthcare professional to identify non-verbal cues, to tease out information which a patient had forgotten or was unable to explain within the program's rigid parameters. The development of a rapport between the nurse and the patient can instil a sense of confidence in the planned surgical journey and maintain the caring touch in modern health-care.

REFERENCES

1. D.L. Crosby, G.H. Griffith, J.R.E. Jenkins, R. Real, B.C. Roberts and A.P.M. Forrest (1972). General surgical pre-admission clinic *British Medical Journal* **3**:157–9.

2. V. Newton (1996). Care in pre-admission clinics. *Nursing Times* **92**(1): 27–8.

3. S. Nelson (1995). Pre-admission clinics for thoracic surgery. *Nursing Times*, April 12, **91**(15): 29–31.

4. M.S.C. Malkin (2000). Patients' perceptions of a pre-admission clinic. *Journal of Nursing Management* **8**(2): 107.

5. L. Graineer (1995). Evaluating pre-operative care. *Nursing Times* **91**(15): 31–2

6. D. Bond and K. Barton (1994). Patient assessment before surgery. *Nursing Standard* **8**(28): 23–8.

7. R. Kerridge, A. Lee, E. Latchford, S.J. Beehan and K.M. Hillman (1995). The perioperative system: A new approach to managing elective surgery. *Anaesthesia and Intensive Care* **23**(5): 591–6.

8. The National Confidential Enquiry into Perioperative Deaths (NCEPOD) (2002). *Functioning as a Team?* NCEPOD. http://www. ncepod.org.uk/pdf/2002/02full.pdf (Accessed 23.02.2007).

9. C. Gannon (2005). Will the lead clinician please stand up? *British Medical Journal* **330**: 737.

10. L. Pearce (2004). Safe Admission. *Nursing Standard* **19**(8): 14–15.

11. D. Casey and G. Ormrod (2003). The effectiveness of nurse-led pre-assessment clinics. *Professional Nurse* **18**(12): 685–7.

12. J. Haddock and C. Burrows (1997). The role of the nurse in health promotion: an evaluation of a smoking cessation programme in surgical pre-admission clinics. *Journal of Advanced Nursing* **26**: 1098–110.

13. L. Wolfenden, J. Wiggers, J. Knight, E. Campbell, A. Spigelman, R. Kerridge and K. Moore (2005). Increasing smoking cessation in a preoperative clinic: a randomized controlled trial. *Preventative Medicine* **41**(1): 284–90.

14. H. Scott (2005). Nurses' work must be recognised and rewarded. *British Journal of Nursing* **14**(11): 593.

15. P.J. Thomson, I.R. Fletcher and C. Downey (2004). Nurses versus clinicians? Who's best at preoperative assessment? *Ambulatory Surgery* **11**(1-2): 33–6.

16. M. Radford, A. Abbassi, A. Williamson and P. Johnston (2003). Redefining perioperative advanced practice – the nurse specialist in anaesthesia and emergency surgery. *British Journal of Perioperative Nursing* **13**(11): 468–71.

17. G. Ormrod and D. Casey (2004). The educational preparation of nursing staff undertaking pre-assessment of surgical patients – a discussion of the issues. *Nurse Education Today* **24**: 256–62.

18. J. Neasham (1996). Nurse led pre assessment clinics. *British Journal of Theatre Nursing* **6**(8): 5–10.

19. H. Walsgrove (2005). Putting education into practice for pre-operative patient assessment. *Nursing Standard* **20**(47): 35–40.

20. E. Janke, V. Chalk and H. Kinley (2002). *Preoperative Assessment: Setting a Standard through Learning.* NHS Modernisation Agency. University of Southampton.

21. H. Walsgrove (2006). Putting education into practice for pre-operative patient assessment.
Nursing Standard 20(47): 35–9. Available on-line at:
http://www.nursing-standard.co.uk/archives/ns/vol20-47/pdfs/v20n47p3540.pdf (Accessed 15.05.2007)

22. W.A. van Klei, P.J. Hennis, J. Moen, C.J. Kalkman and K.G. Moons (2004). The accuracy of trained nurses in pre-operative health assessment: results of the OPEN study. *Anaesthesia* **59**: 971–8.

23. H. Kinley, C. Czoski-Murray, S. George, C. McCabe, J. Primrose, C. Reilly, R. Wood, P. Nicolson, C. Healy, S. Read, J. Norman, E. Janke, H. Alhameed, N. Fernandes and E. Thomas (2002). Effectiveness of appropriately trained nurses in preoperative assessment: randomized controlled equivalence/non-inferiority trial. *British Medical Journal* **325**: 1323–6.

24. L. Wadsworth, A. Smith and H. Waterman (2002). The nurse practitioner's role in day case preoperative assessment. *Nursing Standard* **16**(47): 41–4.

25. H. Rushforth, A. Bliss, D. Burge and A. Glasper (2000). Nurse-led pre-operative assessment: a study of appropriateness. *Paediatric Nursing* **12**(5): 15–21.

26. S.P. Fischer (1996). Development and effectiveness of an anaesthesia preoperative evaluation clinic in a teaching hospital. *Anesthesiology* **85**(1): 196–206.

27. B. Guido (2004). The role of the nurse practitioner in an ambulatory surgery unit. *Association of Operating Room Nurses (AORN) Journal* **79**: 606–14.

28. Association of Anaesthetists of Great Britain and Ireland (AAGBI) (2001). *Preoperative Assessment: the Role of the Anaesthetist.* AAGBI. http://www.aagbi.org/publications/guidelines/docs/preoperativeass01.pdf
(Accessed 15.05.2007)

29. W. Hilditch, A.J. Asbury and J.M. Crawford (2003). Preoperative screening: criteria for referring to anaesthetists. *Anaesthesia* **58**: 117–24.

30. P.K. Barnes, P.A. Emerson, S. Hajnal, W.J. Radford and J. Congleton (2000). Influence of an anaesthetist on nurse-led, computer-based, pre-operative assessment. *Anaesthesia* **55**: 576–89.

31. M. Reed, S. Wright and F. Armitage (1997). Nurse-led general surgical pre-operative assessment clinic. *Journal of the Royal College of Surgeons in Edinburgh* **42**: 310–13.

32. J. Bramhall (2002). The role of nurses in preoperative assessment. *Nursing Times* **98**(40): 34–5.

33. J. Smith and C. Rudd (1998). Streamlining pre-operative assessment in orthopaedics. *Nursing Standard* **13**(1): 45–8.

34. C.A. Clinch (1997). Nurses achieve quality with pre-assessment clinics. *Journal of Clinical Nursing* **6**: 147–51.

35. C. Jay (1998). The role of the pre-admissions pharmacist. *The Hospital Pharmacist* **5**: 105–6.

36. H.L. Hick, P.E. Deady, D.J. Wright and J. Silcock (2001). The impact of the pharmacist on an elective general surgery pre-admission clinic. *Pharmacy World and Science* **23**(2): 65–9.

37. C.B. Koay and N.J. Marks (1996). A nurse-led preadmission clinic for elective ENT surgery: the first 8 months. *Annals of the Royal College of Surgeons for England* **78**: 15–19.

38. M.S. Whiteley, K. Wilmott and R.B. Offland (1997). A specialist nurse can replace pre-registration house officers in the surgical pre-admission clinic. *Annals of Royal College of Surgeons of England* **79**: 257–60.

39. A. Jones, P. Penfold, M. Bailey, C. Charig, D. Choolun and A.M. Rollin (2000). Pre-admission clerking of urology patients by nurses. *Professional Nurse* **15**(4): 261–6.

40. M.R. Rail and J.J. Pandit (2003). Day of surgery cancellations after nurse-led pre-assessment in an elective surgical centre: the first two years. *Anaesthesia* **58**(7): 692.

41. K. Spilsbury and J. Meyer (2001). Defining the nursing contribution to patient outcome: lessons from a review of the literature examining nursing outcomes, skill mix and changing roles. *Journal of Clinical Nursing* **10**: 3–14.

42. J.E. Hartley *et al* (1997). Nurse-led pre-admission clinics in general surgery provide major cost benefits. *British Journal of Surgery* **84** Supplement 1: 41–2.

43. J.B. Pollard and L. Olsen (1999). Early outpatient preoperative anesthesia assessment: does it help to reduce operating room cancellations? *Anesthesia and Analgesia* **89**: 502–5.

44. D. Wilson-Nunn (2005). *Rewriting protocols, reducing cancellations at Cromer Hospital.* Available on-line at: http://www.cgsupport.nhs.uk/Resources/Eurekas/Secondary_Care/Rewriting_Protocols_at_Cromer_Hospital.asp (Accessed 28.01.2007)

45. World Health Organisation (2005). *eHealth: proposed tools and services.* Available on-line at: http://www.who.int/gb/ebwha/pdf_files/EB117/B117_15-en.pdf (Accessed 18.01.2008)

46. http://www.connectingforhealth.nhs.uk (Accessed 18.01.2008)

47. http://www.prompte.com/ (Accessed 10.01.2008)

48. D.J. Mingay, M.F. Roizen, M Belkin, L. Headley and J.F. Foss (2000). Evaluation of Touchtone Telephone for In-home Completion of HealthQuiz™ Preoperative Assessment Questionnaire. *The Internet Journal of Anesthesiology.* **4**(1) Available on-line at: http://www.ispub.com/ostia/index.php?xmlFilePath=journals/ija/vol4n1/healthquiz.xml (Accessed 18.1.2008)

49. http://www.informatics.co.uk/synopsis_homepage.html (Accessed 10.01.2008)

50. AnaesthesiaUK (2004). *Goldman Cardiac Risk Index* Available on-line at: http://www.frca.co.uk/article.aspx?articleid=100187 (Accessed 10.01.2008)

51. Vascular Anaesthesia Society of Great Britain and Ireland (VASGBI) (undated). Detsky and Goldman calculators. Available on-line at: http://www.vasgbi.com/riskdetsky.htm (Accessed 10.01.2008)

52. http://en.wikipedia.org/wiki/Telemedicine (Accessed 18.01.2008)

53. S. Hornby (1993). Collaborative Care Interprofessional, Interagency and Interpersonal. Oxford: Blackwell Scientific Publication.

54. L.M. Plauntz (2007). Preoperative assessment of the surgical patient. Nursing Clinics of North America. **42**: 361–77.

55. J. Bell (2005). The impact of the agenda for change on preoperative assessment nurses. *Abstract Book – The Preoperative Association 2nd National Conference.* Abstract No. 031.

2 Preoperative estimation of survival and mortality risk

John Carlisle

SUMMARY

This chapter will describe:

- how to estimate the chances of survival and death and methods to reduce risk
- how to decide whether to proceed with surgery and to help minimise risk
- a step-by-step sequence to determine risk and review other risk scores
- how information from a fitness test increases the precision of the survival estimate.

INTRODUCTION

A common question from patients is 'what are my chances of survival (my risk of dying) if I have surgery?' More specifically, what happens to my chances if I have *this* surgery? Researchers have tried to answer this question by looking at populations having surgery and recording who is alive and who is dead one month after surgery (actually the outcome has usually been cardiac complication rather than death). Some people are more likely to die and some types of surgery are more likely to kill. Researchers recorded before surgery whether or not patients have a factor that they (the researchers) thought might influence the risk of dying, for instance whether the patient had had a heart attack. Researchers also recorded what surgery the patient had. Then, usually one month after surgery, the researcher recorded whether or not the patient had experienced the outcome(s) of interest – usually heart attack, stroke or 'cardiac' death. In this way researchers could see whether or not the presence of a variable was associated with the outcome and by how much (using multivariate logistic and linear regression statistics). Different researchers have generally associated similar patient and surgical variables with the same (or similar) outcomes. I list later some of the scoring systems that have resulted from these associative studies.

However, there are sources of survival data that until now preoperative services have not used. In this chapter I will describe how to use these sources of information. The benefits of using previously untapped information sources are:

- the precision and reliability of risk estimates will be better (data derived from a bigger population)
- you can estimate preoperative mortality risk as well as the postoperative risk (putting the latter into context to facilitate decision-making)
- you can estimate survival chances for anybody having any operation, not just people similar to those assessed by the perioperative researchers.

Once a patient knows the likelihood of good and bad outcomes, before and after surgery, with and without surgery, they can decide what to do. We can plan how to make their hospital stay safe, using resources, like intensive care, efficiently.

Assessing risk

To make an informed decision as to whether or not to have surgery one needs to know: what the risk is for good and bad outcomes without surgery (see below); what the risk is for long-term (more than one month) good and bad outcomes after surgery. Most published scoring systems do not provide this information.

This chapter will provide you with a template for risk assessment for one outcome – death. This template is based upon a logical sequence of steps for risk calculation, which can also be used to determine the risks for other specific outcomes (such as myocardial infarction, cardiac arrest, cardiac death, deep vein thromboses). The first stage in this process is to start with the average risk of dying for a population with a given age and sex. Population risks, published by the United Kingdom government, are derived from all deaths in the UK and are therefore precise. Other scoring systems derive risk from relatively small surgical populations, numbering in total a few thousand. These systems do not assess the preoperative risk. There are much larger survival studies of people not having surgery. These provide more precise estimates of the preoperative association of a variable, such as heart failure, and survival. The preoperative risk for an outcome such as death illustrates to patients and clinicians the likelihood of an outcome *without* surgery. The final step in the sequence is to estimate the effect of a particular operation on a person's risk (of death), i.e. the postoperative risk. Once you have followed these steps and calculated the postoperative risk, you can compare it with the risk quoted by published scoring systems. One caution is that the scoring system you are comparing with is for the same outcome (this chapter describes death – although many scoring systems are for cardiovascular events). If the two estimates are particularly different you should recalculate and try and determine whether your patient is particularly different from the patients used to calculate the risks in the surgical scoring system.

The importance of fitness

To predict survival from surgery you need to measure the fitness of the patient as best you can.

The four variables that together predict survival in people without disease are:

- age
- sex
- socioeconomic status
- fitness.

These variables also form the basis of survival prediction for people with systemic diseases: a few diseases independently increase risk above and beyond their effect on fitness (see below). If you assess fitness by history alone you will be unable to predict survival as well as you could if you measured fitness directly, no matter how many other variables you take into account.

Calculating the preoperative risk of dying

Four variables, described in Step one, Step two and Step three, determine the risk of dying in the healthy patient. Five additional variables determine the risk of dying in patients with disease. Each variable is independent, so multiply the risk you have calculated in preceding steps by the value in the next step.

Step one: Age and sex *(www.gad.gov.uk)*

In the United Kingdom all deaths are recorded and used to calculate age-specific and sex-specific survival. These figures are updated every year and can be downloaded in spreadsheet form giving survival for men and women. Table 2.1 lists examples of mortality risk and median life expectancy for men and women. These data provide a precise but average risk of dying. **The risk of death doubles about every seven years**. For instance, the risk that a 58-year-old woman will die in the next month is 1 in 2500, the risk that a 65-year-old woman will die is 1 in 1250. **The risk that a man will die is 1.7 times the risk that a woman will die**. Steps two onward determine how average a patient is.

Table 2.1 Examples of UK monthly mortality and median years left

Deaths per 10 000	Survivors per 10 000	One death in:	Survivors per death	Female age (years left)	Male age (years left)
1 in 10,000	9999 in 10,000	10,000	9999	**42** (40)	**35** (36)
2 in 10,000	9998 in 10,000	5000	4999	**49** (33)	**45** (30)
4 in 10,000	9996 in 10,000	2500	2499	**58** (25)	**53** (22)
8 in 10,000	9992 in 10,000	1250	1249	**65** (19)	**60** (17)

16 in 10,000	9984 in 10,000	625	624	**71** (15)	**67** (12)
32 in 10,000	9968 in 10,000	313	312	**77** (11)	**73** (9)
64 in 10,000	9936 in 10,000	157	156	**84** (7)	**80** (6)
128 in 10,000	9872 in 10,000	79	78	**90** (4)	**87** (5)
256 in 10,000	9744 in 10,000	40	39	**97** (3)	**95** (3)

Http://www.gad.gov.uk/Demography_Data/Life_Tables/Interim_life_tables.asp

Step two: Wealth

The impoverished are twice as likely to die as the wealthy. This association is reasonably consistent using occupation, educational qualification or income as the measurement of wealth. Ethnicity is not an independent risk factor: poverty, and the risk factors listed below, account for differences in all-cause mortality between ethnic groups. Regional mortality rates account for some geographical variation in wealth. Multiply the average regional mortality rate by 1.5 for the impoverished and by 0.7 for the wealthy.[1,2]

Step three: Aerobic fitness

Fit people are more likely to survive than unfit people, for both healthy and diseased populations. Traditional assessment is based upon the maximum work (power) that someone says they can achieve, usually in terms of day-to-day activities, like walking or going upstairs. The approximate power required to achieve these activities is listed in tables as the number of METs (metabolic equivalents). One MET is the internal power used at rest. The MET scale of daily activities was not intended to be a prognostic measure and imprecisely stratifies risk. Fitness assessment by history, using the MET scale and others, is unreliable.

Bodies are powered by oxidising food. Food oxidation at rest is often quoted as using 3.5 millilitres of oxygen every minute for every kilogram of body mass (3.5 ml O_2/kg per min). This is the value most MET scales assume as one MET and the value used by treadmill studies of fitness and survival. When fitness is tested by observation, rather than relying upon how fit people say they are, the following relationships apply between fitness and survival for men and women:

- The expected peak power (in METs) for men[3] is 18.4 – (0.16 x age).
- The expected peak power (in METs) for women[4] is 14.7 – (0.13 x age).
- The risk of dying is more for unfit people – multiply the risk (from Step one and Step two) by **1.19** for every MET short of the expected peak power (for age). The risk of dying is less for fit people – multiply the average risk by **0.84** for every MET in excess of the expected peak power.[5-11]

Incidentally the value used in the MET scale for oxygen consumption at rest is incorrect. The correct average adult resting oxygen consumption is 2.6 ml O_2/kg per min, with 95% of adults consuming between 2.0 and 3.4 ml O_2/kg per min.[12]

Fitness testing provides precise prognostic information and replaces risk based upon historical factors, such as hypertension and diabetes (see pages 23–4). However historical risk factors can help one decide which test to do: the incremental shuttle walk test (ISWT) or cardiopulmonary exercise testing (CPX). CPX is more complex than the ISWT. In the CPX test peak oxygen consumption (and therefore METs) are *measured* directly, whereas the ISWT *estimates* peak METs (and oxygen consumption). CPX testing provides the most precise prognostic information, but it is too labour-intensive a method to use in every preoperative patient, unlike the ISWT. This assessment in relation to cardiac disease and management is discussed in more detail in Chapter 5.

Measuring fitness, part one: incremental shuttle walk test (ISWT)

The ISWT is better than many other fitness tests, such as the distance walked in 6 or 12 minutes, or the number of stair flights ascended, because it requires the participant to increase power throughout the test. The ISWT is a slower version of the 'shuttle' or 'bleep' test used in sport. In the ISWT you have to keep travelling to and fro 10 metres, around two cones 9.5m apart (figure 2.1). In the first minute of the ISWT, participants are usually asked to complete three 10m lengths, four lengths in the next minute and so on.[13-16] In Table 2.2, (see page 20) I have illustrated the power levels that men and women of different ages are expected to achieve, using the relationships between age and expected peak power that I have described above. I have added two levels, so that if you started at level one you would have to complete one length in the first minute and two in the second minute. These two (new) levels allow the elderly and infirm to start very slowly. I have suggested faster starting levels for fitter and younger men and women. I have assumed that people start to jog above a speed of 130m/min (level 13) when I calculated oxygen consumptions and METs: the relationship between speed and work is different for walking and running.[17-23]

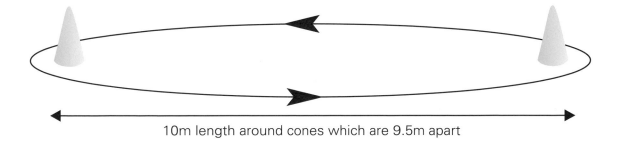

10m length around cones which are 9.5m apart

Figure 2.1 Incremental shuttle walk test course

Table 2.2a Predicted fitness for men

	L1	L2	L3	L4	L5	L6	L7	L8	L9	L10	L11	L12	L13	L14	L15	L16	L17	L18	L19	L20	L21	L22	L23	L24	L25	L26	L27	L28
New level	1	2	3	4	5	6	7	8	9	10	11	12	13	14	15	16	17	18	19	20	21	22	23	24	25	26	27	28
Old METs	1.2	1.6	2.0	2.4	2.8	3.3	3.7	4.1	4.6	5.0	5.6	6.1	6.6	7.1	7.6	8.0	8.6	9.1	9.6	10.0	10.6	11.1	11.6	12.0	12.6	13.1	13.6	14.1
Distance × 100m	0.1	0.3	0.6	1	1.5	2.1	2.8	3.6	4.7	5.7	6.8	7.9	9.2	10.6	12.1	13.7	15.4	17.2	19.1	21.1	23.2	25.4	27.7	30.1	32.6	35.2	37.9	41.7
Speed (m/min)	10	20	30	40	50	60	70	80	90	100	110	120	130	140	150	160	170	180	190	200	210	220	230	240	250	260	270	280
New METs	1.6	2.2	2.7	3.2	3.8	4.4	5.0	5.6	6.2	6.7	7.5	8.2	8.9	9.6	10.2	10.8	11.6	12.3	12.9	13.5	14.3	14.9	15.6	16.2	17.0	17.6	18.3	19.0
VO2 (ml/kg/min)	4	6	7	8	10	12	13	14	16	18	20	22	23	25	27	28	30	32	34	35	37	39	41	42	44	46	48	50

AGE (years) / Peak for age (men): 90, 80, 70, 60, 50, 40, 30.

Table 2.2b Predicted fitness for women

	L1	L2	L3	L4	L5	L6	L7	L8	L9	L10	L11	L12	L13	L14	L15	L16	L17	L18	L19	L20	L21	L22	L23	L24	L25	L26	L27	L28
New level	1	2	3	4	5	6	7	8	9	10	11	12	13	14	15	16	17	18	19	20	21	22	23	24	25	26	27	28
Old METs	1.2	1.6	2.0	2.4	2.8	3.3	3.7	4.1	4.6	5.0	5.6	6.1	6.6	7.1	7.6	8.0	8.6	9.1	9.6	10.0	10.6	11.1	11.6	12.0	12.6	13.1	13.6	14.1
Distance × 100m	0.1	0.3	0.6	1	1.5	2.1	2.8	3.6	4.7	5.7	6.8	7.9	9.2	10.6	12.1	13.7	15.4	17.2	19.1	21.1	23.2	25.4	27.7	30.1	32.6	35.2	37.9	41.7
Speed (m/min)	10	20	30	40	50	60	70	80	90	100	110	120	130	140	150	160	170	180	190	200	210	220	230	240	250	260	270	280
New METs	1.6	2.0	2.4	2.8	3.3	3.7	4.1	4.6	5.0	5.5	6.2	6.7	7.5	8.2	8.9	9.6	10.2	10.8	11.6	12.3	12.9	13.5	14.3	14.9	15.6	16.2	17.0	17.6
VO2 (ml/kg/min)	4	6	7	8	10	12	13	14	16	18	20	22	23	25	27	28	30	32	34	35	37	39	41	42	44	46	48	50

AGE (years) / Peak for age (women): 90, 80, 70, 60, 50, 40, 30, 20.

Table 2.2

New level: number of lengths each minute in the ISWT. **Distance:** cumulative distance if one started at level 1. **Old MET:** multiples of resting oxygen consumption estimated as 3.5ml O_2/kg per min. **New MET:** multiples of resting oxygen consumption estimated as 2.6ml O_2/kg per min. **VO2:** oxygen consumption.

Looking at Table 2.2a, a 60-year-old man of average fitness would start at new level five and would be expected to reach level 17 (indicated by a black box). A 60-year-old man who continued to level 24 (indicated by an unshaded box) would have **half** the average risk of dying. A 60-year-old man with **double** the average risk of dying would stop at level 11 (indicated by a dark grey box) having also started at level five. A 60-year-old man with four times the average risk would not exceed level 3 (another unshaded box). You may need to start patients at a lower level than I have indicated if you think they are particularly unfit, so that they walk at least five minutes before stopping.

Measuring fitness, part two: cardiopulmonary exercise testing (CPX)

Only the distance (and time) walked (or run) is recorded by the ISWT. This is used to estimate the peak power and oxygen consumption achieved. How well someone's body copes up to the time they stop is not measured: with the ISWT this information cannot be used to improve prognostication.

Cardiopulmonary exercise testing (CPX or CPET), unlike the ISWT, directly measures the aerobic capacity of someone whilst they exercise, usually either on a treadmill or bicycle[24] (see Figure 2.2, page 22). The CPX test measures the breath volume, oxygen consumption and carbon dioxide production during exercise. An ECG with ST segment analysis and pulse oximetry is recorded throughout, along with intermittent non-invasive blood pressures. Rarely, arterial blood gases are sampled. As in the ISWT, power increases throughout the CPX test until the person stops, by increased braking on the bicycle and by increased speed and gradient on the treadmill. Incremental exercise should last at least five minutes, and preferably ten minutes, to accurately gauge prognosis.

The expected peak powers (and related peak oxygen consumptions) for men and women of different ages, are the same for CPX as for ISWT. Combinations of CPX variables that improve prognostic precision include: the amount of breathing needed to get oxygen in ($\dot{V}_E/\dot{V}_{O_2}$) and carbon dioxide out ($\dot{V}_E/\dot{V}_{CO_2}$); the amount of oxygen used to fuel increasing power ($\dot{V}_{O_2}/W$); and the threshold above which aerobic respiration alone cannot meet metabolic demand – the 'anaerobic threshold' (AT).[25-31] Heart rate during exercise and recovery also supply additional prognostic information.[32] Changes in the ECG complex, for instance ST depression or elevation, do not usually increase prognostic precision. Patients with hip and knee osteoarthritis or claudication who find walking painful may prefer bicycle CPX to either the ISWT or treadmill CPX. The more complete prognostic information provided by CPX tests is probably of use if it:

● helps clinicians determine whether surgery is more likely to harm or benefit a patient

● helps patients determine whether to have surgery

● helps determine the efficient use of scarce resources (critical care, transplants)

● helps determine the likelihood that interventions could improve outcomes.

Readers interested in using CPX results should refer to specialist texts listed on page 32.

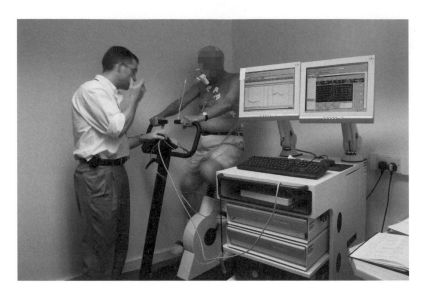

Figure 2.2 CPX testing

Step four: Heart, brain, kidneys and legs

Steps one, two and three calculate the preoperative risk of dying in someone without disease. Five diagnoses independently increase the risk already calculated using age, sex, wealth and fitness.

Histories of peripheral vascular disease (PVD), stroke, heart failure, myocardial infarction or renal failure (creatinine concentration more than 150μmol/L) each independently increase the risk of dying by about **1.5**. Temporary ischaemia, instead of tissue infarction, in the heart (angina) or brain (TIAs) increases the risk of dying by **1.2** rather than **1.5**. The elevated risk following infarction is maintained over decades, whilst the lesser risk from stable temporary ischaemia falls over time.[1,2, 33-44]

How to use Steps one to four

Step one: Determine baseline risk with age and sex.

Step two: Multiply baseline risk from Step one by **1.5** for poorest, **0.7** for wealthiest.

Step three: Multiply risk from Step two by the relative risk associated with the peak power achieved in the ISWT or CPX test.

Step four: Multiply risk from Step three for a history of each of the following – myocardial infarction (**1.5**); heart failure (**1.5**); stroke (**1.5**); peripheral vascular disease (**1.5**); creatinine concentration more than 150μmol/L (**1.5**).

An example is shown in Box 2.1(opposite).

Box 2.1 Example of risk assessment process in surgery

What is the (preoperative) risk that a 54-year-old woman, who smokes and is treated for hypertension and type 2 diabetes, who had a heart attack four years ago, and who can reach new level 10 in the ISWT, will die in the next month?

Step one: average risk of dying for a 54-year-old woman is 1 in 3418.

Step two: estimate unchanged as no socioeconomic information.

Step three: estimate multiplied by relative fitness. Average peak power (in old METs) expected for a 54-year-old woman is 14.7 − (0.13 x 54) = 7.7 old METs. This is new level 15 (or old level 13) in the ISWT. She reached new level 10, or about 5.6 old METs. The difference is 7.7 − 5.6 = 2.1 METs. The relative risk is 1.19 x 2.1 = **2.5**. So the new estimate is 2.5 in 3418.

Step four: estimate multiplied for previous heart attack (**1.5**) = 1.5 x 2.5 = 3.75 in 3418.

In other words, her approximate risk of dying in the next month is 1 in 910, and her approximate chance of survival is 909 in 910.

Smoking, diabetes, blood pressure and cholesterol

These risk factors for cardiovascular disease do not alter risk if fitness has been measured. Calculation of the preoperative risk of dying is complete with Steps one to four using nine variables: age, sex, wealth, fitness, five diseases (listed on page 25). The effect on survival of the background risk factors that I discuss here, and that occupy the time of primary care, is detected through these nine variables. These variables are only independent risk factors if fitness has not been measured.[1,2,33-44] Smoking, diabetes, hypertension and hypercholesterolaemia increase the risk of death, mainly through atherosclerotic disease. I have simplified the relationship between these variables and death. There is no blood pressure, cholesterol 'threshold' or smoke exposure for which the risk of death suddenly increases. The relationship is a gradual increase in risk with higher values, or a decrease in risk with lower values.

Smoking

In the United Kingdom about one in four adults smoke. Someone who smokes (or who has stopped in the last five years) is about **1.5** times as likely to die as average. Someone who has not smoked in the last 5 years is about **0.8** times as likely to die as average. The risk of dying increases by **1.2** for every 10 pack-years. One pack-year is smoking 20 cigarettes each day for one year or ten cigarettes each day for two years (and so on).

Diabetes

About one in 20 adults in the UK have a diagnosis of diabetes, of whom 10% have Type 1 diabetes and 90% have Type 2 diabetes. Type 1 diabetes increases the risk of dying **3** times; Type2 diabetes increases the risk of dying **2** times. Non-diabetics have about an average risk of dying.

Hypertension

About one in three adults are either already treated for hypertension, or consistently have a systolic blood pressure (SBP) above 140mmHg when it is measured in primary care. Adults treated for hypertension, or who have a SBP in primary care above 160mmHg, are about **1.5** times as likely to die as average. Untreated adults with systolic blood pressures in primary care below 130mmHg are about **0.7** times as likely to die as average. Adults with SBP between 130mmHg and 160mmHg have an average risk of dying. Use the blood pressure recorded in primary care to guide your risk calculations. Do not use blood pressure measured in hospital to calculate risk. Blood pressures measured in hospital clinics are usually higher and do not correlate with outcome as well as those measured in primary care.

Hypercholesterolaemia

The average adult cholesterol level is about 5.5mmol/L (220mg/dL). Lipidaemic atherosclerotic risk is also measured as the ratio of total cholesterol to high density cholesterol, the average of which is about 4.5. People with total cholesterol concentrations at least 8mmol/L (350mg/dL), or total:HDL ratios at least 7, are **1.25** times as likely to die as average. People with total cholesterol concentrations less than 4.1mmol/L (150mg/dL), or total:HDL ratios less than 3.1, are **0.8** times as likely to die as average. The risk of dying is about average for values in between these. Lipidaemic atherosclerotic risk is calculated on more than one blood sample. So, as with blood pressures, prognosis should use serum lipid measurements taken in primary care.

How to use Steps one, two and four without fitness

If you do not measure fitness (Step three) you have to calculate risk of dying using histories of smoking, diabetes, blood pressure, and cholesterol concentration. This risk estimation will be less accurate than risk estimates using results from the ISWT or CPX.

Step one: Determine baseline risk with age and sex.

Step two: Multiply baseline risk from Step one by **1.5** for poorest, **0.7** for wealthiest.

Smoking, diabetes, blood pressure, cholesterol: Multiply risk from Step two for smoking (**1.5**) or non-smoking (**0.8**), diabetes (**3** for Type 1 or **2** for Type 2), treated hypertension or SBP more than 160mmHg (**1.5**) or SBP less than 130mmHg (**0.7**), and cholesterol high (**1.25**) or low (**0.8**).

Step four: multiply this risk for a history of each of the following: myocardial infarction (**1.5**); heart failure (**1.5**); stroke (**1.5**); peripheral vascular disease (**1.5**); creatinine concentration more than 150µmol/L (**1.5**).

An example is shown in Box 2.2.

Box 2.2 Example of risk assessment process in surgery

What is the (preoperative) risk that a 54-year-old man, who smokes and is treated for hypertension and type two diabetes, and who had a heart attack four years ago, will die in the next month?

Step one: average risk of dying for a 54-year-old man is 1 in 2235.

Step two: estimate unchanged as no socioeconomic information.

Smoking, diabetes, blood pressure, cholesterol: estimate multiplied for smoking (1.5), Type 2 diabetes (2) and hypertension (1.5) = 2 x 1.5 x 1.5 = 4.5 in 2235.

Step four: estimate multiplied for previous heart attack (1.5) = 4.5 x 1.5 = 6.75 in 2235.

In other words, his approximate risk of dying in the next month is 1 in 330, and his approximate chance of survival is 329 in 330.

Step five: the effect of surgery

In the preceding steps we have calculated the preoperative risk of dying per month, using a measure of fitness and eight other variables, or 12 variables and no fitness measurement. To calculate the postoperative risk of dying (in the month after surgery) we need to estimate what effect, if any, surgery has upon the risk of dying.

Because information is scarce for most operations, the risk estimate we calculate for dying in the month after surgery will be more uncertain than the estimate of the preoperative risk of dying. Most people feel worse for some time after surgery than they did before surgery. Similarly most people are probably more likely to die in the month after elective surgery than if they had not had surgery. Elective operations are performed to prolong life, and make it better, but these effects can only be detected when patients are followed up for longer than one month. How much surgery extends life and improves its quality remains unknown for most operations. Although longer-term quality of life has been assessed in some postoperative patients, particularly after operations for cancer, randomised controlled trials that can determine benefit and harm are largely confined to surgery for coronary artery disease.

The risk of dying is increased more by major surgery than by minor surgery. Major surgery includes operations on arteries and intra-abdominal and intrathoracic viscera. Postoperative inflammatory responses increase oxygen demand, acid production and blood coagulability. This response peaks about two days after surgery and, in uncomplicated cases, gradually diminishes over subsequent days and weeks. The risk of dying parallels these changes, although there are additional risks that may not parallel the postoperative inflammatory response, for instance drug administration errors and hospital-acquired infections. The risk of dying should be the same as being at home if the body's physiological state is unchanged by surgery, as long as miscellaneous risks from being hospitalised are minimal. Indeed, home is not a risk-free environment and it is easy to imagine someone whose risk of dying may be less, while having elective surgery, than when pursuing their normal activities. On average the risk of dying will be unchanged by minor surgery, such as cystoscopy. The risk of dying increases most, about **12** times, in the month following open abdominal aortic aneurysm repair.[45] Other major surgeries, such as anterior resections, may increase the risk about **5** times. The risk following elective knee or hip replacement may increase about **3** times.

Calculate the risk of dying in the month following surgery by multiplying the figure you have calculated (in Steps one to four) by the relative risk associated with the proposed surgery. It is possible that this risk estimation could be made more accurate by factoring in additional anaesthetic or surgical factors, and perhaps some residual patient factors, but it is unclear what factors to include and whether they increase or decrease the relative risk of surgery (see below).

Other scoring systems

The American College of Cardiology/American Heart Association (ACC/AHA) guideline on perioperative cardiovascular evaluation and care for noncardiac surgery references 12 scoring systems.[46] I discuss this guideline in more detail in Chapter 5. The ACC/AHA guideline is extensive and well-referenced but it does not provide a template for calculating risk. It is primarily concerned with determining what perioperative interventions to use, such as beta-blockade and coronary artery bypass grafting, when and in whom. In this section I will concentrate on the risk score published in 1999 that the ACC/AHA recommends and that is currently most popular – the revised cardiac risk index (RCRI),[47] a revision of the original Goldman score published 22 years previously.[48]

Revised Cardiac Risk Index (RCRI)

You could use the RCRI in addition to the risk calculation tool I have described. When you use the RCRI remember the following.

- The RCRI cannot be used to estimate preoperative risk – it is a tool for estimating postoperative risks. The RCRI was derived from a population older than 49 with planned admissions of at least two days.

- The RCRI cannot be used to estimate risk in populations having minor or moderate surgery.

- The RCRI cannot be used to estimate the risk of postoperative death – it is a tool for estimating the risk that a patient will experience one or more of four 'major cardiac complications': myocardial infarction (MI); complete heart block; ventricular fibrillation or primary cardiac arrest; pulmonary oedema.

- The RCRI estimates the risk of one of these outcomes occurring within five days of surgery and would estimate less well the risk during a longer period (such as a month). As I have mentioned, the RCRI cannot be used to estimate the risk of dying: the RCRI was not designed to predict the two-thirds of the deaths (31/43) that the authors categorised as not associated with a 'major cardiac complication'.

- The RCRI assigned the same risk – one point – to each factor. The authors reported that the odds ratios for the six factors ranged from 1.9 to 3.0 in the multivariate analysis. The authors justified using one point, instead of the odds ratios for each factor, because the areas under the receiver operating characteristic (ROC) curves were similar. There are two general problems. Comparison of the ROC curves of six factors cannot be relied upon to detect important differences between the two scoring systems. The second problem is that values of odds ratios (as opposed to risk ratios) are sensitive to the pretest probability: factors that affect the rate of postoperative complications but were not assessed by the authors (or could not be assessed by the authors). Odds ratios cannot be used for other patients unless the effects of these factors are the same, unlike risk ratios.

- The number of participants that contributed to the derivation and validation of the RCRI is far smaller than the populations used to calculate the preoperative risk sequence I have described (above). For instance the RCRI was developed from 108 major cardiac complications that occurred in 92 patients in a surgical population of 4315 participants. The national life tables (www.gad.gov.uk) that form Step one in the risk calculation I have described used 1.72 million deaths that occurred over a three-year period (2004–6) in the UK population of 62.3 million.

Keeping in mind these limitations, the RCRI found that 'major postoperative cardiac complications' were associated with four preoperative factors:

- Ischaemic heart disease, defined as: previous MI (including Q waves on ECG), positive ECG exercise test, angina, GTN use.

- Heart failure, defined as: previous history, nocturnal dyspnoea, third heart sound gallop, bilateral crackles or CXR pulmonary oedema.

- Cerebrovascular disease, defined as: transient ischaemic attack or stroke.

- High-risk elective surgery, defined as: abdominal aortic aneurysm repair, intrathoracic surgery, intraperitoneal surgery.

Two other variables associated with major cardiac complications in the derivation cohort (2893 participants) were not associated with major cardiac complications in the validation cohort (1422 participants).

- Renal impairment, defined as creatinine concentration greater than 177μmol/L.
- Insulin therapy for diabetes.

It is unclear whether one should use these two risk factors to estimate the postoperative risk of a major cardiac complication, but most subsequent researchers have applied the six derivation RCRI variables, not the four validation RCRI variables. The rate of postoperative major cardiac complications was associated with the number of risk factors. The complication rate was 1/200 for participants with no risk factor; 1/100 with one risk factor; 1/20 with two risk factors; 1/10 with more than two risk factors. If you want to use the RCRI you need to remember that this is a score for cardiac complications after major surgery.

Modified Cardiac Risk Index (MCRI)

The starting point for this 1986 score, like the RCRI, was Goldman's original 1977 score and it was incorporated into the 1997 American College of Cardiology's guideline for assessing and managing perioperative risk from coronary artery disease.[49,50] The MCRI authors added some risk factors and removed others. The MCRI also changed the values assigned to risk factors common to the 1977 score, as the RCRI was to do 13 years later. The MCRI has similar shortcomings to the RCRI and uses a more complicated scoring system. One attractive aspect of the MCRI's Bayesian methodology is that the risk is calculated by multiplying the pretest (average) probability for a postoperative complication by the MCRI score (or more exactly, the likelihood ratio). Unfortunately, ironically, the 'pretest' probability in the MCRI is not a preoperative probability. It cannot help the patient put the risk into context.

Customised Risk Index

This risk index used the RCRI as the starting point and was derived for patients undergoing vascular surgeries.[51] This risk score was developed using total mortality within 30 days of surgery (153/2310) as the outcome, instead of cardiac complications, which I think is more useful. This scoring system identified similar mortality risk factors to the other risk indices, but gives more detail of the absolute and relative risks associated with different types of vascular surgeries, from carotid endarterectomy to ruptured aortic aneurysm.

Reducing the risk of dying

Reducing the relative operative mortality risk

Most research has tried to reduce the relative risk of a given operation by preoperative, intraoperative and postoperative monitoring, fluid and drugs. These interventions attempt to reduce the risk calculated in Step five. Although most research only measured survival up to one month following surgery, it seems reasonable to suppose that the measured reductions in mortality would have persisted. The preoperative assessment of risk, as I've described above, can help to identify which patients are more or less likely to benefit from such perioperative interventions.

Reducing the preoperative mortality risk

Reducing the relative risk of operations with intensive methods of risk-reduction uses critical care resources that are scarce and expensive, so they will only be used for the highest-risk cases. There are more low-risk than high-risk surgical patients. Although their individual risks of dying are lower, the total burden of postoperative low-risk death is substantial. Lives can be saved more often by making patients fitter before their operations. So what can one do to reduce preoperative and long-term risk? Long-term survival is increased mainly by reducing the risk of atherosclerotic ischaemic disease.

1. Stopping smoking
Preoperative risk is less for non-smokers, although it may take months or years before the risk of dying falls after stopping smoking.

2. Getting fitter
Fitter people live longer. Fitter people have lower blood pressure and lower cholesterol. People who exercise have less 'sticky' blood and are less stressed than people who do not.

3. Take drugs if you're healthy
Drugs can further reduce blood coagulability, blood pressure and cholesterol, such as aspirin, 'statins', diuretics, beta-blockers, calcium-channel blockers and ACE (angiotensin converting enzyme) inhibitors. Survival is probably slightly prolonged in any population that takes these drugs. Prescription of these drugs has only traditionally been considered worthwhile in populations that have a risk of a cardiovascular event above 1 in 10 over the next 10 years (a cardiovascular event is stroke, acute coronary syndrome or death due to either). More recently a proposal has been made to prescribe a concoction of six drugs to everyone older than 54 years.

4. Take drugs if you're unhealthy
People who have had strokes and acute coronary syndromes are much more likely to experience a(nother) cardiovascular event in the next 10 years than people who have not – which is why they are prescribed the drugs I've listed above. But kidney failure, heart failure and some cancers may also be made less likely by drugs (and fitness).

It is not clear how long these interventions – stopping smoking, exercise, drugs – take to reduce the preoperative risk of dying. After myocardial infarction (or other acute coronary syndromes) the risk of dying falls within days and is further reduced within days of starting protective drugs. But drugs further reduce risk (compared to placebo) over the following weeks and months. It makes sense to use as much time as is available preoperatively to get people fitter and to optimise their preoperative, long-term, survival in order to reduce postoperative mortality.

CONCLUSION

Postoperative risk of death and morbidity is most effectively prevented by reducing the preoperative risk of death and morbidity. Postoperative risk is best estimated by precisely calculating the preoperative risk, then multiplying by a factor that reflects the severity of the operation. Preoperative mortality risk is most accurately assessed by incorporating a measure of fitness either the ISWT or a CPX test.

Preoperative services can help primary care practitioners ensure that patients are offered the most effective current drug combination. The risk of dying will be least for patients who have had the longest preoperative time getting fitter, not smoking and taking the best drugs.

REFERENCES

1.J. Hippisley-Cox, C. Coupland, Y. Vinigradova, J. Robson, M. May and P. Brindle (2007). Derivation and validation of QRISK, a new cardiovascular disease risk score for the United Kingdom: prospective open cohort study. *British Medical Journal* **335**: 136–48.

2. D.A. Alter, A. Chong, P.C. Austin, C. Mustard, K. Iron, J.I. Williams et al. (2006). Socioeconomic status and mortality after acute myocardial infarction. *Annals of Internal Medicine* **144**: 82–93.

3. J. Myers, M. Prakash, V. Froelicher, S. Partington and J.E. Atwood (2002). Exercise capacity and mortality among men referred for exercise testing. *New England Journal of Medicine* **346**: 793–801.

4. M. Gulati, H.R. Black, L.J. Shaw, M.F. Arnsdorf, C.N.B. Merz, M.S. Lauer et al. (2005). The prognostic value of a nomogram for exercise capacity in women. *New England Journal of Medicine* **353**: 468–75.

5. S. Lai, A. Kaykha, T. Yamazaki, M. Goldstein, J.M. Spin, J. Myers et al. (2004). Treadmill scores in elderly men. *Journal of the American College of Cardiology* **43**: 606–15.

6. T. Yamazaki, J. Myers and V.F. Froelicher (2004). Effect of age and end point on the prognostic value of the exercise test. *Chest* **125**: 1920–8.

7. J.A. Laukkanen, S. Kuri, R. Salonen, R. Rauramaa and J.T. Salonen (2004). The predictive value of cardiorespiratory fitness for cardiovascular events in men with various risk profiles: a prospective population-based cohort study. *European Heart Journal* **25**: 1428–37.

8. S. Mora, R.F. Redberg, Y. Cui, M.K. Whiteman, J.A. Flaws, A.R. Sharrett and R.S. Blumenthal (2003). Ability of exercise testing to predict cardiovascular and all-cause death in asymptomatic women. *Journal of the Americal Medical Association* **290**: 1600–7.

9. M.K. Aktas, V. Ozduran, C.E. Pothier, R. Lang and M.S. Lauer (2004). Global risk scores and exercise testing for predicting all-cause mortality in a preventive medicine program. *Journal of the Americal Medical Association* **292**: 1462–8.

10. M. Prakash, J. Myers, V.F. Froelicher, R. Marcus, D. Do, D. Kalisetti and J.E. Atwood (2001). Clinical exercise test predictors of all-cause mortality: Results from > 6,000 consecutive referred male patients. *Chest* **120**: 1003–13.

11. S. Mora, R.F. Redberg, R. Sharrett and R.S. Blumenthal (2005). Enhanced risk assessment in asymptomatic individuals with exercise testing and Framingham risk scores. *Circulation* **112**: 1566–72.

12. N.M. Byrne, A.P. Hills, G.R. Hunter, R.L. Weinsier and Y. Schutz (2005). Metabolic equivalent: one size does not fit all. *Journal of Applied Physiology* **99** 1112–19.

13. S.J. Singh, M.D.L. Morgan, S. Scott, D. Walters and A.E. Hardmann (1992). The development of the shuttle walking test of disability in patients with chronic airways obstruction. *Thorax* **47**: 1019–24.

14. F.J. Morales, A. Martínez, M. Méndez, A. Agarrado, F. Ortega, J. Fernández-Guerra et al. (1999). A shuttle walk test for assessment of functional capacity in chronic heart failure. *American Heart Journal* **138**: 292–8.

15. M.E. Lewis, C. Newall, J.N. Townend, S.L. Hill and R.S. Bonner (2001). Incremental shuttle walk test in the assessment of patients for heart transplantation. *Heart* **86**: 183–7.

16. T. Win, A. Jackson, A.M. Groves, L.D. Sharples, S.C. Charman and C.M. Laroche (2006). Comparison of shuttle walk with measured peak oxygen consumption in patients with operable lung cancer. *Thorax* **61**: 57–60.

17. R.D. Hagan, T. Strathman, L. Strathman and L.R. Gettman (1980). Oxygen uptake and energy expenditure during horizontal treadmill running. *Journal of Applied Physiology* **49**: 571–5.

18. R.C. Browning and R. Kram (2005). Energetic cost and preferred speed of walking in obese vs. normal weight women. *Obesity Research* **13**: 891–9.

19. R.C. Browning, E.A. Baker, J.A. Herron and R. Kram (2006). Effects of obesity and sex on the energetic cost and preferred speed of walking. *Journal of Applied Physiology* **100**: 390–8.

20. T. Shono, K. Fujishima, N. Hotta, T. Ogaki and K. Matsumoto (2001). Cardiorespiratory response to low-intensity walking in water and on land in elderly women. *Journal of Physiological Anthropology and Applied Human Science* **20**: 269–74.

21. D. Malatesta, D. Simar, Y. Dauvilliers, R. Candau, F. Borrani, C. Préfaut and C. Caillaud (2003). Energy cost of walking and gait instability in healthy 65- and 80-yr-olds. *Journal of Applied Physiology* **95**: 2248–56.

22. P.E. Martin, D.E. Rothstein and D.D. Larish (1992). Effects of age and physical activity status on the speed-aerobic demand relationship of walking. *Journal of Applied Physiology* **73**: 200–6.

23. S.E. Turner, P.R. Eastwood, N.M. Cecins, D.R. Hillman and S.C. Jenkins (2004). Physiologic responses to incremental and self-paced exercise in COPD. *Chest* **126**: 766–73.

24. M. Maeder, T. Wolber, R. Atefy, M. Gadza, P. Ammann, J. Myers et al. (2005). Impact of the exercise mode on exercise capacity: bicycle testing revisited. *Chest* **128**: 2804–11.

25. H. Tsurugaya, H. Adachi, M. Kurabayashi, S. Ohshima and K. Taniguchi (2006). Prognostic impact of ventilatory efficiency in heart disease patients with preserved exercise tolerance. *Circulation* **70**: 1332–6.

26. A. Koike, H. Itoh, M. Kato, H. Sawada, T. Aizawa, L.T. Fu and H. Watanabe (2001). Prognostic power of ventilatory responses during submaximal exercise in patients with chronic heart disease. *Chest* **121**: 1581–8.

27. M. Robbins, G. Francis, F.J. Pashkow, C.E. Snader, K. Hoercher, J.B. Young et al. (1999). Ventilatory and heart rate responses to exercise: better predictors of heart failure mortality than peak oxygen consumption. *Chest* **100**: 2411–17.

28. L.C. Davies, R. Wensel, P. Georgiadou, M. Cicoira, A.J.S. Coats, M. Piepoli et al. (2006). Enhanced prognostic value from cardiopulmonary exercise testing in chronic heart failure by non-linear analysis: oxygen uptake efficiency slope. *European Heart Journal* **27**: 684–90.

29. U. Corrà, A. Mezzani, E. Bosimini and P. Giannuzzi (2004). Cardiopulmonary exercise testing and prognosis in chronic heart failure: a prognosticating algorithm for the individual patient. *Chest* **126**: 942–50.

30. A.K. Gitt, K. Wasserman, C. Kilkowski, T. Kleemann, A. Kilkowski, M. Bangert et al. (2002). Exercise anaerobic threshold and ventilatory efficiency identify heart failure patients for high risk of early death. *Circulation* **106**: 3079–84.

31. M. Guazzi, J. Myers and R. Arena (2005). Cardiopulmonary Exercise Testing in the clinical and prognostic assessment of diastolic heart failure. *Journal of the American College of Cardiology* **46**: 1883–90.

32. T. Bilsel, S. Terzi, T. Akbulut, N. Sayar, G. Hobikoglu and K. Yesilcimen (2006). Abnormal heart rate recovery immediately after cardiopulmonary exercise testing in heart failure patients. *International Heart Journal* **47**: 431–40.

33. P. Brindle, A. Beswick, T. Fahey and S. Ebrahim (2006). Accuracy and impact of risk assessment in the primary prevention of cardiovascular disease: a systematic review. *Heart* **92**: 1752–9.

34. S.G. Wannamethee, A.G. Sharper and L. Lennon (2004). Cardiovascular disease incidence and mortality in older men with diabetes and in men with coronary heart disease. *Heart* **90**: 1398–1403.

35. J.P. Empana, P. Ducimetière, D. Arveiler, J. Ferrières, A. Evans, J.B. Ruidavets et al. (2004). Are the Framingham and PROCAM coronary heart disease risk functions applicable to different European populations? The PRIME study. *European Heart Journal* **24**: 1903–11.

36. P. Brindle, J. Emberson, F. Lampe, M. Walker, P. Whincup, T. Fahey et al. (2003). Predictive accuracy of the Framingham coronary risk score in British men: prospective cohort study. *British Medical Journal* **327**: 1267–73.

37. R.M. Conroy, K. Pyörälä, A.P. Fitzgerald, S. Sans, A. Menotti, G. De Backer et al. (2003). Estimation of ten-year risk of fatal cardiovascular disease in Europe: the SCORE project. *European Heart Journal* **24**: 987–1003.

38. F.C. Lampe, P.H. Whincup, S.G. Wannamethee, A.G. Shaper, M. Walker and S. Ebrahim (2001). The natural history of prevalent ischaemic heart disease in middle-aged men. *European Heart Journal* **21**: 1052–62.

39. D.A. Alter, A. Chong, P.C. Austin, C. Mustard, K. Iron, J.I. Williams et al. (2006). Socioeconomic status and mortality after acute myocardial infarction. *Annals of Internal Medicine* **144**: 82–93.

40. T.C. Clayton, J. Lubsen, S.J. Pocock, Z. Vókó, B-A. Kirwan, K.A.A. Fox et al. (2005). Risk score for predicting death, myocardial infarction, and stroke in patients with stable angina, based on a large randomised trial cohort of patients. *British Medical Journal* **331**: 869–74.

41. H. Hemingway, A. McCallum, M. Shipley, K. Manderbacka, P. Martikainen and I. Keskimäki (2006). Incidence and prognostic implications of stable angina pectoris among women and men. *Journal of the American Medical Association* **295**: 1404–11.

42. T.G. Clark, M.F.G. Murphy and P.M. Rothwell (2003). Long term risks of stroke, myocardial infarction, and vascular death in 'low risk' patients with a non-recent transient ischaemic attack. *Journal of Neurology Neurosurgery and Psychiatry* **74**: 577–80.

43. P.E. Norman, J.W. Eikelboorn and G.J. Hankey (2004). Peripheral arterial disease: prognostic significance and prevention of atherothrombotic complications. *Medical Journal of Australia* **181**: 150–4.

44. R.J. McManus, J. Mant, C.F.M. Meulendijks, R.A. Salter, H.M. Pattison, A.K. Roalfe et al. (2002). Comparison of estimates and calculations of risk of coronary heart disease by doctors and nurses using different calculation tools in general practice: cross sectional study. *British Medical Journal* **324**: 459–64.

45. J. Carlisle and M. Swart (2007). Mid-term survival after elective abdominal aortic aneurysm surgery predicted by cardiopulmonary exercise testing. *British Journal of Surgery* **94**: 966–9.

46. L.A. Fleisher, J.A. Beckman, K.A. Brown, H. Calkins, E. Chaikof, K.E. Fleischmann et al. (2007). ACC/AHA 2007 guidelines on perioperative cardiovascular evaluation and care for noncardiac surgery: a report of the American College of Cardiology/American Heart Association task force on practice guidelines. *Journal of the American College of Cardiology* **50**: 159–241.

47. T.H. Lee, E.R. Marcantonio, C.M. Mangione, E.J. Thomas, C.A. Polanczyk, E.F. Cook et al. (1999). Derivation and prospective validation of a simple index for prediction of cardiac risk of major noncardiac surgery. *Circulation* **100**: 1043–9.

48. L. Goldman, D.L. Caldera, S.R. Nussbaum, F.S. Southwick, D. Krogstad, B. Murray et al. (1977). Multifactorial index of cardiac risk in noncardiac surgical procedures. *New England Journal of Medicine* **297**: 845–50.

49. A.S. Detsky, H.B. Abrams, J.R. McLaughlin, D.J. Drucker, Z. Sasson, N. Johnston et al. (1986). Predicting cardiac complications in patients undergoing non-cardiac surgery. *Journal of General Internal Medicine* **1**: 211–19.

50. American College of Physicians (1997). Guidelines for assessing and managing the perioperative risk from coronary artery disease associated with major noncardiac surgery. *Annals of Internal Medicine* **127**: 309–12.

51. M.D. Kertai, E. Boersma, J. Klein, H. van Urk and D. Poldermans (2005). Optimizing the prediction of perioperative mortality in vascular surgery by using a customized probability model. *Archives of Internal Medicine* **165**: 898–904.

FURTHER READING

Communicating risks: illusion or truth? *British Medical Journal* **327** (2003), themed issue 7417.

G. Gigerenzer (2003). *Reckoning with Risk: Learning to Live with Uncertainty* (London: Penguin).

J. A. Paulos (2001). *Innumeracy: Mathematical Illiteracy and its Consequences*, 1st edn (New York, NY: Hill and Wang).

P. Older and A. Hall (2002). Preoperative assessment of elderly surgical patients. (In K. Wasserman (ed.), *Cardiopulmonary Exercise Testing and Cardiovascular Health*. Armonk, NY: Futura Publishing Company.)

P. Older and A. Hall (2003). Myocardial ischemia or cardiac failure: Which constitutes the major perioperative risk? (In J.-L.Vincent (ed.), *Year Book of Critical Care and Emergency Medicine*. Berlin, Heidelberg, New York: Springer-Verlag.)

P. Older and A. Hall (2007). The role of cardiopulmonary exercise testing in preoperative evaluation of surgical patients. (In *Recent Advances in Anaesthesia and Intensive Care* **24** Cambridge: Cambridge University Press.)

Chapter 3 History taking

Hilary Walsgrove

SUMMARY

This chapter will describe:

- the purpose of taking a health history at preoperative assessment
- various methods of obtaining a health history
- the preoperative assessment history taking consultation
- functional assessment and systems inquiry
- recording a clinical health history assessment.

INTRODUCTION

The importance of obtaining an accurate and comprehensive patient history should not be under-estimated. It is the baseline upon which appropriate diagnostic reasoning and clinical decision-making can be made in order to optimise the patient's health prior to surgery and anaesthesia.

History taking should not be viewed in isolation. The communication skills and consultation techniques required to extract relevant information from a patient, and/or relative, should be a core component of the practice of healthcare professionals and need to be considered as essential. A reliable and clear record of the patient's medical history, to serve as a foundation for creating a plan of care, will ensure that the patient's surgical journey is effective, reducing the risk of suboptimal management and increasing safety with the least possible distress for the patient and their significant others. For the history taking process to be executed well, a number of essential elements should be considered, such as the environment. The knowledge and expertise of the healthcare professional and the required information should create a complete and thorough assessment.

The essential elements of history taking include a medical, surgical and anaesthetic history; general and focused system review health history; social history, including recreational activities; psychological/emotional issues. This is described in further detail later in this chapter. Details of the information exchange between the patient and the assessor should be recorded and addressed to ensure patients' expectations are understood and aligned with the anticipated plan of care and course of recovery including discharge from the hospital. There are a number of additional considerations dependent on the individual patient, for example, whether the patient is a child or elderly, their sexual history, any learning disability, as well as cultural and religious considerations (these areas are beyond the scope of this chapter).

Once the history has been obtained, the ensuing clinical examination can be focused accordingly (see Chapter 4). Relevant investigations and observations, including vital signs, can be undertaken depending upon the systemic disease/co-morbidity identified (seeChapters 5–12).

The aims of taking a preoperative assessment history

Preoperative optimisation can decrease the risk to the patient, improve surgical outcomes, and ensure effective and timely use of healthcare resources, whilst also ensuring the implementation of preventative and precautionary interventions prior to surgery for patients who are potentially at risk.[1] The patient history is also useful for establishing a baseline for postoperative evaluation.[1] Effective preoperative preparation and education have been shown to aid recovery and reduce postoperative morbidity.[2]

Methods of preoperative assessment history taking

Preoperative assessment aims to identify level of fitness for surgery and anaesthesia, with particular emphasis on the cardiovascular and respiratory systems and potential airway difficulties. However, a whole systems approach is required to assess and identify disease processes or other factors that may impact on the patient's surgical and anaesthetic course. The organisation of preoperative assessment varies according to local policies/practices and, therefore, how the patient history is obtained varies accordingly. The assessment should be relevant and effective according to patient need, method of anaesthesia planned and the severity of the surgical procedure.

Preoperative assessment questionnaires

Self-completed questionnaires can be sent by post or electronically[3] or completed at the time of the surgical outpatient appointment. In recent years, use of computer-interpreted screening questionnaires has increased.[3] Such questionnaires extract information from patients, and are reviewed by appropriately trained clerical, nursing or other members of staff, invariably using a specific protocol. This method identifies patients with problems who may need more formal preoperative assessment within a clinic setting. It enables useful information to be obtained about the patient in a relatively simple manner and is especially useful for fit patients, such as those in ASA 1 and 2 grading categories requiring minor and/or intermediate type surgical procedures.[4]

Preoperative assessment by direct contact

Obtaining patient information for preoperative assessment via telephone interview can decrease visits to hospital. It can be performed in the community such as by the general practitioner or other community care practitioner or at a designated preoperative assessment clinic based in the community or hospital. This model of care enables more comprehensive information to be gathered about the patient by a healthcare professional experienced in undertaking consultations of this type (rather than by the self-reporting method identified above) and allows patients to ask questions and share concerns on a more personal level. These more direct methods of preoperative assessment will provide the main focus for the rest of this chapter. There is an increasing trend towards optimisation by the primary care provider, prior to referral for surgery for the patient undergoing an elective procedure.

The preoperative assessment consultation

Setting the scene

The creation of the right environment can play a vital part in the success of a consultation.[5] Ideally a quiet, private, comfortable place should be allocated for this purpose, where patient privacy, confidentiality and dignity can be maintained throughout and where interruptions are kept to a minimum. It is suggested that extraneous noises may distract, intrude and raise stress levels for the patient as well as the assessor.[6] If possible, seating should be arranged in a non-confrontational manner. If a computer is used, the screen and keyboard should not get in the way or create a distraction/barrier.[7] Within a more open area, such as a hospital ward, this may be very difficult to achieve. The assessor within the ward environment should pull up a chair next to the patient's bed or bedside chair and sit level with the patient so that they can clearly see them and maintain eye contact.

Preparation for the consultation

First impressions play an important role, with the assessor's demeanour, attitude and dress having an influence.[8] The maintenance of a professional, neutral attitude and showing concern and understanding for the patient's situation are key to the conduct of the consultation.[7] A supportive, encouraging approach that is unbiased and non-judgemental will make the patient more forthcoming in terms of sharing personal information.[9] Establishing contact with the patient by shaking their hand during the opening of the consultation may help to establish a rapport and put them at ease,[10] as well as addressing the patient by name and the assessor introducing him/herself and explaining what is going to happen during the consultation.

The assessor should ensure that they are consulting with the correct patient. A prior review of the patient's medical notes and/or screening questionnaire is valuable, as it allows the assessor to build up an initial picture of the patient.[11] If the patient senses that the assessor has some knowledge of them at the outset, this can inspire confidence and demonstrate that the assessor has a personal interest in them. It is suggested that lack of interest in a patient, remoteness or a distant manner or a superior professional attitude are unhelpful in a relationship, such as one that is built between preoperative assessor and patient.[12]

Communication skills

Non-verbal communication, as well as verbal communication can be used to gain further information pertaining to the patient's health status. It is the medium through which relationships begin and develop, and the quality of the communication directly influences the quality of the relationship between the assessor and the patient. Thus barriers to the communication process should be kept to a minimum.[13] The lack of active participation in listening has been described as a key barrier in this process. Egan[14] uses the acronym SOLER as a prompt to encourage active listening by health professionals, which would be useful in a preoperative assessment (see Box 3.1).

Box 3.1 SOLER[14]

- Sitting **S**quarely in relation to the patient
- with an **O**pen stance
- **L**eaning slightly forward and maintaining
- **E**ye contact in a
- **R**elaxed manner indicates attention to what the patient is saying

Other points to note, in relation to non-verbal communication, include the assessor's use of reassuring gestures, ensuring he/she is not crossing his/her arms, looking bored or rushed. Observing the patient for non-verbal cues will elicit important information within the consultation. For example, if the patient is uncomfortable or unsure about answering a question, they may lower their voice or glance around uneasily.[9]

Verbal communication skills should be considered and used appropriately, e.g. silence, facilitation, confirmation, reflection, clarification, summary and conclusion.[9] Open-ended questions allow the patient to respond freely and to express feelings, opinions and ideas and to provide more detailed information. Closed questions help to gain clear, concise feedback on specific points. It may be pertinent to alternate between both questioning styles.

A skilled healthcare professional will adapt to the patient's style of communication and the use of broad questions followed by more focused questions will elicit as much information as possible in the patient's own words.[15] Any questions need to be asked in a manner the patient understands and in the language they speak. Patients are often not familiar with healthcare terminology and jargon, which should be avoided, as it can lead to confusion and misinterpretation of information.[16] The accuracy and completeness of the patient's answers largely depend on the skills of the assessor.[9]

The content of the history taking episode should give consideration to the following areas, in a structured approach:

- Presenting complaint and its symptoms
- Diagnosis (if relevant)
- Past medical history
- Previous surgical experiences
- Anaesthetic history, including problems experienced and family history of anaesthetic problems
- Medications
- Allergies
- Family history
- Social and psychological history
- Activities of daily living
- Systems enquiry

There is evidence to suggest that the patient's history contributes to approximately 60–80% of data required for focused examination and any subsequent clinical decision-making and diagnosis.[17]

Biographical data

Biographical data is usually gathered at the start of the patient's surgical journey and may be recorded by a member of clerical staff, such as the clinic receptionist or by a healthcare assistant. This is vital information to help ensure that the patient's surgical journey runs smoothly and efficiently, that channels of communication are maintained and the patient is cared for in accordance with individual, religious and cultural needs.

Presenting complaint

When obtaining information about the presenting complaint, it is useful to ask the patient to discuss the issue in their own words, using open-ended questions. This will ascertain their knowledge and understanding of the situation and of the planned surgery and guide the assessor with regard to the focus of the remainder of the consultation. The assessor is thus able to ensure that the patient's interpretation of the situation is accurate and to check that the patient is presenting for the correct procedure, depending on the nature of their presenting problem/s. If the preoperative assessment appointment is not 'one-stop', at the same time as the patient's consultation with the surgeon when the decision to treat has been made, the assessor needs to check whether the patient's symptoms have altered since the initial consultation with the surgeon.

Most patients will have been through an initial healthcare consultation, leading to a diagnosis of for the presenting complaint which, in turn, led to the decision to operate and the proposed surgical procedure. Other patients will be presenting at preoperative assessment for an investigative procedure to ascertain the nature of their problem. It is important for the preoperative assessor to ensure the patient is fully aware of the planned procedure, to check this with the patient, and to ensure that this information correlates with the medical notes. This corresponds with initiating the process of informed consent for the patient, in relation to the surgery and/or anaesthetic technique that will be employed.

The assessor has the opportunity to discuss the patient's symptoms, the impact on their life and ability to function.[9] All of this information will help with the organisational aspects involved in planning the patient's surgery, i.e. operating theatre scheduling, equipment required and the patient's perioperative and postoperative care needs.

The acronym OLDCART (Box 3.2) is a useful tool to aid assessment of the patient's physical complaint/s.

Box 3.2 Physical Complaint/Pain Assessment: 'OLDCART' acronym

O = Onset
- When did it start?

L = Location
- There may be multiple sites

D = Duration
- How long does the complaint/pain last?
- Is it constant?
- Is it intermittent?

C = Characteristics/causative factors (e.g. of pain)
- Neuropathic or nerve (sharp, shooting, burning, electrical)
- Somatic – bone pain is one example (dull, aching)
- Visceral (cramping, squeezing)

A = Aggravating factors
- Moving, walking, sitting, turning, chewing, swallowing, breathing, defecating, urinating

R = Relieving factors
- What makes the problem better?
- What medical and non-medical interventions relieve the complaint/pain?

T = Treatment
- Medications
- Non-pharmacological interventions (e.g. heat, cold, massage, distraction, etc.)

Past medical history

The medical history should comprise all medical problems the patient has experienced to date, including any chronic and episodic illnesses.[18] Any relevant medical history should be explored with the patient to ascertain whether or not it is likely to have an impact on the patient's surgical experience. Previous serious illnesses, treatments and any consequences, hospitalisations or frequent visits to a healthcare professional should be recorded. Patients often underestimate their morbidity, particularly if there has been a gradual deterioration over time, or they may consider their condition to be a part of the normal ageing process. For example, a patient who is being treated for an under-active thyroid may not consider that they have a medical condition and may not see the importance of informing the preoperative assessor of this issue. The availability of a current medication list from the GP can provide some insight into their current, as well as past, health history.

Surgical history

Any surgical procedure the patient has undergone, both major and minor, including dates performed should be recorded, including the type of anaesthesia involved if applicable. It should also be ascertained whether the patient experienced any complications or had any bad experiences from undergoing the surgery and anaesthetic. Any reactions or complications should be explored and considered in future planning of care, e.g. postoperative nausea and vomiting, suboptimal pain control. Knowledge of such problems can help with planning the treatment and care of a patient to ensure that the experience that they have this time is as satisfactory as possible.

This will also assist the assessor to gauge the patient's level of anxiety and any particular fears they may have. A comprehensive surgical history provides information about previous pathology and potential problems that may be encountered such as presence of scar tissue that may hinder the procedure to be undertaken.

Anaesthetic history

An anaesthetic history is more focused on specific aspects of relevance to perioperative management than a general medical history as outlined in (see Box 3.3).[19]

Box 3.3 Anaesthetic history pertinent to preoperative assessment

- Cardiac disease: cardiac failure, angina
- Respiratory disease: breathlessness, stridor, wheeze, smoking history
- Exercise tolerance: on flat surfaces and stairs

- Renal disease
- Liver disease
- Gastric reflux
- Dental conservation work: Bridges, crowns, false teeth
- Pregnancy or the use of oral contraception
- Drug/food allergy or intolerance: nature of food allergy, possible latex allergy
- Potential airway concerns such as facial surgery

Risk assessment tools

The American Society of Anaesthesiologists (ASA) Physical Status Classification is an established scoring tool and is useful for determining patient risk in relation to existing conditions. It can be used as a guide for the patient undergoing anaesthesia and is strongly predictive of peri- and postoperative complications[20] (see Box 3.4). The classification system subjectively categorises patients into five groups by preoperative physical fitness. Originally devised in 1961, it does have limitations; for example, it does not allow for adjustment regarding age, sex, weight or pregnancy or reflect the nature of the planned surgery.[20] Further analysis of risk assessment can be found in Chapter 2.

Box 3.4 ASA grade		
Class	Physical status	Example
I	A completely healthy patient	A fit patient with an inguinal hernia
II	A patient with mild systemic disease	Essential hypertension, mild diabetes without end organ damage
III	A patient with severe systemic disease that is not incapacitating	Angina, moderate to severe COPD
IV	A patient with incapacitating disease that is a constant threat to life	Advanced COPD, cardiac failure
V	A moribund patient who is not expected to live 24 hours with or without surgery	Ruptured aortic aneurysm, massive pulmonary embolism
E	Emergency case	

As outlined above, in the United Kingdom patients are usually coded according to their ASA grade but the NCEPOD[21] (National Confidential Enquiry into Peri-operative Deaths) scores can be used to assess the severity of the planned surgery, with the NCEPOD banding denoting the urgency of the surgery (see Box 3.5).

Box 3.5 NCEPOD grades	
Immediate	Immediate life- limb- or organ-saving intervention – resuscitation simultaneous with intervention. Normally within minutes of decision to operate. A) Life-saving B) Other, e.g. limb- or organ-saving.
Urgent	Intervention for acute onset or clinical deterioration of potentially life-threatening conditions, for those conditions that may threaten the survival of limb or organ, for fixation of many fractures and for relief of pain or other distressing symptoms. Normally within hours of decision to operate.
Expedited	Patient requiring early treatment where the condition is not an immediate threat to life, limb or organ survival. Normally within days of decision to operate.
Elective	Intervention planned, or booked, in advance of routine admission to hospital. Timing to suit patient, hospital and staff.

Cardio-pulmonary exercise testing (CPX), is increasingly the investigation of choice used to stratify the risk of patients undergoing major surgery by measuring their anaerobic threshold.[19] This can be used as an aid in decision-making in consultation with the patient to determine whether surgery should proceed and to predict patient management decisions, such as intensive care requirement postoperatively. It is discussed in detail in Chapters 2 and 5.

Exercise tolerance

The patient's degree of exercise tolerance provides an indication of their fitness for surgery and anaesthesia. Evidence demonstrates that patients with poor exercise tolerance have more perioperative complications.[22] In the absence of formal exercise testing, the preoperative assessor can ascertain the patient's exercise tolerance from the patient history. Questions regarding the nature and frequency of their physical activities, alongside other available information, for example their Metabolic Equivalent Task Score (METs), can assess the patient's ability to undergo surgery safely.

Questioning to establish a patient's exercise tolerance can include the following:

- How far can you walk on the flat?
- How far can you walk uphill?
- How many stairs can you climb before stopping?
- Could you run for a bus?
- Are you able to do the shopping?
- Are you able to do the housework (e.g. hoovering)?
- Are you able to care for yourself?

One way of making questioning more objective is through the use of the New York Heart Association (NYHA) Classification.[23] This specific activity scale grades common physical activities in terms of their MET score and classifies patients according to how many 'METS' they can achieve (Box 3.6). A detailed comparison of risk and METS is also made in Chapter 2.

Box 3.6 New York Heart Association Classification – METS	
NYHA Class	METS
Class I	Can perform activities requiring more than 7 METS
Class II	Can perform activities requiring more than 5 METS but less than 7 METS
Class III	Can perform activities requiring more than 2 METS but less than 5 METS
Class IV	Patient cannot perform activities requiring more than 2 METS

Previous anaesthetic issues

If difficulty with previous anaesthesia is noted, detail of such events should be obtained from the patient or from the anaesthetic record. Individual needs should be identified, particularly issues such as problems with either mask ventilation and/or endotracheal intubation, as this would indicate concern with regard to the patient's airway. Adverse respiratory events are a major cause of injury in anaesthetic practice, with inadequate ventilation being the largest category of adverse events.[2] This can lead to an unplanned admission to a critical care facility, which may be traumatic for the patient who is not expecting it, as well as causing organisational and planning difficulties for the hospital.

Airway assessment

Protection of the airway throughout anaesthesia is essential. Thus a detailed airway assessment should be made, based on information from the patient, their records and a thorough examination. Predictive factors for a potential difficult airway include a past history of a 'difficult airway' and any congenital, acquired or anatomical features. The Mallampati scoring system allows assessment of the oropharyngeal structures including the size and position of the tongue in relation to that of the soft palate, while the tongue rests on the floor of the mouth.[24] Further information on airway assessment can be found in Chapter 7.

A patient who meets the criteria for a potential 'difficult airway' may be less of a challenge to the anaesthetist than the patient with an unrecognised difficult airway, highlighting the importance of accurate and comprehensive history taking in relation to airway management issues.[2]

There are some rare medical conditions that can cause life-threatening anaesthetic problems. Identification at preoperative assessment can decrease the risk and ensure appropriate management is planned.

Malignant hyperthermia (MH)

Malignant hyperthermia is a genetic condition where individuals are predisposed to a potential life-threatening condition when exposed to either volatile anaesthetic agents such as halothane or isoflurane or certain drugs such as succinylcholine (suxamethonium). Individuals in whom no response is triggered initially may develop malignant hyperthermia with subsequent anaesthetic administration.[2] Clinical features of hypermetabolism, such as tachycardia, hypertension, metabolic acidosis, muscle rigidity are indicative and hyperthermia and death may occur if the condition remains untreated.[2,25]

Pseudocholinesterase deficiency

This condition affects the quality or quantity of plasma cholinesterase, an enzyme responsible for metabolism of certain muscle relaxants used in general anaesthesia, such as succinylcholine and mivacurium. It can lead to prolonged apnoea in the anaesthetised patient. Pseudocholinesterase deficiency can be genetically determined or acquired in association with various disease processes, such as liver failure, acute myocardial disease, malnutrition, myxoedema or by certain drugs, such as oral contraceptives, phenylzine, cyclophosphamide and chlorpromazine.[2,25] A line of questioning that may be useful when ascertaining whether the patient has this deficiency would include the following.[26]

- What type of anaesthetic has the patient had (i.e. general or local)?
- Did the patient have any adverse reactions?
- Does the patient have a family history of adverse reactions to anaesthetic?
- Did the patient require mechanical ventilation during postoperative period?
- Was the patient unable to lift their head postoperatively?
- Has the patient been tested for this deficiency (blood sampling for pseudocholinesterase levels)?

Family history

Details of the health of family members can assist in identifying risk factors that may or may not become apparent during the rest of the history taking process. If the patient does not have any previous history of anaesthesia and surgery it may provide an indication of underlying genetic conditions such as those discussed above. A family history of cardiovascular and respiratory disease may also be of significance.

Medication history

Past and current consumption of medications, including prescription, over-the-counter, vitamins/supplements, lotions and alternative remedies as well as recreational drug use should be explored and recorded, including any recently stopped medication. Most medicines taken for chronic conditions should continue as usual, up to and including the day of surgery. However, it may be necessary to omit certain medications or amend the dose of others, such as anticoagulant therapy or steroids. There is a risk of drug interactions with certain medications. Thus drugs used during anaesthesia, peri- and postoperatively should be considered in the light of the patient's regular medication use, including any medication that may be required in an emergency or rescue situation.

A comprehensive medication history should also include use and potential abuse of over-the-counter and prescription medications, the use and abuse of alcohol and other recreational substances, whether legal or illegal and a past and current smoking history. This can be a challenging route of questioning but it is important to stress the value of gaining such information in relation to maintaining their safety during the surgical/anaesthetic process. The patient should be reassured that information remains confidential and withholding information may be detrimental to their health or may delay treatment.[18] More detail of medications management can be found specifically in Chapter 12, and other clinical systems in Chapters 5–11.

Allergies

Establishing a patient's allergy status is key to maintaining patient safety and should include allergies to medications, foods and animals as well as environmental allergens, such as latex.[18] It may be necessary to provide a latex-free environment within the ward and theatre areas and to avoid the use of certain medications or products in order to prevent an adverse event caused by an allergic reaction. A record should be made of the type and severity of the reaction the patient has experienced and any local guidance should be followed.[27]

Functional assessment and activities of living

The patient's perception of their general state of health, including questions about a patient's usual lifestyle and activities of daily living, can provide a baseline for determining their overall health status, exercise tolerance and suitability for surgery and anaesthesia. Details of the patient's home life, such as housing, economic situation, living arrangements and so on, particularly if they live alone or have dependants to care for, should be obtained. This will inform the discharge planning process which should commence at the time of preoperative assessment. An enquiry about occupation, if they are employed, is also important. This may identify areas of risk in their occupation which may influence their recovery and daily activity in the future. Social and sporting activities should also be considered, as they may impact on the patient's recovery postoperatively.

By establishing the patient's normal self-care practices, a plan of care can be developed to optimise the patient's health status and level of independence and to identify realistic health outcomes, relating to their surgical pathway and recovery.[28] Exploration of the patient's activities of living including diet and fluid intake, activity and exercise, sleep patterns, elimination, sexuality, menstrual cycle (if relevant), communication patterns and difficulties, mood and behaviour, coping and stress management, will help build up a picture of the patient's functional capacity and expectations.[27] It will provide a guide for the preoperative assessor of how well the patient will cope postoperatively and any arrangements that may be required for safe and effective discharge from hospital.

System review

This section provides an overview of the system review. Greater depth is available in the relevant chapters.

Cardiovascular

Review of the cardiovascular system requires an understanding of the extent and stability of any disease factors and specific questions regarding cardiovascular status are important for planning perioperative management. Identification of any unstable symptoms, associated with high perioperative risk will influence the decision-making process. Pre-existing cardiovascular conditions, such as previous myocardial infarction, ischaemic heart disease, angina, arrhythmias, heart murmurs, hypertension and heart failure, increase morbidity and mortality from anaesthesia and surgery. Key symptoms of cardiac malfunction to look out for during cardiovascular history taking include breathlessness, chest pain, palpitations, fatigue, syncope and claudication.

Shortness of breath on exertion or lying flat (orthopnoea), is indicative of heart failure. Paroxysmal nocturnal dyspnoea is suggestive of pulmonary oedema.

Questions to be asked with regard to breathlessness include: Do you ever feel short of breath? Does this happen on exertion? How much can you do before getting breathless? Do you ever wake up gasping for breath? If so, do you have to sit up or get out of bed? How many pillows do you sleep on? (If more than two pillows, establish if this is for comfort or due to breathing difficulties.) Are you able to lie flat?

- Do you cough or wheeze when you are short of breath?

When cardiac output fails to provide adequate delivery of oxygen to the tissues, the patient may experience otherwise unexplained fatigue and weakness. Chest pain due to cardiac disease is typically brought on by exertion, cold weather or anxiety and may be relieved by rest or the use of nitrates. It is usually experienced in the retro-sternal region as crushing, squeezing or constricting in nature.[23]

Useful questions to ask include:

- Do you get pain in your chest on exertion (e.g. climbing stairs)?
- Where in the chest do you feel it?
- Is the pain referred anywhere else? For example your left arm, jaw?
- Is it worse in cold weather?
- Is it worse if you exercise after a big meal?
- Is it bad enough to stop you exercising?
- Does it go away when you rest?
- Do you ever get similar pain when you get excited or upset?

If a patient has had a previous myocardial infarction, specific information is required:

- when the attack occurred
- its severity and complications
- treatment received
- duration of hospital stay.

Studies have shown an increased incidence of re-infarction if a patient has had a myocardial infarction within 3 months, or even 1 month of surgery.[29]

Palpitations can be an indicator of the presence of arrhythmias and episodes of syncope can be indicative of heart block. Questions to ask include:

- Is it regular or irregular?
- Is there anything that sets off an attack?
- Can you do anything to stop an attack?
- What do you do when you have an attack?
- Are there any foods that seem to make symptoms worse?
- What medications are you taking?

It can be useful to ask the patient to tap out rate during an attack.

A patient who has a pacemaker in situ is likely to have underlying pathology, usually ischaemic heart disease or arrhythmia. Details of the type of pacemaker, the reason for pacemaker insertion and date of last pacemaker check should be obtained. The check should have been within the last year and a record of the settings noted.

The automatic implantable cardioverter defibrillator (AICD) is now more frequently used for patients with refractory malignant ventricular arrhythmias.[30] Preoperative assessment of patients with an AICD includes details of the underlying cardiac disease (ischaemic or valvular heart disease, cardiomyopathy), and the status of the patient's ventricular function. Such patients should be receiving optimal medical therapy; thus preoperative investigations should focus on detecting any electrolyte imbalance or drug toxicity. Knowledge of the model of AICD is important, as there is wide variation in the functional characteristics of different models.

The presence of coronary artery disease is higher in patients with diabetes mellitus than non-diabetics and there is a higher incidence of both silent myocardial infarction and myocardial ischaemia.

Most hypertensive disease is idiopathic but approximately 10% of patients suffer from hypertension caused by renal, endocrine or pregnancy-related disease. Hypertension needs to be viewed within the context of the patient's general medical condition to determine the need for further evaluation of the cardiac status. Liaison with the primary care team is necessary, particularly if the patient is receiving ongoing management of their hypertension or if a newly diagnosed hypertension is detected at the time of preoperative assessment.

Hypertension is usually symptomless but, if untreated, it may result in enlargement of the heart and failure, renal dysfunction and cerebrovascular accidents. It is important to look for such problems, as they may influence the choice of anaesthetic technique. Patients with untreated or inadequately treated hypertension developed marked swings in blood pressure with situations such as anaesthesia, blood loss or pain.

Management of hypertension should concentrate on methods to reduce perioperative risk. Determinants of risk include the level of the blood pressure, duration of treatment, degree of end organ damage and the type of surgery planned. In relation to the level of hypertension, severe hypertension increases the risk of perioperative blood pressure lability, myocardial ischaemia and myocardial infarction, pulmonary oedema, arrhythmias, renal failure and neurological damage. Patients with any form of preoperative hypertension, treated or untreated, have an increased risk of postoperative hypertension.

Methods to reduce perioperative risk include adequate preoperative blood pressure control. The patient should be advised to continue all hypertensive medications up to and including the day of surgery, with the exception of diuretics. Local guidelines outlining medicine management in relation to continuing and discontinuing medications preoperatively should be referred to. Elective surgery should be delayed if the systolic blood pressure is above 200mmHg or if the diastolic BP is above 120mmHg, preferably lowered to 140/90mmHg over several weeks. Acute control within hours of surgery is inadvisable. Again, local guidelines for the accepted parameters for blood pressure readings and surgery/anaesthesia, should be adhered to.

Respiratory

Lung disease can complicate anaesthesia and influence the postoperative outcome following surgery. Perioperative complications include intubation difficulties, a need for re-intubation, laryngospasm, bronchospasm, aspiration, hyperventilation and hypoxia. The frequency of postoperative respiratory problems necessitates the identification of those patients who are particularly at risk. Patients who present with respiratory problems may need referral to a respiratory physiotherapist preoperatively, depending on the nature and severity of their disease and in relation to the planned surgery and anaesthesia.

It is possible to observe the patient for signs of respiratory distress during the consultation, particularly while talking. Assessment of exercise tolerance, using the 'METS' system described in Box 3.6(see page 42), can be a helpful indicator of the extent of the disease process and risk factors with regard to surgery and anaesthesia.

The presence of key symptoms such as dyspnoea, cough, sputum production and wheeze should be explored in greater detail as discussed below.

Dyspnoea

Dyspnoea is subjective but can indicate the severity of the respiratory disease in terms of exercise tolerance. Dyspnoea at rest represents a serious anaesthetic challenge. The preoperative assessor should enquire about shortness of breath using the line of questioning outlined as part of the cardiovascular system enquiry above (see pages 45–6).

Cough

Cough may indicate a hyper-responsive respiratory tract with increased susceptibility to laryngeal spasm and coughing during induction of anaesthesia. Cough after exercise or at night may be indicative of asthma; a cough following meals may indicate aspiration of gastric contents due to oesophageal abnormalities and a barking cough may be a sign of laryngeal nerve injury. A cough accompanied by sputum may indicate the presence of infection and/or inflammation and may contraindicate elective surgery or require a regional anaesthetic technique, as this enables the preservation of the cough reflex. Some medications, such as ACE inhibitors can induce a cough, due to the bradykinin pathway and it may be appropriate to change these to angiotensin II receptor blockers, which block the bradykinin pathway so a cough is avoided.

Asthma

Asthma can present a number of risks during the perioperative period. Variable airway obstruction, accompanied by a wheeze, can be precipitated by anaesthesia. Manipulation of the airway can cause bronchospasm. Drugs used in anaesthesia release histamine, which can further complicate the management of asthmatic patients. Details of current management of the patient's asthma, along with concordance with any treatments should be obtained. Oral steroid therapy, especially recent changes, periods of hospitalisation and critical care admissions as a result of asthma should be noted and the potential need for additional steroid cover should be assessed. By ascertaining the severity of the patient's disease process, how it is managed and potential risk factors relating to surgery and anaesthesia, the preoperative assessor can ensure safe and effective care is planned.

Upper respiratory tract infection

Symptoms of upper respiratory tract infection with pyrexia are a contraindication to elective surgery. They can lead to airway obstruction, laryngospasm with the postoperative risk of atelectasis and chest infections.

Obstructive sleep apnoea

Patients with obstructive sleep apnoea are particularly vulnerable during anaesthesia and sedation. They may present with a difficult airway and are at increased risk of developing respiratory and cardiopulmonary complications postoperatively.[31] Undiagnosed sleep apnoea is common. An awareness of the symptoms associated with the condition is essential to inform the questioning and history taking process (see Box 3.7).[31] The symptoms and physical characteristics associated with sleep apnoea and other respiratory conditions are discussed further in Chapter 6.

Box 3.7 Symptoms and physical characteristics associated with obstructive sleep apnoea

Symptoms:

Heavy persistent snoring

Excessive daytime sleepiness (somnolence)

Apnoea as observed by sleeping partner

Choking sensations while waking up

Gastro-oesophageal reflux

Reduced ability to concentrate

Memory loss

Personality changes

Mood swings

Night sweating

Nocturia

Dry mouth in the morning

Restless sleep

Morning headache

Impotence

Physical characteristics

Nasal obstruction

Oedematous or long soft palate or uvula

Hypertrophic tongue

Narrow oropharynx (large tonsils, redundant pharyngeal arches)

Adiposity or large neck circumference

Retrognathia

Maxillary hypoplasia

Opiate analgesia may exacerbate this condition with arterial de-saturation being accompanied by cardiac arrhythmias.

Gastro-intestinal conditions, liver disease, renal disease

Conditions associated with the gastro-intestinal tract can increase risk factors for patients undergoing surgery.

Gastric problems

Patients with a history of dyspepsia, acid reflux and recurrent regurgitation, hiatus hernia or increased intra-abdominal pressure (such as occurs in an acutely distended abdomen, intestinal obstruction, morbid obesity or pregnancy), are more susceptible to pulmonary aspiration of gastric contents. Many drugs, including H2-receptor antagonists, proton-pump inhibitors and antacids have been used to reduce and/or eliminate the risk of pulmonary aspiration by decreasing the acidity and volume of gastric fluid. Thus, management of these susceptible patients, using a preoperative medication, including a proton-pump inhibitor is desirable.

Liver disease

Patients with liver disease are complex and may present significant anaesthetic and surgical risk.[25] Liver disease can lead to impaired metabolism of anaesthetic drugs and reduced hepatic clearance of uploads can result in prolonged sleepiness after anaesthesia. Coagulopathies, if unrecognised, may result in unexpectedly heavy intraoperative bleeding or even spinal haematoma after regional block.

Renal disease

The main perioperative risk is deterioration of renal function, which may lead to acute renal failure, which can be fatal if left untreated.[25] Renal disease can be exacerbated by anaesthesia and surgery, with the potential reduction of renal blood flow and drug-induced nephrotoxicity. Patients with renal disease are commonly hypertensive and have a hyperdynamic circulation. Increased serum urea level associated with renal conditions can delay gastric emptying and increase acid secretion in the stomach, thus increasing the risk of aspiration at anaesthetic induction. This may be an indication for preoperative intervention, such as the administration of a proton-pump inhibitor. Further detailed assessment is considered in Chapter 8.

Endocrine disorders

Thyroid disease and diabetes mellitus are probably the most common endocrine disorders encountered at preoperative assessment. The difficulty with diseases such as these is that they are likely to lead to the patient having a plethora of systemic problems that may be exacerbated by anaesthesia and surgery, increasing peri- and postoperative risks. Evaluation of the impact of the disease process on the individual patient is crucial and such patients may need to be optimised prior to anaesthesia. Patients with endocrine disease are likely to be taking medications that should not be omitted pre- and postoperatively and need a plan of pre-, peri- and postoperative management of their disease and medication (further details can be found in Chapter 8). Any clinically evident disease needs to be controlled prior to elective surgery.[25] Patients presenting with thyroid disease may have a goitre, which may potentially compromise the airway, as well as cardiac arrhythmias.

Neurological

The scope of neurological diseases and their anaesthetic implications is broad and beyond the scope of this chapter. Each neurological condition requires careful consideration and individual evaluation to ensure the safety of the patient during surgery and anaesthesia. Documentation of preoperative neurological deficits is essential and a full anaesthetic assessment may be required preoperatively. Attention should be paid to a history or presence of cerebrovascular disease, pituitary adenomas, seizure disorders, such as epilepsy, myopathies, multiple sclerosis, myasthenia gravis and dementia.[2] These are discussed in more detail in Chapter 9.

Musculo-skeletal

Common musculo-skeletal diseases that are autoimmune in nature can have significant implications in relation to surgery and anaesthesia. Such systemic diseases have numerous clinical manifestations that require palliative treatment aimed at suppressing inflammatory or immunological processes to improve symptoms and prevent progressive damage. This group of diseases includes rheumatoid arthritis, ankylosing spondylitis, systemic lupus erythematosus, scleroderma and polymyalgia rheumatica. Significant toxicity is associated with the drug therapies used for their management and this necessitates careful evaluation. The impact of these diseases on perioperative risk and complications relates to the drug therapy used, the type of surgery/anaesthesia planned as well as the disease itself. As a general rule, these patients have a better tolerance of surgery if the disease is optimally controlled preoperatively.[2] It is also important to ascertain key factors relating to the patient in general such as lifestyle, degree of disability and exercise tolerance.

Osteoarthritis does not involve systemic factors in the way that the autoimmune diseases do, but the degree of disability and functional impairment should be noted, especially in relation to the range of movement of the neck and spine with regard to airway management, regional anaesthetic techniques as well as positioning during surgery. Severe functional impairment may mask cardiac and other symptoms that would be significant risks during anaesthesia and surgery.

Completing the history taking process

To conclude, a succinct summary of the main points should be recorded to ensure that the patient is in agreement with the information gathered. The art of history taking is to be thorough without being interrogative and to actively listen to the patient's responses and encourage them to tell their story. Closure of the history taking component of the preoperative assessment can be followed by transition to relevant physical examination, investigations and observations.

Documentation

Accurate and comprehensive documentation provides the principal source of information about the patient, a vital source of inter-professional communication for practitioners caring for and treating the patient and acts as a means of ensuring continuity of care and decreased risk to the patient.[32] All aspects of the patient assessment should be recorded systematically.[25] This should be available to all members of the healthcare team caring for the patient. Comprehensive and accurate documentation aids a smooth process, helping to minimise risks to both patients and staff, as well as being the best form of defence if and when anything goes wrong.[28]

CONCLUSION

This chapter has provided an overview of the history taking element of the preoperative assessment consultation and the different aspects involved in this process. Each patient's history should be considered from an individual perspective. Some key general factors to consider during preoperative assessment history taking have been included. Although it is beyond the scope of this chapter to consider a detailed systems inquiry in relation to all disease processes related to surgery and anaesthesia, the structure and process of history taking in preoperative assessment has been described. The preoperative assessor should consult relevant medical, nursing and anaesthetic texts for further detail of systems evaluation and seek out guidance and advice from clinical colleagues with relevant experience as well as using local guidance and policy to support practice.

REFERENCES

1. M.J. Evans and M.A. Black (1990). *Surgical Nursing*. Pennsylvania: Springhouse Corporation.

2. B.J. Sweitzer (2000). *Handbook of Pre-operative Assessment and Management*. Philadelphia: Lippincott, Williams and Wilkins.

3. J.N. Cashman (ed.) (2001). *Pre-operative Assessment*. London: BMJ Books.

4. R. Kerridge, A. Lee, E. Latchford, S.J. Beehan and K.M. Hilman (1995). The peri-operative system: a new approach to managing elective surgery. *Anaesthesia and Intensive Care* **23**: 591–6.

5. H. Paniagua (1997). Consultations in practice. *Practice Nursing* **8**(8): 20–2.

6. R. Newell (1994). *Intervention Skills for Nurses and Other Health Professionals*. London: Routledge.

7. D. Snadden, R. Laing, G. Masterton and N. Colledge. *History taking and general examination (section 1)* (available at www.acumedic.com/books/bk3944.pdf last accessed 29 March 2010).

8. T. Foster and J. Hawkins (2005). The therapeutic relationship: dead or merely impeded by technology? *British Journal of Nursing* **14**(13): 698–702.

9. D. Beverage and Margaret Eckman (eds) (2005). *Assessment made Incredibly Easy* (3rd edn). London, Philadelphia: Lippincott, Williams and Wilkins.

10. B. Hutchisson, M.L. Phippen and M.P. Wells (2000). *Review of Peri-operative nursing*. Philadelphia: WB Saunders Co.

11. A. Faulkner (1998). *Effective Communication with Patients* (2nd edn). London: Churchill Livingstone.

12. A. Rogers (1989). *Teaching Adults*. Milton Keynes: Open University Press.

13. L. Bernstein and R. Bernstein (1985). *Interviewing: A Guide for Health Professionals* (4th edn). Norwalk, Connecticut: Appleton-Century Crofts.

14. G. Egan (1998). *The Skilled Helper: A Problem Management Approach to Helping* (6th edn). California: Brooks/Cole Publishing company.

15. M. Walsh, A. Crumbie and S. Reveley (2005). *Nurse Practitioners: Clinical Skills and Professional Issues* (2nd edn). Oxford: Butterworth-Heinemann.

16. L. Markenday (ed.) (1997). *Day Surgery for Nurses*. London: NHURR Publishers.

17. J. Silverman, S. Kurtz and J. Draper (1998). *Skills for Communicating with Patients* (2nd edn). Oxford: Radcliffe Publishing.

18. M.E. Zator Estes (2002). *Health Assessment and Physical Examination* (2nd edn). New York: Delmar.

19. A. Minchom (2006). Preoperative assessment. *Anaesthesia and Intensive Care Medicine* **7**(12): 437–41.

20. Anon. (1963). New classification of physical status. *Anesthesiology* **24**: 111.

21. N. Buck, H.B. Devlin and J.N. Lunn (1987). *The Report of a Confidential Enquiry into Peri-operative Deaths*. London: The Nuffield Provincial Hospitals Trust and Kings Fund.

22. D.F. Reilly, M.J. McNeely, D. Doerner, D.L. Greenberg, T.O. Staiger, M.J. Geist, P.A. Vedovatti, J.E. Coffey, M.W. Mora, T.R. Johnson, E.D. Guray, G.A. Van Norman and S.D. Fihn (1999). Self-reported exercise tolerance and the risk of serious perioperative complications. *Archives of Internal Medicine* **159**: 2185–92.

23. C.G. Winnutt (2004). *Lecture Notes: Clinical Anaesthesia* (2nd edn). Oxford: Blackwell Publishing.

24. O. Langeron, E. Masso, C. Huraux, M. Guggiari, A. Bianchi, P. Coriat and B. Riou (2000). Prediction of difficult mask ventilation. *Anesthesiology* **92**: 1229–36.

25. E. Janke, V. Chalk and H. Kinley (2002). *Pre-operative Assessment: Setting a Standard through Learning*. Southampton: Southampton University.

26. D.R. Alexander (1997). Pseudocholinesterase deficiency. *Anaesthesia* **52**: 244–60.

27. J.R. Weber (2001). *Nurses' Handbook of Health Assessment* (4th edn). Philadelphia: Lippincott.

28. M. Hind and P. Wicker (eds) (2000). *Principles of Peri-operative Practice*. London: Churchill Livingstone.

29. S.L. Cohn, G.W. Smetana and H.G. Harrison (2006). *Perioperative Medicine. Just the Facts*. New York: Mc-Graw Hill.

30. P.C.A. Kam (1997). Anaesthetic management of a patient with an automatic implantable cardiovertor defibrillator in situ. *British Journal of Anaesthesia* **78**: 102–6.

31. C. den Herder, J. Schmeck, D.J.K. Appelboom and N. de Vries (2004). Risks of general anaesthesia in people with obstructive sleep apnoea. *British Medical Journal* **329**: 955–9.

32. V. Corben (1997). The Buckinghamshire nursing record audit tool: a unique approach to documentation. *Journal of Nursing Management* **5**: 289–93.

4 Clinical examination

Helen Pickard

SUMMARY

This chapter will describe:
- the process of clinical examination
- the techniques and tools used in examination
- specific examination process of the cardiovascular, respiratory and abdominal systems.

INTRODUCTION

The aim of this chapter is to consider clinical examination using a body systems approach which enables the practitioner to undertake a comprehensive examination in a logical fashion. In conjunction with the clinical history, this allows the practitioner to make a diagnosis and work out a clinical management plan. The chapter will focus on the three main systems which are of primary importance to the preoperative assessment clinician: the respiratory system, the cardiovascular system and the abdomen, to illustrate the systematic approach. These principles can then be applied to other body systems. Such skills have traditionally been the remit of medically trained clinicians but, as discussed in previous chapters, nurses and other Allied Health Professionals (AHPs) are increasingly being asked to develop their roles to include these skills. This chapter is aimed at re-familiarising those who have the skills and need to apply them to the preoperative patient and those who are new to the role and require direction. It is important that those new to these skills are prepared for the new responsibilities and accountability that arise from expansion into this area of clinical practice so that they feel competent and confident to meet these new challenges. Thus, familiarising oneself with the medical model approach will facilitate the cohesive work required to function as an effective team.

Of paramount importance is the ability to scrutinise the minute detail in order to reach a diagnosis and yet also understand which clinical signs are significant and which are not. With practice and experience it is possible to incorporate a holistic perspective, which considers psychological, spiritual and social wellbeing in addition to physiological processes, in order to establish a management plan that is truly patient-centred.

For the novice the most effective method of learning such skills is to practise. Once a basic understanding of the process has been established, it is advisable to link up with an experienced clinician and work alongside them for as long as required to gain confidence and competence. Agreeing a programme of mentorship and supervision is essential if novice practitioners are to become effective and safe practitioners.

Approximately 70 per cent of the information needed to make a diagnosis comes from the history-taking process (see Chapter 3). The subsequent clinical examination is designed to confirm the diagnosis suggested by the history, and therefore determine the plan of care. It is essential that the practitioner maintains an open mind during the process of examination so that the discovery of an unexpected finding does not confuse or obliterate the initial impression. There is often more than one diagnostic possibility and the clinical examination can help to determine the most likely option.

Indeed, the most difficult part of any assessment is making sense of the clinical findings. The examination itself is a relatively simple process that can be learnt. The interpretation and analysis of examination results is less straightforward and requires knowledge of normal and abnormal physiology, in order that clinical findings can be explained and a diagnosis reached. Accurate clinical examination is important but it forms only a small part of the diagnostic and clinical decision making process. The need for underpinning knowledge must not be overlooked. This can only be acquired from relevant experience and extensive reading.

Terminology

An important part of clinical examination involves the accurate documentation of findings. The record of the consultation is likely to be accessed by numerous health professionals and will stand as a legal record of the care given. It is worth taking the time to document findings accurately using appropriate terminology. It should be comprehensive but succinct and should utilise appropriate anatomical descriptions wherever possible. For example, it is much better to write 'right medial malleolus' than 'inner ankle on right foot', as it more clearly describes the site in question. Moreover, such language helps to ensure that non-medical practitioners are better able to communicate unambiguously with their medical colleagues and to demonstrate their clinical credibility, which will ensure that their professional opinion is taken seriously.

The location of body structures is always described in relation to other structures and these terms are used in pairs. They are:

- anterior – nearer the front surface of the body
- posterior – nearer the back surface of the body

- superior – nearer the crown of the head
- inferior – nearer the soles of the feet

- medial – nearer the midline of the body
- lateral – further from the midline of the body

- proximal – nearer to the trunk
- distal – further from the trunk

The terms 'superficial' and 'deep' specify distance from the surface of the body.

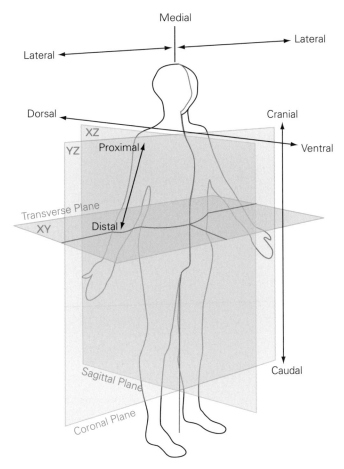

Figure 4.1 Anatomical planes

It is important to understand and become familiar with these terms, as they are extensively used in clinical examination and pathophysiology textbooks.

Before you start

When embarking upon a clinical examination it is important to build a rapport with the patient so they trust you and feel able to cooperate. It is necessary to explain what is going to happen so that the patient knows what to expect and is able to assist during the examination. If the practitioner is calm, relaxed and unhurried, the patient will be reassured. A relaxed patient is easier to examine than a tense patient and the clinical findings will be more accurate. The examination should take place in a warm, well-lit environment that is as private as possible to maintain comfort and dignity for the patient.

The practitioner should try to avoid asking the patient to undergo unnecessary physical effort during the examination, especially if they are feeling breathless or unwell. For this reason it is important to work out an examination sequence that does not overtire the patient.

Box 4.1 Examination sequence

1. Greeting and introduction
2. Note general appearance
    - AVPU, MEWS, GCS (see page 59) as appropriate
    - Hands and nails
    - JVP (see page 62)
    - Face and eyes
    - Mouth
3. Anterior chest
    - Lungs
    - Heart
    - Breasts
4. Posterior chest and back
    - Lungs
    - Spine and sacral area
5. Abdomen
6. Lower limbs
    - Oedema
    - Circulation and pulses
    - Movement
    - Neurology
7. Upper limbs
    - Circulation and pulses
    - Movement
    - Neurology

Examination sequence

Adopting a systematic approach is the key to effective clinical examination, as it reduces the possibility of missing important findings. Box 4.1 gives an example of an examination sequence that may be used, although each clinician will establish their personal preferences in accordance with their particular clinical specialty. A generalised assessment should always be undertaken even if the patient's abnormality seems to be localised to a specific area. The temptation to 'cut corners' in an effort to be more efficient should be resisted in order to minimise the risk of forgetting to ask an important question, which could hold the key to the diagnosis.

First impressions

The examination begins as soon as the practitioner meets the patient. Clinical information is continually gathered throughout the consultation. For example, if the patient walked into the room, were there any problems with their gait? Do they walk with a stick? Do they need help from someone else? Are they able to stand up? Do they appear to be breathless? Can they complete sentences when they talk? Does their facial expression or body position suggest they are in pain? Such unobtrusive observation ensures that a clinical impression begins to form even before the history-taking process is started.

This type of clinical information should not, however, be gathered in a haphazard way. The practitioner must know what to look for and must consciously observe and record findings in a logical way in order to inform their final diagnosis and treatment plan. It is also worth utilising specific tools to establish the status of the patient. For example the AVPU score is a very quick assessment and can be used to describe the patient's conscious level:

A = alert and orientated

V = responsive to voice or speech

P = responsive to pain

U = unresponsive.

There are many other such tools, including the Modified Early Warning Score (MEWS)*, which consider the standard observations of pulse, blood pressure, respiratory rate and temperature, alongside other parameters such as oxygen saturation and urine output, added together to produce a score which gives the practitioner an indication of the severity of the presenting condition. With MEWS, a score of 4 or more is usually indicative of a more serious condition requiring early intervention (see Table 4.1). The Glasgow Coma Scale (GCS) is another tool that considers level of consciousness and measures responses to stimulation in terms of eye opening, best verbal response and best motor response (see Box 4.3). The GCS gives a reliable and standardised assessment of level of consciousness and should always follow if there are any concerns with the AVPU assessment. Documenting such scores during the assessment will allow a baseline to be established and indicate the urgency of the care/treatment required.

* Modified Early Warning score (MEWS) systems employed have local hospital variation for physiological triggers of each parameter.

Table 4.1 Modified Early Warning Score[1]

Score	3	2	1	0	1	2	3
Pulse Rate	<40	–	40–50	51–100	101–110	111–129	=130 or >130
Resp Rate	<8	–	–	8–20	21–25	26–30	>30
Temp °C	–	=35 or <35	–	35.1–37.9	38–38.4	=38.5 or >38.5	–
AVPU	New weakness	New confusion	–	Alert	Voice	Pain	Unresponsive
Systolic BP	<80	80–89	90–109	110–160	161–180	181–200	>200

Source: C.P. Subbe, M. Kruger, L. Gemmel (2001)

Box 4.2 Glasgow Coma Scale[2]

Best eye response (E) – 4 grades starting with the most severe:

1. No eye opening
2. Eye opening in response to pain. (Patient responds to pressure on the patient's fingernail bed; if this does not elicit a response, supraorbital and sternal pressure or rub may be used.)
3. Eye opening to speech. (Not to be confused with the awaking of a sleeping person; such patients receive a score of 4, not 3.)
4. Eyes opening spontaneously.

Best verbal response (V)– 5 grades starting with the most severe:

1. No verbal response.
2. Incomprehensible sounds. (Moaning but no words.)
3. Inappropriate words. (Random or exclamatory articulated speech, but no conversational exchange.)
4. Confused. (The patient responds to questions coherently but there is some disorientation and confusion.)
5. Oriented. (Patient responds coherently and appropriately to questions such as the patient's name and age, where they are and why, the year, month, etc.)

Best motor response (M) – 6 grades starting with the most severe:

1. No motor response.
2. Extension to pain (adduction of arm, internal rotation of shoulder, pronation of forearm, extension of wrist, decerebrate response).
3. Abnormal flexion to pain (adduction of arm, internal rotation of shoulder, pronation of forearm, flexion of wrist, decorticate response).
4. Flexion/Withdrawal to pain (flexion of elbow, supination of forearm, flexion of wrist when supraorbital pressure applied; pulls part of body away when nailbed pinched).
5. Localises to pain. (Purposeful movements towards painful stimuli; e.g., hand crosses mid-line and gets above clavicle when supraorbital pressure applied.)
6. Obeys commands. (The patient does simple things as asked.)

Source: G. Teasdale and B. Jennett (1974)

There is no single correct way to carry out a physical examination and each practitioner over time develops his or her own style. The most common examination sequence is:

- inspection
- palpation
- percussion
- auscultation.

This sequence can be utilised for most of the major body systems. In general the clinician stands to the right of the patient during clinical examination.

NB. Sternal pressure or rub is not recommended in some organisations and suborbital pressure is not recommended in suspected/confirmed facial fracture.

Cardiovascular examination

Inspection

Hands
This section will attempt to separate the clinical signs according to the body system in question, although in reality most clinicians complete their inspection of the hands at the beginning of the examination process. Examination of most body systems starts with inspection of the hands, from a cardiovascular perspective, looking for signs of nicotine staining which will demonstrate a smoking habit. Check for signs of clubbing, characterised by an increase in the amount of soft tissue in the nailbed and fingertip. This sign can best be detected if the patient aligns one nail from each hand back to back. The normal diamond-shaped gap between the two nails is obliterated in early clubbing. Although the physiological cause of the condition is not

well understood, it is often seen in congenital heart conditions and bacterial endocarditis. It is also common in respiratory conditions including carcinoma of the bronchus, cystic fibrosis and bronchiectasis. It may also be present in patients with gastro-intestinal conditions such as Crohn's disease or ulcerative colitis.

Inspect for signs of **peripheral cyanosis**, a blue discoloration at the peripheries, commonly associated with decreased circulation and increased extraction of oxygen in peripheral tissues. **Pale palmar creases** could suggest anaemia.

Inspection of the nails may reveal **koilonychia**, where the nails become 'spoon shaped', a condition often associated with iron deficiency anaemia. In **leukonychia** the nails become white as a result of low albumin levels or severe anaemia. **Splinter haemorrhages**, lines running lengthways down the nail, are caused by bleeding from small blood vessels under the nails and may be the result of trauma due to heavy manual labour or infective endocarditis. Infective endocarditis may be suspected if either **Osler's Nodes**, characterised by painful lesions on the fingertips, or **Janeway Lesions**, red macules on the palm of the hands, are noted, although these are quite rare.

Yellow-coloured deposits in the tendons of hands and arms, known as **tendon xanthomata**, suggest hyperlipidaemia.

Face

Next observe the face. Check for signs of pallor or cyanosis. **Central cyanosis** is observed as a bluish tinge to the lips and tongue usually caused by cardiovascular or pulmonary disease. Skin pallor could be suggestive of anaemia which is also indicated by pale mucous membranes of the lower eyelid. Rosy cheeks with bluish tinge due to dilation of capillaries known as **mitral facies**, might suggest pulmonary hypertension and low cardiac output typical of severe mitral stenosis.

Observe for signs of pain or discomfort, breathlessness or sweating all of which can be significant indicators of cardiovascular disease.

The presence of **xanthalasma**, yellow deposits on the eyelid can indicate hyperlipidaemia, as can **corneal arcus**, a white line surrounding the iris.

Jugular venous pressure (JVP)

Next inspect the neck for evidence of raised jugular venous pressure (JVP). The internal jugular vein is the vessel used to assess JVP. This enters the neck just behind the angle of the jaw and runs downwards behind the sternomastoid muscle and enters the thorax at the head of the clavicle before draining directly into the right side of the heart. The JVP can only be inspected if the neck muscles are relaxed. It should be assessed from the righthand side whilst the patient relaxes at an angle of 45 degrees (see Figure 4.2).

In normal venous pressure the column of blood in the internal jugular vein, with the patient lying in this position, should not be visible more than 4–5cm above the sternal angle, although the JVP becomes more prominent if the patient lies flat.

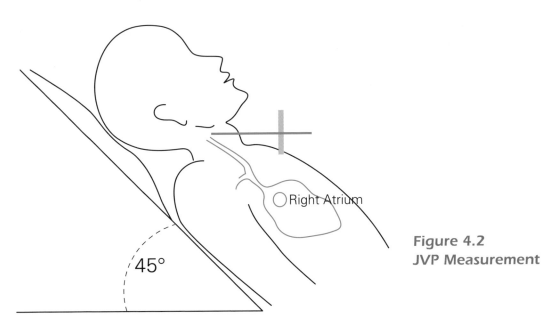

**Figure 4.2
JVP Measurement**

Venous pulses are distinguishable from arterial pulses in the neck because they cannot be palpated and they have two or more flickering movements with each impulse. Each of these flickering waves is associated with specific points in the cardiac cycle. Experienced clinicians can inspect these waves to establish the cause of the raised JVP although it is sufficient to be able to simply identify a raised JVP.

Causes of a raised JVP:

- **Right-sided heart failure** due to the inability of the right side of the heart to cope with the venous blood returning to the heart, causing a backflow and hence raised JVP.
- **Tricuspid valve incompetence** causing a backflow of blood from the right ventricle into the right atrium and then upwards to the jugular vein.
- **Increased blood volume** for example, in patients following excessive intravenous fluid administration.
- **SVC (superior vena cava) obstruction** by a large mass or space occupying lesion which obstructs venous return to the heart. This usually results in a raised JVP, which is static and not pulsatile.

Chest wall inspection

Inspect the chest for any obvious scars, which might suggest previous surgery or trauma, presence of pacemaker or implantable defibrillator, abnormal masses or pulsations and assess the breathing pattern. Skeletal abnormalities such as **pectus excavatum** (funnel chest) and **kyphoscoliosis** (curvature of the spine) can cause a shift in the position of the heart and large vessels, displacing the apex beat.

Palpation

This should begin with examination of the pulses which should consider the following:

- Rate
- Rhythm
- Volume
- Pulse character

Rate

In healthy adults the heart rate is usually between 60 and 100 beats per minute. A rapid pulse rate of 100 or greater can be the result of a variety of physiological situations including exercise, severe haemorrhage, systemic sepsis, severe anaemia and certain cardiac arrhythmias such as atrial fibrillation. Linking the tachycardia with the history that has been discussed can lead to identification of the most likely cause. Bradycardia, a slow pulse rate of 50 beats per minute or less, can be caused by extreme fitness or cardiac problems such as complete heart block, or the effects of drugs such as beta-blockers or digoxin.

Rhythm

The pulse rhythm may be regular or irregular. It is important to feel the pulse for a full minute in order to ascertain the rhythm. In healthy individuals it is described as being **regularly regular** in which the beats are consistently evenly spaced.

A pulse that is **regularly irregular** follows a repetitive pattern of unevenly spaced beats. This is not uncommon where there are regularly occurring ventricular ectopic beats, for example.

An **irregularly irregular** rhythm, where there is no discernible pattern, is most common in atrial fibrillation. A 12-lead ECG should be performed if there is any suspicion of a cardiac arrhythmia. This should always be discussed with another clinician until competence is obtained in ECG interpretation.

Volume

Pulse volume refers to the amount of movement detected by the palpating finger. A small pulse volume is found in conditions where blood flow is reduced. This can include low circulating volume following haemorrhage or conditions in which cardiac output is reduced such as myocardial infarction.

Pulse character

There are a number of different characteristics that can be detected through palpation including a **collapsing pulse**, caused by having a large difference between the systolic and diastolic blood pressure. It can be detected by raising the arm whilst monitoring the pulse. This causes a change in the 'feel' of the pulse so that it appears to 'jerk'. It is commonly found in patients with aortic incompetence, or in any condition necessitating an increase in cardiac output. This includes fever and thyrotoxicosis.

Pulsus paradoxus is a reduction in pulse volume during inspiration. It can be associated with restrictive pericarditis or pericardial effusion. It can also be a normal variant in some individuals, especially children.

Pulsus alternans is characterised by alternating normal and small volume pulses. It is commonly found in left ventricular failure where there is an inability of the left ventricle to contract consistently.

Palpating pulse points

It is important to ensure that you palpate pulse points across a range of anatomical sites in order to ensure that the circulation is adequate (see Figure 4.3). These include:

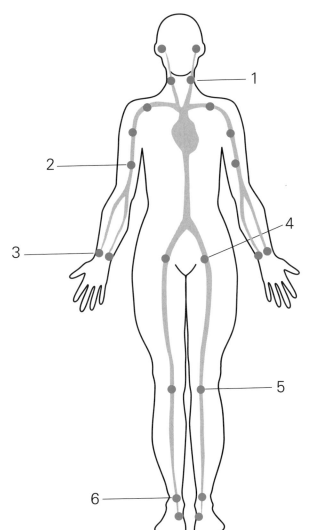

1 Carotid pulse

2 Brachial pulse

3 Radial pulse

4 Femoral pulses

5 Popliteal pulses – located behind the knee and best felt with the leg bent slightly

6 Pedal pulses – dorsalis pedis located on the top (dorsal) surface of the foot – posterior tibialis which is behind the ankle on the medial aspect of the lower leg

Figure 4.3 Pulse pressure points

Check both corresponding pulses to ensure they are consistent with each other but do not occlude both carotid pulses at the same time as this can result in collapse due to reduced cerebral blood flow. There are a number of ways to document findings. One method is to draw findings on a diagram, indicating a '+' for pulses that were present.

Blood pressure

Obtaining the patient's blood pressure will provide further information regarding the patient's cardiovascular status. Do not be tempted to allow the electronic vital signs machine to do all the work. The machine may have difficulty in detecting a reading, as in patients who have compromised circulation or perhaps have a tremor; thus manual equipment and competence in using it is still a necessity. An awareness of white coat hypertension and local guidance regarding parameters of acceptable blood pressure recordings is essential.

Apex beat

The apex beat is usually taken to be the lowest and most lateral point on the chest where the cardiac impulse can be easily palpated. In healthy individuals this is usually at the fifth intercostal space, in midclavicular line (below the fifth rib), found by counting downwards from the sternal angle at the junction of the sternum and second rib (see Figure 4.4). To palpate the apex beat, the practitioner should gently place their fingers along the contour of the ribs, ensuring that the tip of one finger rests over the space below the fifth rib. Gently move the fingers laterally until the apex beat can be palpated. If the apex beat is found to be displaced laterally this suggests that there may be some underlying pathology. Often this indicates cardiac enlargement, which can often be confirmed by a chest X-ray, but it could also be indicative of mediastinal shift as in tension pneumothorax or large pleural effusion.

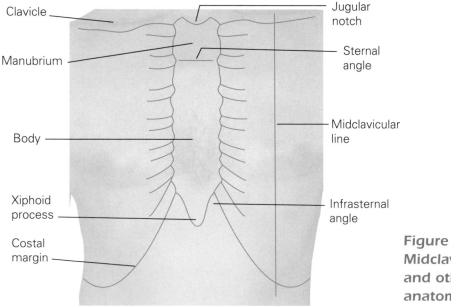

Figure 4.4 Midclavicular line and other chest anatomical points

Character of the apex beat

Palpation of the apex beat can lead to detection of other signs such as heaves or thrills. A **heave** is a strong, thrusting palpable impulse, which lifts your hand from the chest wall, and can indicate left ventricular hypertrophy, which can occur in hypertension or aortic stenosis. If the heave is detected nearer to the sternum than the apex (parasternal heave) it can indicate right ventricular hypertrophy or dilatation such as that found in pulmonary hypertension. A **thrill** is a palpable murmur, the sensation of which is likened to a purring cat. The most common thrill is due to aortic stenosis and is often palpable at the apex. Such findings should be highlighted to ensure further cardiac assessment is undertaken.

Ankles and sacrum

Palpate the lower limbs for signs of pitting oedema. Use the forefinger and thumb to gently squeeze the limb. If the imprint of the digits remains after release then pitting oedema is present. If noted bilaterally this can be a sign of heart failure or hypoproteinaemia. It is important to determine the extent of pitting, as it is not uncommon for it to extend up to the sacral and genital areas. To detect sacral oedema sit the patient forward and press gently onto the sacral area looking for residual indentation of the skin. Unilateral leg pitting is commonly seen in deep vein thrombosis.

Percussion

Percussion of the lung fields is relevant to the cardiovascular status of the patient, as it may elicit the presence of pulmonary oedema caused by heart failure. It is possible to percuss the chest wall to determine the position of the heart but this is not carried out routinely. Further details of percussion are given on pages 75–6.

Auscultation of heart sounds

A good-quality stethoscope is essential and will make cardiac auscultation much easier and more effective. The stethoscope will have a number of components. Firstly it will have two earpieces, which should point forward slightly when inserted into the ears. The tubing should be around 25cm in length and will be attached to the bell and diaphragm at the end. The bell enables the clinician to hear low-pitched sounds such as diastolic murmurs or the third heart sound in cardiac failure. The diaphragm emphasises high-pitched sounds and is useful to identify the second heart sound and early diastolic murmurs.

Some stethoscopes have an integrated bell and diaphragm apparatus whilst others are separate and require the operator to rotate the endpiece through 180 degrees to engage the different components. Some more sophisticated stethoscopes have built-in electronic apparatus so that heart sounds can be enhanced and recorded. Selection of the style is based upon personal preference but it is advisable to select one that is not too complicated initially, as these may be more difficult to use and are certainly more expensive.

Sound is transmitted in the direction of blood flow; therefore specific sounds are best heard in areas where the blood flows after it has passed through a valve or where turbulent flow radiates. For this reason it is important that the stethoscope is aligned to specific landmarks on the chest wall in order to hear all four valves (see Figure 4.5).

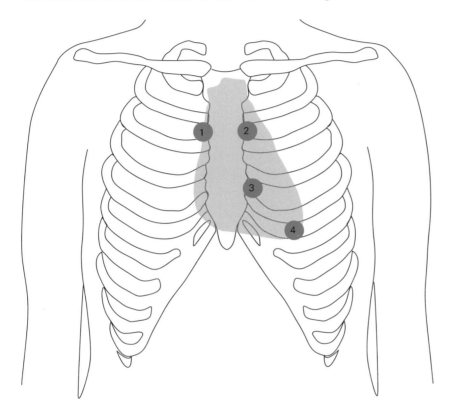

Figure 4.5 Points of auscultation

1. Aortic valve area *2nd intercostal space, right sternal edge*

2. Pulmonary area *2nd intercostal space, left sternal edge*

3. Tricuspid area *4th intercostal space, left sternal edge*

4. Mitral area *5th intercostal space, midclavicular line*

In order to understand the sounds that are heard on auscultation it is necessary to be familiar with the anatomy of the heart, the blood flow and the cardiac cycle.

Cardiac cycle

The heart consists of four chambers, two atria at the top and two ventricles below. These are connected by two sets of valves, the atrioventricular and semilunar valves.

The atrioventricular valves are situated between the atria and the ventricles. The tricuspid valve is on the right and mitral valve on the left.

Atrial and ventricular muscular contractions alternate. The different phases are termed **ventricular systole**, during which the ventricles contract and atria relax, and **ventricular diastole,** characterised by atrial contraction and ventricular relaxation. As ventricular systole begins, ventricular contraction raises the pressure in the ventricles. The leaves of the atrioventricular valves are forced to snap shut, preventing backflow into the atria.

This gives rise to the **first heart sound (S1) characterised by the sound 'lubb'**. It is not usually possible to discern two sounds although there are in fact two valves closing. This is because they close almost simultaneously, giving rise to only one sound (see Figure 4.7).

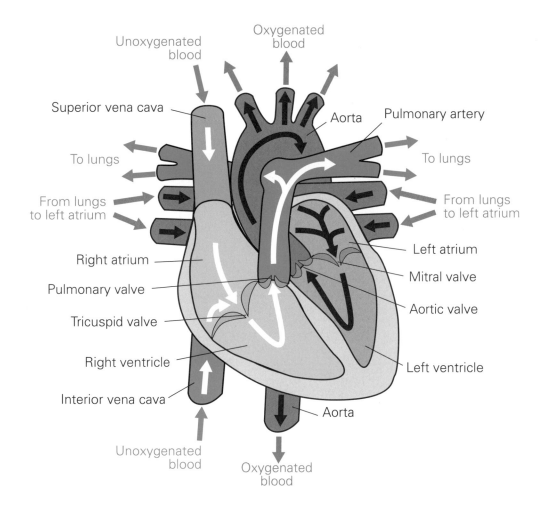

Figure 4.6 Heart anatomy

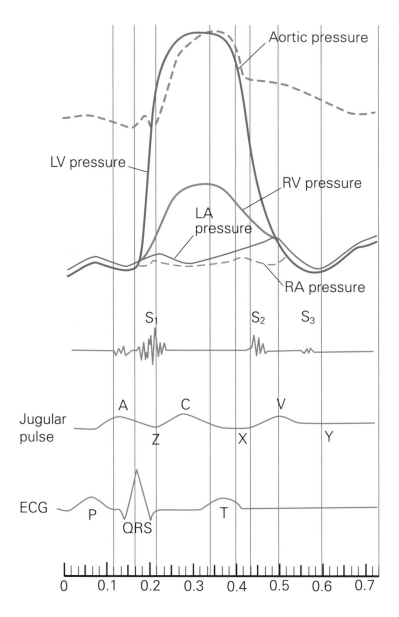

Figure 4.7
Cardiac cycle

Once the mitral and tricuspid valves close, the pressure in the contracting ventricles rises until it exceeds that in the aorta and pulmonary artery.

The second set of valves, the **aortic** and **pulmonary** valves, also termed semilunar valves, separate the right and left ventricles from the pulmonary artery and the aorta respectively. These are forced open by the rising pressure in the ventricles. Blood is squeezed into the pulmonary artery on the right, where it enters the pulmonary circulation in readiness for oxygenation, and the aorta on the left, which enables oxygenated blood to be circulated to the body tissues. Valve opening is usually a silent event and is therefore not usually heard on auscultation.

When the ventricles are almost empty they begin to relax and the pressure within them drops. Eventually the pressure within the two large blood vessels exceeds that in the ventricles and the column of blood forces the semilunar valves shut, preventing backward flow into the ventricles. This gives rise to the **second heart sound (S2) characterised by the sound 'dubb'**.

Once again this normally occurs simultaneously in both ventricles and only one sound is heard on auscultation. However, as the pressure in the right side of the heart is slightly lower than that on the left, the second heart sounds may have two distinct components, the first produced by the aortic valve and the second by the pulmonary valve. The sound of the closing aortic valve tends to mask that of the pulmonary valve so that only one sound is heard. However, during inspiration both components may be heard. This is referred to as a **'split S2'** and can be a perfectly normal variation.

As the ventricular pressure falls below that of the atrial pressure, the mitral and tricuspid valves are forced open to allow blood from the atria to refill the ventricles. The filling of the ventricles sometimes produces a third heart sound **S3**.

The subsequent contraction of the atria, which ensures ejection of the remaining blood into the ventricles, can sometimes be heard as a fourth heart sound **S4**.

In summary:

S1 'Lubb'	Atrioventricular valves close
S2 'Dubb'	Semilunar valves close
S3	Filling of ventricles
S4	Contraction of atria

The cycle then begins again.

Murmurs

Valve disease can often be detected on auscultation. The flow of blood through a narrowed or stenosed valve or indeed a 'floppy', leaky or incompetent valve will sound different from the crisp sharp 'lubb-dubb' elicited by a healthy valve. The distorted 'whooshing' sound is described as a murmur and can be evident at different parts of the cardiac cycle depending upon the valve affected and the valve disorder present.

Murmurs are either systolic or diastolic. When assessing for a murmur it is important to note the:

1. **Site**: The site of the loudest sound will help to identify the valve affected. Also check whether the sound **radiates** anywhere else. Aortic murmurs often radiate to the right side of the neck, whilst pulmonary murmurs radiate to below the clavicle and the neck. Tricuspid murmurs radiate to the lower left sternal border and mitral murmurs radiate to the axilla.

2. **Character:** Whether the sound is loud or soft, early, late or occurring mid cycle.

3. **Relationship to posture**: Sitting forward makes an aortic incompetence louder whilst lying on the left side makes mitral stenosis louder.

4. **Relationship to respiration**: Inspiration increases right heart murmurs, whilst expiration increases left heart murmurs.

5. **Timing**: Every murmur must be timed against the carotid pulse to establish if it is a systolic or diastolic event.

Systolic murmurs are usually soft and are caused either by incomplete closing of mitral or tricuspid valves or poor opening of aortic or pulmonary valves. **Pansystolic murmurs** are caused by leakage of blood through a valve that is meant to be closed during systole. The intensity of the murmur is constant throughout systole. This type of murmur occurs in:

- mitral regurgitation (incompetence)
- tricuspid regurgitation (incompetence).

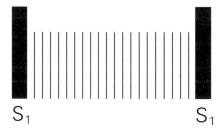

S_1 S_1 S_1

Figure 4.8 Pansystolic murmur

Ejection systolic murmurs are caused by restricted flow through a valve which is normally open in systole but which has become narrowed. The murmur starts quietly and rises to a crescendo mid-systole and then becomes quiet towards the end of systole. This type of murmur occurs in:

- aortic stenosis
- pulmonary stenosis.

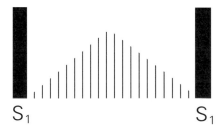

S_1 S_1 S_1

Figure 4.9 Ejection systolic murmur

Diastolic murmurs are usually caused by incomplete closure of the aortic or pulmonary valve or narrowing of the mitral and tricuspid valves. They are not always easy to hear for the novice practitioner.

Early diastolic murmurs are described as a 'whispering letter R' heard loudest at the beginning of diastole. This is caused by aortic or pulmonary incompetence. It is heard best if the patient is asked to sit forward and hold their breath at the end of expiration. It is heard best at the left sternal edge.

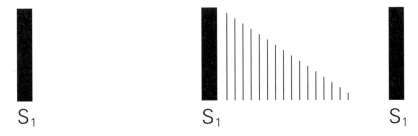

Figure 4.10 Early diastolic murmur

Mid-diastolic murmur is described as a low-pitched rumbling throughout diastole. It is caused by blood flow through a narrowed mitral or tricuspid valve and is best heard with the patient lying in the left lateral position, using the bell at the apex.

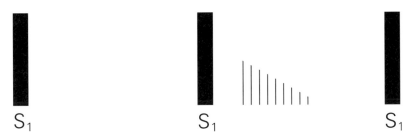

Figure 4.11 Mid-diastolic murmur

Additional heart sounds

Pericardial rub – caused by inflammation of the pericardial sac. It occurs in both systole and diastole. It sounds like creaking leather and is widely heard but more distinct at the apex.

Ejection click – occurs during systole and is a high-pitched ringing which follows S1. It is a feature of aortic and pulmonary valve stenosis.

Opening snap – a diastolic sound occurring after S2. It occurs in mitral stenosis and is caused by the movement of the rigid valve.

Such sounds can be difficult for novice practitioners to discern and describe, but any unusual or unexpected sounds should be noted, even if they cannot be immediately identified, so that more extensive investigations can be arranged. It is likely that patients presenting with unexpected anomalies on auscultation may require an echocardiogram to further assess their cardiac status.

Respiratory examination

Inspection and general observation

Begin with the hands. This should be done at the same time as the cardiovascular examination to avoid repetition for the patient.

The presence of **clubbing** can suggest bronchial cancer, lung abscess cystic fibrosis and bronchiectasis, whilst **nicotine staining** alerts the clinician to the likelihood of a significant smoking habit. **Tremor** of the hands can indicate stimulation of beta receptors in skeletal muscle caused by the administration of bronchodilators. A **flapping tremor** could suggest carbon dioxide retention in type 2 respiratory failure. **Peripheral cyanosis** is once again significant as it may suggest a diminished oxygen supply to the tissues caused by respiratory inadequacy.

Evidence of **cachexia** characterised by muscle wasting, evidence of weight loss, dry and wrinkled skin could be a sign of an underlying malignancy, neurological condition or chronic disease, all of which can involve dyspnoea.

Observe the patient at rest and also whilst talking to assess the severity of any **dyspnoea**. Listen for evidence of **wheeze** or **stridor** and for **cough**, observing whether this is dry or productive. Observe **sputum** colour and quantity. Also listen to voice quality. Hoarseness can indicate recurrent **laryngeal** nerve problems.

Central cyanosis can be present in either diseases of the lungs or heart. Check for evidence of **Horner's syndrome**, characterised by a slight drooping of one of the upper eyelids (ptosis) and pupillary constriction of the affected eye. The patient may also report impaired sweating on the same side of the face (ipsilateral side). These signs can be caused by paralysis of the cervical sympathetic nerve, one of the causes of which is a tumour in the lung apex.

Next inspect the chest and thorax as previously mentioned. Look for evidence of scars, which might suggest previous pulmonary surgery including chest drains and deformities of the spine or chest wall. A **pigeon chest** (pectus carinatum) is characterised by an outward bowing of the chest, often the result of chronic childhood respiratory illness, whilst a **funnel chest** (pectus excavatum) is a developmental defect resulting in a depression of the lower part of the sternum. In severe cases this can result in restriction of lung capacity. Spinal deformities include **kyphosis**, a forward bending of the spine, and **scoliosis**, a lateral bending of the spine. These can lead to asymmetry of the chest and can restrict lung movement. They can be simultaneously present in a condition known as **kyphoscoliosis**.

Observe chest movements for **symmetry**. Unilateral diminished chest movements will provide a clue as to which side the abnormality is located. **Intercostal recession**, characterised by a drawing in of the tissue above the intercostal spaces with respiration, may indicate severe upper airway obstruction. Also look for rate, rhythm, depth and effort of respiration. Respiratory rate should always be timed for one full minute. Normal respiratory rate at rest is 14–16 breaths per minute. **Tachypnoea** is an increased respiratory rate, whilst **apnoea** means cessation of breathing.

Palpation

Start by feeling for the position of the trachea. This is done by placing two fingers either side of the trachea and judging whether the distances between the trachea and the sterno-mastoid tendons are the same on either side. This should be done gently as it can be uncomfortable for the patient. Deviation of the trachea in either direction is an indication of underlying disease, e.g. a pneumothorax can displace the mediastinum and therefore the trachea towards the affected side although a tension pneumothorax can displace the trachea away from the affected side, especially as the pressure increases within the chest cavity. Consolidation and subsequent lung tissue collapse caused by pneumonia can also cause tracheal deviation towards the affected side. Masses in the region of the neck, e.g. thyroid enlargement can also displace the trachea. If tracheal deviation is suspected a chest X-ray is vital to help identify the underlying cause.

The chest wall should be gently palpated to ascertain any areas of tenderness which may indicate disease or inflammation in muscle, bone or cartilage which are often characterised by localised areas of tenderness. It is important to be careful when identifying tender areas, as it is likely to cause discomfort to the patient.

Observe for symmetrical chest expansion by palpation. This is usually performed from behind the patient by placing the hands either side of the chest, ensuring the palms and fingers are firmly in contact with the chest wall. The thumbs should be fairly closely aligned in the middle of the chest and should be pointing upwards free from the chest wall. Ask the patient to take a deep breath in. The thumbs should move apart equally if both sides of the chest are expanding equally.

Chest expansion can be reduced on one side more than the other for a number of reasons. For example in pneumothorax, pleural effusion (a collection of fluid in the pleural space) and pneumonia where there is a large amount of collapse or consolidation and therefore very little air entering the lung tissue. Reduced movement on both sides suggests a chronic respiratory problem such as chronic obstructive pulmonary disease or pulmonary fibrosis. If there is any concern about lung expansion a chest X-ray should be undertaken to seek further clarification.

Percussion

The purpose of percussion is to detect 'hollowness' of the chest, which is termed the 'percussion note', and to compare it with the reciprocal area on the opposite side of the chest. Differences in the 'note' detected will give clues to the underlying pathology, which can then be considered with other findings to enable the clinician to establish the most likely diagnosis. This is a new skill for most non-medical practitioners that requires practice in order to obtain competence and confidence in the clinical situation.

The practitioner should place the outstretched hand (left hand for a right-handed practitioner) on the chest wall, ensuring that the middle finger is firmly placed in an intercostal space. Lift the other fingers up off the chest wall slightly, as they may absorb some of the sound and make it more difficult to distinguish the note.

Using the tip of the middle finger on the right hand, strike the middle phalanx of the middle finger of the left hand as it lies on the chest wall, using a loose swing action from the wrist. The percussing finger should be quickly moved out of the way so that it does not dampen the sound generated. The note generated by this action is quite subtle and can only be appreciated if it is compared with the note generated in a similar position on the other side of the chest wall.

For this reason it is important to identify several complementary points on either side of the chest, both front and back, to percuss.

By moving from the left to the right and comparing one side to the other, it is possible to detect subtle changes in the percussion note that can give clues to the underlying pathology. It is important to percuss the lung apices, which can be done by directly striking the clavicles rather than the left hand.

Avoid percussing the midline over the sternum or the region overlying the scapulae at the back, as these bony structures will prevent any meaningful assessment of the lung fields.

The percussion note will vary subtly depending on the underlying structure. In normal lung fields the percussion note elicited is described as **resonant**. This suggests that the underlying healthy tissue is a mixture of air-filled sacs, lung tissue and blood vessels. A **hyper-resonant** percussion note, which sounds drum-like, is usually suggestive of an air-filled cavity as in pneumothorax.

A **dull** percussion note indicates that the underlying structure is rather more solid. This could be suggestive of an underlying organ such as liver, which is often detectable anteriorly at the level of the fifth intercostal space in the right midclavicular line. This would be a normal finding. However, an area of consolidation or a tumour could also be detectable from a dull percussion note.

If the percussion note is extremely dull or **stony dull**, such as the sound that would be heard if a stone were percussed, it is likely that there is underlying fluid such as that found in a pleural effusion or haemothorax.

Auscultation

Breath sounds are auscultated using the bell of the stethoscope. As with percussion of breath sounds, it is important to assess the lung fields anteriorly and posteriorly in a systematic way, comparing one side with the other.

Place the stethoscope firmly on the chest wall and ask the patient to breathe in and out slowly through the mouth. Listen carefully to the complete breath sound. There are different components to the breath sound, which will vary according to the position of the stethoscope. Listen to the quality of the sound and its intensity. Also make note of any added sounds that may be heard. Try to avoid rapid breathing or prolonged examination as the patient may begin to feel light headed.

Breath sounds

In order to interpret what is heard on auscultation an understanding of the origin and variation of breath is required. Breath sounds are generated by turbulent airflow in the large airways. Normal breath sounds have distinctive inspiratory and expiratory phases that vary slightly depending upon the area being auscultated. If the stethoscope is placed over the trachea the sounds will be loud with a blowing quality. The sounds are similar in length and are separated by a pause. These are known as **bronchial breath sounds**. In contrast normal breath sounds heard at the lung bases are known as **vesicular breath sounds**, and have a quieter rustling quality. They have a long inspiratory phase and a shorter expiratory phase that follows immediately with no gap in between. These sounds are transmitted from the upper airways to the alveolar sacs or vesicles, hence their name. The sound is different at the bases because lung tissue is largely air filled and, in accordance with the laws of physics, air is not as good at transmitting sound as solid matter. The importance of this is that in the presence of consolidation, such as pneumonia, a lung abscess or a tumour, breath sounds will be transmitted much more easily. The result is that bronchial breath sounds will be heard at the bases. This alerts the clinician that there may be some abnormal pathology requiring further investigation.

The **absence** of breath sounds suggests that there is no airflow in the underlying tissue. This can be due to the presence of pneumothorax or a pleural effusion (fluid in the pleural space) and warrants further investigation.

Vocal resonance

If the clinician suspects some abnormal underlying pathology it can be further assessed using a technique known as vocal resonance. With the stethoscope on the chest wall the clinician asks the patient to say '99'. The sound heard can be compared with a reciprocal site on the other side of the chest. If the sound is clearer on one side than the other, very likely the same side as the bronchial breath sounds were heard, this supports the clinician's suspicion that there may be some underlying pathology. The clarity of the sound will vary depending on the underlying tissue and will again be louder where there is solid matter underlying.

Added sounds

In addition to breath sounds it is often possible to hear other sounds that may help the clinician to reach a diagnosis. For example **wheezes** are continuous sounds that have a musical quality, usually louder on expiration. They are abnormal sounds suggestive of airway narrowing and may be high pitched or low pitched depending upon the diameter of the airway from which they originate. High-pitched sounds originate in smaller airways and low-pitched suggest larger airway narrowing. Inspiratory wheeze suggests severe airway narrowing or partial airway obstruction. Wheeze is common in conditions such as asthma and COPD. In contrast **crackles** (sometimes referred to as crepitations or rales) are interrupted non-musical sounds usually caused by collapsing peripheral airways on expiration. They vary in quality and can be described as being coarse or fine. Fine crackles are said to sound like hair being rubbed between the fingers, whereas coarse crackles are more like the sound made by blowing air through a liquid with a straw. It is important to note the timing of crackles as well as their quality, since this can give a clue as to their origin. Fine crackles occurring late in inspiration may suggest pulmonary fibrosis, whereas pulmonary oedema or bronchial secretions may cause coarse crackles heard in the middle of the expiratory phase. Crackles heard throughout both inspiratory and expiratory phases are characteristic of bronchiectasis. A **pleural rub** is said to sound like creaking leather on auscultation and is heard when there is a problem with the outer layers of the lungs. Normally the pleura are separated by a lubricating liquid and therefore slide over each other during respiration. However, the pleura can become inflamed and stiff, giving rise to a rub. The patient may complain of pleuritic chest pain, which has a sharp, stabbing quality and is worse on movement or deep inspiration.

Putting it all together

It is worth remembering that findings, either from percussion or auscultation, can be very subtle and it is important that the clinician pieces together all the bits of the jigsaw to help them make sense of their findings and reach a differential diagnosis. Table 4.2 is used to demonstrate this. It is, however, worth bearing in mind that not all clinical presentations follow textbook rules and that in some situations one or more signs may be absent, and indeed additional or contradictory signs might be present. This can make diagnosis challenging, emphasising the need for an accurate clinical history. Often the history can provide information to confirm the diagnosis despite apparent anomalies on examination. Clinical judgement and decision making in such circumstances require experience and practice.

Table 4.2 Respiratory examination findings and diagnosis

	Tracheal deviation	Chest wall movement	Percussion note	Breath sounds	Added sounds
Normal lung tissue	None	Equal bilaterally	Resonant	Vesicular	None
Pleural effusion	Possible	Reduced on affected side	Stony dull	Absent over fluid	Possible rub
Consolidation	None	Reduced on affected side	Dull	Bronchial	Crackles
Asthma	None	Decreased symmetrically	Resonant	Normal or reduced	Wheeze
Pneumothorax	Possible	Reduced on affected side	Hyper-resonant	Absent	None

Abdominal examination

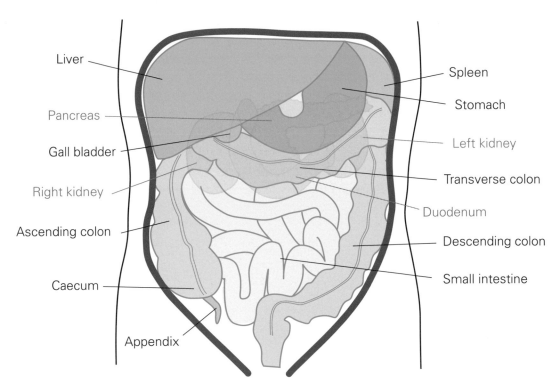

Figure 4.12 Abdominal organs

Since there are a great many different structures within very close proximity in the abdominal cavity, diagnosis of abdominal complaints can be very difficult. This is compounded by the fact that very few of the organs in the abdomen have their own sensory nerve supply, which makes it difficult for the brain to accurately distinguish the source of the pain. The patient is not always able to give a very clear description of their pain, although other symptoms may indicate which organ system is involved. Clinical examination is required to help establish the source of the pain. However, the clinician must also acknowledge that some organs are not easily accessible to palpation because they are situated behind other organs or are protected by bony structures such as the rib cage or pelvis. Because of these restrictions, correct positioning of the patient and clinical examination technique are of vital importance if the clinician is to succeed in obtaining necessary information.

Before embarking on abdominal examination it is essential to obtain a clear understanding of the anatomical position of the many organs and their relationships to each other.

Much of the liver, stomach and all of the spleen are protected by the rib cage. The duodenum and the pancreas lie deep in the upper abdomen, where they are not normally palpable. The kidneys are posterior organs, lying behind and outside the peritoneal cavity (retroperitoneal).

The upper portions of the kidneys are protected by the rib cage and because the right kidney is slightly lower than the left, being displaced by the liver, it is sometimes possible to palpate its lower pole on examination in a healthy individual. The pelvis protects the bladder and reproductive organs, which means they are not usually palpable, although a very full bladder can often be palpated above the level of the pelvis. The area between the ribs and the pelvis contains the large and small intestines and the major blood vessels including the aorta and inferior vena cava.

Abdominal examination is best carried out with the patient lying flat on the examination couch or bed. If this is uncomfortable, begin the examination with the patient sitting and lay the patient flat when the abdomen is being examined. One pillow under the head for comfort and also one pillow under the knees to ensure the abdominal muscles are relaxed can be helpful. Ideally patients should have their arms by their sides, be warm, comfortable and the room well lit. It is difficult to elicit any clinical signs if the abdominal muscles are tense.

Inspection

It is important to look for any clinical signs that may suggest an abdominal problem so once again the examination begins with general observation. Note whether the patient looks to be in pain. Also look for evidence of weight loss and muscle wasting, sweating and bruising. Look at skin colour for evidence of jaundice. Jaundice can be seen as a yellow discoloration of the skin or the sclera and can indicate obstruction of the common bile duct by either a gallstone or mass, or liver disease.

Once again the presence of **clubbing** could suggest an inflammatory bowel disorder such as Crohn's disease. **Koilonychia** or spoon-shaped nails could suggest iron deficiency anaemia whereas **leukonychia** or white nails could indicate hypoproteinuria often associated with liver disease. The presence of **liver palms**, which is a reddening of the palm due to peripheral vasodilatation, can be associated with liver disease, pregnancy or thyrotoxicosis. Also look for **spider naevi**, which are small red vascular malformations easily identifiable because they fill from a central arteriole. They characteristically blanche from the middle when gentle pressure is applied. They are commonly distributed on the hands, face, upper chest and back and if seen in excess (i.e. more than five) are frequently associated with chronic liver disease.

Next look at the mouth, for signs of inflammation, **ulceration** or **bleeding**. This could be caused by malnourishment but is also found in immuno-suppressed patients, or those with inflammatory bowel disease. Occasionally ulcers can indicate oral cancer, especially if they persist for several weeks. The tongue should be observed for abnormalities such as **thrush**, white patches caused by candidal yeast infection. These can be easily scraped off with a tongue depressor. If they are not easily removed, the cause of the white patches could be **leukoplakia**, a premalignant condition requiring further investigation. A **smooth red tongue** may be caused by iron or vitamin B12 deficiency.

Abdominal inspection
Look at the abdomen from the right side of the bed, observing for scars, and note their location.

Also note any old silver stretch marks, which could suggest previous weight loss or often pregnancy. The presence of purple stretch marks (striae), may be suggestive of Cushing's syndrome.

Check for evidence of dilated veins, which could be indicative of obstruction in the inferior vena cava or portal systems. Obstruction in the inferior vena cava or common iliac veins usually causes longitudinally aligned veins to appear at the sides of the abdomen. This is the result of blood flow bypassing the obstruction and travelling from the lower limbs to the thorax via the superficial veins of the abdominal wall. If the obstruction is in the portal circulation of the liver, which may be caused by cirrhosis, the engorged veins are more centrally placed and can form a cluster of vessels flowing in all directions away from the umbilicus. This is termed caput medusa and is the result of the reopening of the umbilical vein.

Note the shape of the abdomen and observe for distension, which may be generalised or caused by a localised swelling. Asymmetry caused by localised swelling is best seen from the foot of the bed. Look for rashes or lesions and note the presence of stomas.

Palpation

There are nine named regions, which should be referred to when describing any clinical findings. The anatomical quadrants and regions, used in the examination to describe areas in the clinical record and as an aid to diagnosis, can be seen in Figure 4.13.

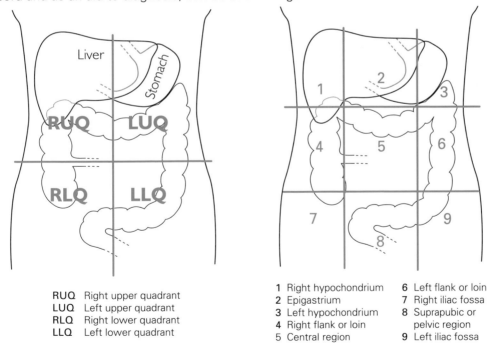

RUQ Right upper quadrant
LUQ Left upper quadrant
RLQ Right lower quadrant
LLQ Left lower quadrant

1 Right hypochondrium
2 Epigastrium
3 Left hypochondrium
4 Right flank or loin
5 Central region
6 Left flank or loin
7 Right iliac fossa
8 Suprapubic or pelvic region
9 Left iliac fossa

Figure 4.13 Anatomical quadrants and regions

Abdominal palpation should take each of the areas into account. Palpation is usually done from the patient's right side and with the examiner's right hand. Before starting, check whether the patient has any tender areas and start in an area where tenderness is not reported.

Light palpation

Start by gently palpating all nine regions with the right hand, whilst at the same time trying to visualise the underlying organs. Use the flat of the hand and the fingers rather than the fingertips. Note the patient's facial expression, which might indicate the presence of any tenderness. If tenderness is elicited assess the extent and whether there is any guarding present (guarding occurs when the overlying abdominal muscles contract). This can be a voluntary response in an anxious patient, but in the presence of underlying inflammation, such as in peritonitis, reflex muscle contraction occurs (involuntary guarding). Observe for rebound tenderness, which can indicate intra-abdominal disease, by gently pressing the abdomen with the hand, then quickly removing it. If rebound tenderness is present the pain will be worse as the hand is removed. Note the site of tenderness as this can indicate the organ responsible. For example, right iliac fossa pain can often indicate appendicitis, whereas tenderness in the right hypochondrium may suggest cholecystitis. However, it is not impossible for pain to be referred from one area to another so tenderness can be felt some distance away from the cause.

Deep palpation

Provided the patient is not too uncomfortable, proceed to deeper palpation in order to ascertain whether any abnormal mass or swelling is present. Place the left hand over the right and allow the right hand to feel the abdomen using a slow rocking motion, whilst the left hand applies pressure. Again examine all the different areas, taking note of the location of masses or swellings that may be present and identify the presenting characteristics. The checklist below is pertinent to any swelling or 'lump', not only abdominal abnormalities. Such characteristics may be present in a breast or testicular lump.

Characteristics of a 'lump'

1. Note the anatomical site of the swelling and the depth in relation to the skin surface.
2. Record the size in centimetres and the shape of the swelling.
3. Is the surface of the swelling smooth or irregular on palpation? Does it have a clearly defined edge?
4. Is there any trans-illumination? You can check this by shining a light through the swelling to ascertain whether the lump is fluid filled or solid. This technique is particularly useful in testicular examination. Abdominal masses rarely trans-illuminate unless they are very superficial.
5. Check whether the skin temperature at the site of the swelling is raised. Does the local area feel hot? Is the skin superficial to the swelling red or discoloured?
6. Ascertain whether there is localised tenderness. Is the lump painful?
7. What is the consistency of the lump? Is it hard or soft and pliable?

8. Is the swelling fixed or does it move around when palpated?
9. Is the mass pulsatile? If the swelling is due to an aneurysm caused by a weakened arterial wall it may be possible to feel it pulsate under the fingertips. A pulsatile mass should be very carefully palpated in order to minimise the risk of damaging it.
10. Is there any fluctuation in the characteristics of the swelling? Does the patient report intermittent coming and going of the swelling, or does it appear to have changed on repeat examination?
11. Is it possible to reduce the swelling by applying gentle pressure to it?
12. Is there any obvious lymph node enlargement in the local area, for example in the groin?
13. Does the patient look unwell?

It is possible that swelling may be caused by stools in the colon, in which case it may appear to have changed or resolved on repeated examination. An area of localised infection such as an abscess is likely to be hot to touch, red and tender. The patient may also appear systemically unwell. In contrast a well patient with a painless lump may have a malignancy. A comprehensive description of the characteristics of the swelling helps to identify the cause and will direct the practitioner towards the process of further investigation. Specific organs within the abdomen should be located and features noted.

Liver
The liver extends from the fifth intercostal space on the right of the midline down to the lower edge of the rib cage (costal margin). It can become enlarged in a number of diseases, and thus it is possible to palpate the liver below the costal margin. Hepatic enlargement, or hepatomegaly, may be the result of early cirrhosis, the liver is often shrunken in end-stage cirrhosis and therefore not palpable. It can also be the enlarged due to excess alcohol, fatty liver. Malignancy, either primary or metastatic, can also cause hepatomegaly, as can congestive heart failure, viral hepatitis, haematological conditions such as leukaemia and lymphoma.

As the liver can become excessively enlarged, it is necessary to start the examination at a considerable distance from the edge of the normal liver. Use either the tips of the fingers or the edge of the hand with the fingers parallel to the costal margin and start at the right iliac fossa. Ask the patient to take a deep breath in and apply gentle pressure upwards towards the liver. As the patient breathes out, lift the hand and move further up towards the costal margin. Repeat this process until the costal margin is reached. If the liver is enlarged it will move downwards on inspiration to meet the hand, allowing the practitioner to identify the position of the liver edge. This can be described in terms of centimetres or finger widths from the costal margin. If the liver is identified, it is important to ascertain its texture. It may be described as smooth, irregular, firm or nodular. Check whether the patient experiences pain or discomfort on palpation, as some conditions give rise to a tender liver.

Spleen
The spleen lies against the diaphragm at the level of the ninth to the eleventh ribs, mostly

posterior to the mid-axillary line. It is lateral to the stomach and just above the left kidney. It is not usually possible to palpate the spleen; however, in some conditions the spleen can become grossly enlarged and it may extend across the abdomen towards the umbilicus. Causes of splenic enlargement include portal hypertension, infections such as glandular fever and malaria, haematological conditions including leukaemia, lymphoma and haemolytic anaemia.

For this reason it is important to start palpation, using the fingertips, from the right iliac fossa, moving diagonally across the abdomen towards the left costal margin. This time, because of the posterior-lateral position of the spleen, a bimanual technique is used (this uses both hands). It is helpful to support the left flank with the left hand as this moves the spleen gently towards the costal margin. Once again move the palpating hand gradually across the abdomen in time with the patient's respiration 2cm at a time. If the spleen edge is felt, note its position. In general if the spleen is enlarged it may be difficult to get one's fingers underneath the costal margin, due to the abnormal position of the spleen.

Kidneys

The kidneys lie towards the posterior of the abdomen. Thus any tenderness is often felt in the back. The area between the spine and the lower border of the twelfth rib, the costovertebral angle, defines the region to assess for kidney tenderness. The kidneys are not usually palpable on examination as they are retroperitoneal organs (lying towards the back of the abdomen behind the peritoneal cavity which contains the gut and most of the other organs of the abdomen), and are protected by the rib cage. The right kidney is slightly lower than the left as it is slightly displaced by the liver. It is possible to palpate the kidneys if they become abnormally enlarged, for example, in the presence of renal tumours, hydronephrosis and polycystic kidney disease. If the latter is present the kidney surface will have a distinctive nodular surface that can be detected on palpation.

Once again a bimanual technique is needed to palpate kidneys. To palpate the right kidney, place the left hand at the back, just below and parallel to the twelfth rib, with the fingertips just reaching the costovertebral angle. Gently push upwards, trying to displace the kidney anteriorly. At the same time place the right hand gently in the right upper quadrant. Ask the patient to take a deep breath. At the peak of inspiration press the right hand firmly and deeply into the right upper quadrant, just below the costal margin, and try to capture the kidney between the two hands. If it is palpable it should be possible to 'ballot', or bounce, the kidney between the upper and lower hands, taking care not to cause any damage. As the patient breathes out, the kidney may be felt to slide back into its original position. The same process is used to palpate the left kidney, by repositioning the hands in the corresponding positions on the opposite side.

Aorta

The aorta is the main artery running from the heart, carrying oxygenated blood to the extremities. It lies slightly to the left of the mid-line and is situated deep within the abdomen and the width can be assessed by pressing deeply in the upper abdomen with one hand either side of the aorta. Use the fingertips to detect the pulsations. This is particularly important in patients over the age of fifty who may be susceptible to vascular disease. The normal aorta should be about 3cm in diameter. If it feels wider than this and pulsates outwards towards the fingers it is possible that the patient has an aortic aneurysm. The ease with which aortic pulsations are felt varies greatly with the thickness of the abdominal wall. In slim people it is not uncommon to see the abdomen pulsate, due to the relative closeness of the aorta to the body surface. Examination of the aorta should be undertaken with care in order to prevent damage to delicate structures. If an aneurysm is suspected it might be preferable to avoid palpation but to alert a vascular expert.

Percussion

Percussion of the abdomen is performed using a two-handed technique similar to chest percussion. General percussion over the abdomen will detect abnormal gas, fluid collection or possibly masses.

In the abdomen the percussion note is predominantly tympanic or drum-like in character because of the distribution of gas in the gastrointestinal tract, but scattered areas of dullness due to faeces and fluid are also typical. Note any large areas of dullness that may indicate an underlying mass or enlarged organ. Always try to percuss from an area of resonance to the area of dullness to identify the position of the underlying organ or mass accurately. Try to establish the position of the liver through percussion; the upper border is usually identified at the fifth intercostal space in the midclavicular line on the right. Start at the third intercostal space and gradually percuss downwards to identify the upper border of the liver. The lower border is usually in line with the costal margin. Percuss upwards from the right iliac fossa to ensure any enlargement is accurately detected. Ask the patient to breathe in and the dullness should move down as the liver descends.

Because enlargement of the spleen occurs anteriorly and medially, it can produce a dull percussion note that replaces the tympany of the stomach and colon which it overlies. Percuss downwards from the left lower anterior chest wall, around the ninth intercostal space, between lung resonance above and the costal margin below (Traube's Space), noting any dullness. Percussion alone cannot usually confirm splenomegaly but it can raise the examiner's suspicions of it. Once again, a full and thorough examination is needed to build up a complete picture.

Shifting dullness

This is a test to demonstrate the presence of free fluid or ascites in the abdominal cavity. Ascites can be caused by a number of conditions, for example alcoholic liver disease, and can cause severe abdominal distension due to the many litres of fluid that have accumulated.

Percussion for ascites depends upon detecting shifting dullness on change of position. Start with the patient lying flat. Percuss from the midline to the flank until the note becomes dull, suggesting the presence of fluid. Keep the hand on the abdomen at that point and ask the patient to roll over to the opposite side. Wait for about 10 seconds until any fluid present resettles with the new position, then percuss again over the marked area. If this now elicits a tympanic note then 'shifting dullness' has been demonstrated and the presence of ascites confirmed.

Auscultation

With the patient lying flat, listen for bowel sounds by placing the diaphragm of the stethoscope slightly to the right of the umbilicus and wait for up to a minute until you hear gurgling noises, which are caused by peristaltic activity in the gut. The pitch of the sound depends upon the distension of the bowel and the proportion of gas and fluid. Normal bowel sounds are low-pitched gurgles occurring every few seconds. In intestinal obstruction the frequency of the sounds increases and they are usually described as 'tinkling'. An absence of bowel sounds can suggest paralytic ileus or peritonitis.

Listen over the major vessels for bruits, or turbulent blood flow, indicating narrowing of the vessel. Listen just above the umbilicus for the aorta, and 2–3cm above and lateral to the umbilicus for the renal arteries to establish whether there is evidence of renal artery stenosis. Listen over the liver for bruits associated with hepatic disease and for friction rubs which are sometime associated with inflammation.

This essentially completes the abdominal examination apart from a rectal examination, which is not described here.

CONCLUSION

This chapter aims to provide an insight into the knowledge and detail required to undertake a clinical examination. It is essential that the clinician has a sound understanding, not only of the examination technique but also the pathophysiology of diseases and conditions within their scope of practice.

There is clearly a great deal not covered in this chapter, including neurological examination, examination of the eye, ear, nose and throat, lymph nodes, breast and musculoskeletal system, to name but a few. However, it is hoped that the systematic approach demonstrated illustrates the process that can be applied to other body systems.

Learners are advised to invest in a detailed clinical examination textbook, of which there are many examples. This will provide a detailed explanation and description of all the required skills, regardless of specialist interest. However, learners are also advised to seek mentorship and support from medical colleagues to enable them to become competent in their field.

REFERENCES

1. C.P. Subbe, M. Kruger and L. Gemmel (2001). Validation of a Modified Early Warning Score in medical admissions. *Quarterly Journal of Medicine* **94**: 521–6.

2. G. Teasdale and B. Jennett (1974). Assessment of coma and impaired consciousness. A practical scale. *The Lancet* **13**(2) (7872): 81–4.

Further reading

G. Douglas, F. Nicol and C. Robertson (2005). *Macleod's Clinical Examination* (11th edn). Edinburgh: Churchill Livingstone.

O. Epstein, G.D. Perkin, J. Cookson and D.P. De Bono (2003). *Clinical Examination* (3rd edn). Oxford: Mosby, Elsevier.

J.T. Talley and S. O'Connor (2006). *Clinical Examination. A Systematic Guide to Physical Diagnosis* (5th edn). Edinburgh: Churchill Livingstone.

5 Preoperative assessment of cardiovascular system and management of concurrent disease

John Carlisle

SUMMARY

This chapter will describe:

- **cardiovascular disease**
- **the role of testing in the preoperative phase**
- **the clinical approach to preoperative optimisation of cardiovascular disease**
- **therapeutic treatment of cardiovascular disease and implications for perioperative care.**

INTRODUCTION

One in ten adults in the United Kingdom have chronic cardiovascular disease. The most common disease process is atherosclerosis – fatty scarring within arterial walls. This inflammatory process thickens the arterial wall (throttling blood supply – angina, claudication), which becomes stiff (systolic hypertension) and weak (aneurysm formation and wall dissection). However, arterial narrowing, wall stiffness and weakness do not directly cause blood clots that cause most atherosclerotic deaths. Fat, leaking through scabs (plaques) that cover diseased arterial walls, causes blood to clot. The clot stops blood flow, causing tissue infarction (heart attacks, strokes, black toes) and organ failure (heart failure, dementia and immobility). The risk of infarction is related to this risk of plaque rupture, which in turn depends upon the shape, position, fat and neutrophil content of the plaque. Atherosclerosis affects all arteries: symptomatic (ischaemia, infarction) and asymptomatic (plaques, intima-media thickness, stiffness) disease in one artery, for instance the carotid artery, predicts risk of symptomatic disease in the perfusion territory of other arteries, for instance the coronaries. About 1 in 30 adults have stable angina, 1 in 50 have had a heart attack and 1 in 70 have had a stroke.

Heart attacks and strokes are becoming less common. The age-specific rate of cardiovascular events is 35% of the rate 25 years ago. Each year the rate of cardiovascular events in the population is 96% of the year before.[1] The reduction in the rate of ischaemic death has not been accompanied by an increase in the rate of heart failure.[2] The incidence of cardiovascular events increases with age. The risk parallels the overall risk of dying (see Chapter 2): the risk doubles every 7 years, or is 1.1 times the risk for someone a year younger.

In the preoperative clinic, assessment of cardiovascular disease centres on a targeted history for heart attacks (myocardial infarction (MI)), angina, shortness of breath, stroke, transient cerebral ischaemia and claudication. Assessment is completed by an objective measure of fitness. If history and fitness measures are complete, the only physical examination required is heart auscultation for the murmur of aortic stenosis. Most preoperative assessment clinics would choose to refer patients back to general practitioners if they complain of cardiovascular symptoms that have not been previously addressed (see below).

Cardiovascular disease and cardiovascular outcomes

In Chapter 2 a Step process for calculating mortality risk is described in detail. This method can also be used to assess mortality risk in adult patients with: heart failure,[3-11] valvular disease[12] and acyanotic congenital heart disease.[13-16]

The absolute risk for having a stroke or developing heart disease depends upon age, sex, socioeconomic status and fitness. Smoking, hypertension, hypercholesterolaemia and diabetes may also be used to calculate risk, particularly if fitness has not been objectively measured. These are the same risk factors that predict all-cause mortality. There are various scores and risk calculators that you can use to calculate the risk of cardiovascular events.[17, 18] Fortunately the risk of non-fatal stroke, and the risk of non-fatal myocardial infarction, are each about half the calculated mortality risk.[19] For instance, if the risk of dying per month is 1 in 500, the risk of having a non-fatal stroke will be about 1 in 1000, and the risk of having a non-fatal myocardial infarction will also be about 1 in 1000. So all one need do is calculate the risk of dying – as described in Chapter 2 – and divide by two to determine the risks of stroke and MI. Patients who have had strokes are more likely to have another stroke than an MI and vice versa. To calculate the risks of recurrent strokes, or recurrent MIs, multiply this crude estimate by 1.5.

There are a number of common clinical conditions that are commonly managed in the preoperative clinic and described below.

Hypertension

Hypertension was historically seen as a potentially dangerous risk factor, although in preoperative terms there is little evidence to support cancelling surgery due to the condition.[20] Therefore, the decision whether to proceed with surgery or delay, in an attempt to reduce risk, should be made *with* the patient rather than *on their behalf*. Patients are made to endure painful and distressing symptoms despite their willingness to have surgery sooner, perhaps at slightly higher risk, rather than have surgery later in the hope that risk can be substantially reduced.

Smoking and hypercholesterolaemia increase the risk of death, stroke and acute coronary syndrome by an amount similar to hypertension. But most clinicians do not postpone surgery until the cholesterol is reduced or until the patient has quit smoking for two months. We do not make patients walk, run, cycle or swim daily before surgery, yet fitness is a stronger predictor for death and morbidity than any other modifiable factor!

Preventative medicine considers absolute risk to be much more important than relative risk. People with lower absolute risks are not treated (threshold is currently a 1 in 5 risk for a cardiovascular event over the next 10 years), even though 'normal' cardiovascular risk can also be reduced by lowering blood pressure or cholesterol concentration further. A normotensive man is more likely to die than a hypertensive woman the same age and is more likely to die than a hypertensive man 7 years younger. Normotensive normocholesterolaemic old men will have a greater absolute benefit from antihypertensive medication (and anticholesterolaemic medication) than young hypertensive hypercholesterolaemic women. Preventative medicine also recognises patient autonomy – you don't have to take antihypertensive medication if you don't want it. The common preoperative practice of postponing operations if the diastolic blood pressure exceeds 110mmHg is absurd without reference to absolute risk and patient autonomy. If a patient does not want their blood pressure reduced to limit non-operative long-term risk there is little reason to insist that they have their blood pressure reduced for an operation.

One reason that blood pressure has become a perioperative issue is that it is the only cardiovascular risk factor, apart from fitness, that can be easily measured anywhere. But ironically blood pressure is the only variable that systematically overestimates risk when measured in hospital. The blood pressure measurements that correlate best with cardiovascular events are those taken outside hospital.[21] The other reason that blood pressure has become a preoperative issue above all other cardiovascular risk factors is that it is measured intraoperatively and anaesthetic-induced hypotension is more likely in hypertensive patients. This may be a good reason to alter anaesthetic management for patients with a history of hypertension, but it is not a good reason to cancel hypertensive patients.

Only one in four patients prescribed antihypertensive medication become normotensive.[22] Small reductions in blood pressure can reduce stroke risk, but have little effect on heart attack risk and do not prevent deaths.[23] The absolute benefit from treating hypertension will vary, depending upon patient age, sex, fitness and previous cardiovascular events. Between 5000 and 12,000 hypertensive adults who have not had a cardiovascular event need to be treated to prevent one stroke per month.[24] Beta-blockers decrease blood pressure by 11/6mmHg on average. One stroke per month is prevented for every 12,000 hypertensive patients treated with a beta-blocker.[25] Calcium channel blockers decrease blood pressure by similar amounts but prevent three strokes per month for every 12,000 hypertensive patients treated.[26] One myocardial infarction per month is prevented for every 12,000 hypertensive patients who take aspirin. However, overall mortality is not decreased by aspirin because the risk for fatal haemorrhage is increased by aspirin.[27] Diuretics probably reduce blood pressure the quickest.[28]

The possible reduction in stroke risk provided by preoperative antihypertensive treatment for two months is similar to the increase in stroke risk associated with being two months older. It is time to remove the stigma of elevated blood pressure measured in preoperative assessment clinics. Global cardiovascular and mortality risks for each patient should be calculated without undue emphasis on hypertension.

Myocardial infarction

Myocardial infarction kills, mainly through ventricular fibrillation or heart failure. The risk of dying in the first month after a myocardial infarction is about 50 times the risk of dying in the month before a myocardial infarction, despite treatment (fibrinolysis or angioplasty).[29] The long-term relative mortality risk associated with a previous myocardial infarction is 1.5 times the risk without. The claim – made in many perioperative texts – that risk has returned to 'normal' six months after a heart attack is certainly incorrect. By 12 months, the relative risk has fallen to about three times the risk of someone who did not have an MI. Between one and 12 months after a heart attack, the relative risk probably falls exponentially, so that six months after a heart attack the relative risk may be about 6 (see Chapter 2). The absolute risk of dying – which is the risk that will help the patient and clinicians decide when and whether to proceed with surgery – is calculated by combining the relative risk with the other risk factors described previously in Chapter 2.

Atrial fibrillation

Age, history of cardiovascular events and decreased fitness explain most of the doubled mortality risk associated with atrial fibrillation (AF). Warfarin decreases the risk of dying in patients with atrial fibrillation (relative risk 0.8): if the monthly mortality risk for a hypothetical patient with AF is 5 in 1200, warfarin would reduce the risk to 4 in 1200. Warfarin halves the risk of stroke, for instance from 5 in 1200 per month to 2.5 in 1200 per month. Aspirin is less effective than warfarin, the relative risk for stroke being about 0.8 compared to placebo. Of course the absolute benefit from either warfarin or aspirin depends upon the absolute risk of death or stroke without medication.[30-32] See above and Chapter 2 to calculate this baseline risk.

Prosthetic heart valves

The risk of symptomatic arterial thromboemboli is increased for patients with prosthetic heart valves, particularly within the first three months after valve replacement. But the absolute risk is less for biological valves (as opposed to mechanical valves) and aortic valve replacement (as opposed to mitral valve replacement). Patients with mechanical mitral valves have about a 1 in 1000 monthly risk of thromboemboli whilst taking warfarin. Patients who have biological aortic valves have about a 1 in 2400 monthly risk without any medication, but sometimes take aspirin.[33]

Anticoagulation

Before surgery the questions that have to be answered for patients taking warfarin, aspirin or clopidogrel (see below) for atrial fibrillation, prosthetic heart valves or intracoronary stents are:

● What is the risk of death or disability from enclosed or massive haemorrhage for this surgery, both on medication and off medication?

● What is the risk of death or disability from thromboemboli, both on medication and off medication?

The answers to these questions should inform the decisions:

● whether to stop anticoagulation before surgery;

● whether to start alternative antithrombotic interventions perioperatively;

● when to restart anticoagulation after surgery if it has been stopped.

One typical preoperative protocol for warfarin is: Take the last dose of warfarin five days before all surgeries except dental and cataract extractions.

(1) Start subcutaneous fractionated heparin 36 hours later at home (administered by patient, district nurse or practice nurse) if the clot risk is high; do not start heparin if the clot risk is low. See Table 5.1.

(2) No fractionated heparin in the 12 hours preceding surgery.

(3) Restart warfarin after surgery (the same day or as prescribed by the surgical consultant).

Table 5.1 Factors associated with risk of clot

HIGH risk of clot	LOW risk of clot
Within 30 days of first warfarin dose	At least 60 days after first warfarin dose
Treated for multiple arterial or venous clots	Treated for first clot
Atrial fibrillation with mitral valve disease	Atrial fibrillation without mitral valve disease
History of clot with cancer	
Mechanical mitral valve	Tissue valves and mechanical aortic valve

Further discussion on preoperative haematological management including warfarin can be found in Chapter 11.

Coronary artery bypass and coronary artery stents

For most patients with chronic stable angina, whether mild, moderate or severe, coronary artery bypass grafting (CABG) and percutaneous coronary interventions (PCI) are palliative procedures.

That is, they relieve anginal pain that has not responded to maximal medical therapy but they do not prolong survival.

Most of the evidence comparing medication with CABG comes from 2649 patients recruited into seven randomised controlled trials (RTCs) between 1972 and 1984.[34] Drugs used to reduce cardiovascular risk and techniques used to achieve coronary bypass have changed since 1984 but further RCTs have not been conducted. The median survival was 100 months after CABG and 96 months without (difference unlikely to be less than 50 days), but more people died in the first year with CABG than without. It is not surprising that patients do not benefit from 'prophylactic' CABG before undergoing non-cardiac surgery.[35,36]

Percutaneous coronary angioplasty and stenting, collectively known as 'percutaneous coronary intervention' (PCI), have also been used to treat angina since the CABG studies were published. PCI is less invasive than CABG, but relief from angina is less prolonged.[37-39] PCI, with or without stents, does not prolong survival in patients with stable angina and simple single-vessel disease.[40,41] PCI probably shortens survival in patients with complex multivessel coronary disease: the risk of dying might be increased ten-fold in the first month after stenting and the risk of death remains two to three times expected for more than a year.[42-44] Patients are about 1.2 times more likely to die after PCI (with or without stents) than after CABG.

Angioplasty inflates a balloon to stretch open a narrowed length of coronary artery. The opened artery can narrow, either due to elastic recoil ('rebound') or continued atherosclerotic hypertrophy. Bare metal mesh stents reduce recoil in the short term but wall hypertrophy through the mesh can narrow the vessel lumen. Mesh impregnated with a drug – sirolimus or paclitaxel – slows wall hypertrophy, maintaining coronary arterial blood flow. The risk of dying in the first three months following insertion of drug-eluting stents (DES) is possibly two-thirds the risk of dying after insertion of bare-metal stents (BMS). However, the risk of dying after this initial period is probably three times greater for DES than for BMS.[45-51] This may be related to the effect of stopping clopidogrel, which increases the DES risk of dying four to five times but has little effect on the BMS risk of dying.[52-57] The increased risk of dying in patients with DES who stop clopidogrel can be used to try and calculate the relative merits of continuing or stopping clopidogrel perioperatively.

For example, consider a 67-year-old man who had a single drug-eluting stent inserted 6 months ago in the left anterior descending coronary artery. He has not had a heart attack, a stroke, renal failure or peripheral vascular disease. He achieves a peak oxygen consumption of 21ml/kg per minute (expected 27ml/kg per minute). The average monthly risk of dying for a 67-year-old man is 1 in 600. The reduced exercise capacity increases this risk to about 1 in 300. Because the DES was inserted for simple disease and because he is still taking clopidogrel it is reasonable to assume that his risk of dying is about 1 in 300 per month. If the clopidogrel is stopped his risk of dying increases, perhaps five-fold, to about 1 in 60. The risk of dying in the month following laparoscopic cholecystectomy may be about twice the risk of dying in the month preceding surgery. So, his risk of dying in the month after surgery is about 1 in 150 if clopidogrel is continued and about 1 in 30 if it is stopped, with similar risks for non-fatal myocardial infarction.

Do not refer patients to cardiologists if they think their angina is adequately controlled. Refer patients who think their angina is inadequately controlled if:

- they are not on maximal medical therapy (refer to previous cardiology investigations and documentation);
- they are on maximal medical therapy but they will consider either PCI or CABG.

Do not refer patients who are on maximal medical therapy but will not consider PCI or CABG, or patients whose angiography has already shown anatomy that is not amenable to either technique.

Cardiovascular testing

Coronary angiography

Table 5.2 Matrix for relations between ISWT, CPX and cardiac symptoms

Exercise symptom	ST depression (mm)	ISWT distance (m)	CPX O$_2$ (ml O$_2$/ kg/min)	Old METS
Angina and stops exercise	None	< 320	< 14	< 4
	> 0.9	< 900	< 23	< 6.5
	> 1.9	< 1700	< 32	< 9
	> 2.9	< 3500	< 46	< 13
	> 3.9	< 5000	< 60	< 17
Angina and continues	> 0.9	< 550	< 18	< 5
	> 1.9	< 1050	< 25	< 7
	> 2.9	< 2100	< 35	< 10
	> 3.9	< 3500	< 46	< 13
No angina	> 0.9	< 60	< 7	< 2
	> 1.9	< 550	< 18	< 5
	> 2.9	< 1350	< 28	< 8
	> 3.9	< 2500	< 39	< 11

MET: metabolic equivalent (one MET = 3.5ml O$_2$/kg/min). Modified from Mark *et al*.[59]

Current guidelines recommend angiography for patients with suspected coronary artery disease and a predicted monthly mortality greater than 1 in 400.[58] However, the authors of this guideline had to have considered the fact that most men older than 71 years have at least this mortality risk. Most patients will not experience angina during preoperative exercise testing, including those with ischaemic heart disease and a history of angina – breathlessness is a better predictor for the presence of coronary artery stenoses than angina. The aim is to identify patients more likely to die than the average with ischaemic heart disease. The seven trials I mentioned above found that CABG increased median survival by 9 months, from 7 years 6 months to 8 years 3 months (difference unlikely to be less than 3 months) in the third of patients with higher risk, and by 19 months, from 6 years 9 months to 8 years 4 months (difference unlikely to be less than 5 months) in patients with left main stem coronary artery stenosis of at least 70%.

If a patient fails to achieve the following distances (see Table 5.2, page 95) during the incremental shuttle walk test (ISWT) or the following oxygen consumptions during cardiopulmonary exercise testing (CPX), and has ST changes compared to rest, the guideline suggests referral for coronary angiography.

Again there is little to be gained by cardiological review if the patient has had coronary angiography that has shown that PCI and CABG would not be helpful.

Echocardiograms

Fitness, measured by either ISWT or CPX, predicts survival more accurately than does transthoracic echocardiography. Even dobutamine stress echocardiography, single photon emission computerised tomography or stress scintillography probably add little prognostic information to CPX results.

Patients with left ventricular outflow obstruction, such as severe aortic stenosis, can be anaesthetised for non-cardiac surgery. One might expect that risk could be estimated by fitness tests, because patients whose cardiac output is limited will reach lower power levels. It is unknown whether fitness tests adequately assess both non-operative and operative risks in patients with undiagnosed aortic stenosis. Because the answer is uncertain, and because tailored intraoperative management may reduce risk, it seems reasonable to use echocardiography, in addition to exercise testing, to identify patients with moderate or severe aortic stenosis. I cannot guide readers on how useful different echocardiographic strategies are to measure and limit mortality risk. What follows is a strategy that has not been validated; your local policy will depend upon discussions with cardiologists and echocardiographers.

You could request an echocardiogram for a patient with a heart murmur who meets one or more of the following criteria:

- Left ventricular hypertrophy on a resting 12-lead electrocardiogram
- Inability to achieve 4 old METS or 5.5 new METs (peak oxygen consumption of 14mls O_2/kg per min)
- Faints or angina

- Planned major surgery (if older than 40 years)
- Planned hypotensive anaesthesia (if older than 40 years).

Unprepared elective or scheduled patients

This chapter has concentrated on cardiovascular risk assessment and disease management in patients presenting for elective or scheduled surgery who are under the care of a primary care physician. The principles that have been outlined also apply to patients who are either not registered with, or who have not attended, a primary care service. To assess non-operative risks you will need to spend more time either directly assessing risk or liaising with a primary care service. Unprepared patients are more likely to benefit from delaying surgery to allow risk factors to be assessed and reduced, but perhaps are also less likely to want to do so.

The principles of assessment and preparation of patients for emergency surgery are also the same. But risk reduction will depend upon reducing the relative risk of surgery as there will be no time to reduce non-operative risk.

Management of disease, management of risk

This chapter has discussed aspects of managing cardiovascular disease and reducing risk. It seems reasonable to use the opportunity of the visit to the preoperative assessment clinic to educate the patient about interventions that reduce the risk of death, stroke and heart attack in primary care. It is also right to identify patients who fulfil criteria for primary (or secondary) drug prevention of cardiovascular events but who are not receiving full pharmaceutical protection. At the time of writing there is inadequate evidence to support starting medication (such as beta-blockers or statins) just because the patient is scheduled for surgery.

CONCLUSION

Assessment of cardiovascular disease depends upon a targeted history, a fitness test and cardiac auscultation. Perioperative risk of death and cardiovascular events is calculated from the preoperative risk of death, taking into account the results of assessment. Particular attention should be paid to coronary stent implantation.

For many patients cardiovascular disease is optimally managed, and risk reduced, by primary care. The preoperative clinic can assist primary care by checking that patients are aware of how they can reduce their long-term risk, by stopping smoking, exercise, a balanced diet and drugs (if the 10-year risk for a cardiovascular event exceeds 1 in 5). Of particular note, blood pressure measurements in secondary care are unlikely to realistically reflect long-term cardiovascular risk. Delaying surgery to commence treatment in patients who are truly hypertensive is unlikely to result in significant net perioperative benefit. Delaying surgery to get fitter will be more beneficial.

Stopping clopidogrel increases the risk for postoperative in-stent thrombosis, myocardial infarction and death, by about 1.2 times for bare-metal stents and 5 times for drug-eluting stents.

REFERENCES

1. S.L. Hardoon, P.H. Whincup, L.T. Lennon, S.G. Wannamethee, S. Capewell and R.W. Morris (2008). How much of the recent decline in the incidence of myocardial infarction in British men can be explained by changes in cardiovascular risk factors? *Circulation* **117**: 598–604.

2. M.J. Goldacre, D. Mant, M. Duncan and M. Griffith (2005). Mortality from heart failure in an English population, 1979-2003: study of death certification. *Journal of Epidemiology and Community Health* **59**: 782–4.

3. M. Guazzi, G. Reina, G. Tumminello and M.D. Guazzi (2005). Exercise ventilation inefficiency and cardiovascular mortality in heart failure: the critical independent prognostic value of the arterial CO_2 partial pressure. *European Heart Journal* **26**: 472–80.

4. M. Robbins, G. Francis, F.J. Pashkow, C.E. Snader, K. Hoercher, J.B. Young et al. (1999). Ventilatory and heart rate responses to exercise better predictors of heart failure mortality than peak oxygen consumption. *Circulation* **100**: 2411–7.

5. L.C. Davies, R. Wensel, P. Georgiadou, M. Cicoira, A.J.S. Coats, M.F. Piepoli et al. (2006). Enhanced prognostic value from cardiopulmonary exercise testing in chronic heart failure by non-linear analysis: oxygen uptake efficiency slope. *European Heart Journal* **27**: 684–90.

6. U. Corrà, A. Mezzani, E. Bosimini and P. Giannuzzi (2004). Cardiopulmonary exercise testing and prognosis in chronic heart failure: a prognosticating algorithm for the individual patient. *Chest* **126**: 942–50.

7. P. Agostoni, M. Guazzi, M. Bussotti, S. De Vita and P. Palermo (2002). Carvedilol reduces the inappropriate increase in ventilation during exercise in heart failure patients. *Chest* **122**: 2062–7.

8. A.K. Gitt, K. Wasserman, C. Kilkowski, T. Kleeman, A. Kilkowski, M. Bangert et al. (2002). Exercise anaerobic threshold and ventilatory efficiency identify heart failure patients for high risk of early death. *Circulation* **106**: 3079–84.

9. M. Guazzi, J. Myers and R. Arena (2005). Cardiopulmonary exercise testing in the clinical and prognostic assessment of diastolic heart failure. *Journal of the American College of Cardiology* **46**: 1883–90.

10. T. Bilsel, S. Terzi, T. Akbulut, N. Sayar, G. Hobikoglu and K. Yesilcimen(2006). Abnormal heart rate recovery immediately after cardiopulmonary exercise testing in heart failure patients. *International Heart Journal* **47**: 431–40.

11. M. Arzt, M. Schulz, R. Wensel, S. Montalvàn, F.C. Blumberg, G.A.J. Riegger et al. (2005). Nocturnal continuous positive airway pressure improves ventilatory efficiency during exercise in patients with chronic heart failure. *Chest* **127**: 794–802.

12. D. Messika-Zeitoun, B.D. Johnson, V. Nkomo, J-F. Avierinos, T.G. Allison, C. Scott et al. (2006). Cardiopulmonary exercise testing determination of functional capacity in mitral regurgitation. *Journal of the American College of Cardiology* **47**: 2521–7.

13. K. Dimopoulos, D.O. Okonko, G-P. Diller, C.S. Borberg, T.V. Salukhe, S.V. Babu-Narayan et al. (2006). Abnormal ventilatory response to exercise in adults with congenital heart disease relates to cyanosis and predicts survival. *Circulation* **113**: 2796–802.

14. A. Giardini, S. Specchia, T.A. Tacy, G. Coutsoumbas, G. Gargiulo, A. Donti et al. (2007). Usefulness of cardiopulmonary exercise to predict long-term prognosis in adults with repaired tetralogy of Fallot. *American Journal of Cardiology* **99**: 1462–7.

15. H. Tsurugaya, A. Adachi, M. Kurabayashi, S. Ohshima and K. Taniguchi (2006). Prognostic impact of ventilatory efficiency in heart disease patients with preserved exercise tolerance. *Circulation Journal* **70**: 1332–6.

16. A. Koike, H. Itoh, M. Kato, H. Sawada, T. Aizawa, L. Tai Fu et al. (2002). Prognostic power of ventilatory responses during submaximal exercise in patients with chronic heart disease. *Chest* **121**: 1581–8.

17. J. Hippisley-Cox, C. Coupland, Y. Vinogradova, J. Robson, M. May and P. Brindle (2007). Derivation and validation of QRISK, a new cardiovascular disease risk score for the United Kingdom: prospective open cohort study. *British Medical Journal* **335**: 136–48.

18. R.B. D'Agostino, R.S. Vasan, M.J. Pencina, P.A. Wolf, M. Cobain, J.M. Massaro *et al.* (2008). General cardiovascular risk profile for use in primary care. *Circulation* **117**: 743–53.

19. P.G. Steg, D.L. Bhatt, P.W.F. Wilson, R. D'Agostino, E.M. Ohman, J. Röther et al. (2007). One-year cardiovascular event rates in outpatients with atherothrombosis. *Journal of the Americal Medical Association* **297**: 1197–206.

20. S.J. Howell, J.W. Sear and P. Foëx (2004). Hypertension, hypertensive heart disease and perioperative cardiac risk. *British Journal of Anaesthesia* **92**: 570–83.

21. R.H. Fagard and V.A. Cornelissen (2007). Incidence of cardiovascular events in white-coat, masked and sustained hypertension versus true normotension: a meta-analysis. *Journal of Hypertension* **25**: 2193–8.

22. M. Burnier (2002). Blood pressure control and the implementation of guidelines in clinical practice: can we fill the gap? *Journal of Hypertension* **20**: 1251–3.

23. J.A. Staessen, J.G. Wang and L. Thijs (2003). Cardiovascular prevention and blood pressure reduction: a quantitative overview updated until 1 March 2003. *Journal of Hypertension* **21**: 1055–76

24. A. Quan, K. Kerlikowske, F. Gueyffier, J.P. Boissel, for the INDANA Investigators (2000). Pharmacotherapy for hypertension in women of different races. *Cochrane Database of Systematic Reviews*, Issue 2. Art. No.: CD002146. DOI: 10.1002/14651858. CD002146.

25. C.S. Wiysonge, H. Bradley, B.M. Mayosi, R. Maroney, A. Mbewu, L.H. Opie et al. (2007), Beta-blockers for hypertension. *Cochrane Database of Systematic Reviews*, Issue 1. Art. No.: CD002003. DOI: 10.1002/14651858.CD002003.pub2.

26. B. Dahlöf, P.S. Sever, N.R. Poulter, H. Wedel, D.G. Beevers, M. Caulfield et al. (2005). ASCOT Investigators. Prevention of cardiovascular events with an antihypertensive regimen of amlodipine adding perindopril as required versus atenolol adding bendroflumethiazide as required, in the Anglo-Scandinavian Cardiac Outcomes Trial-Blood Pressure Lowering Arm (ASCOT-BPLA): a multicentre randomised controlled trial. *Lancet* **366**: 895–906.

27. G.Y.H. Lip and D.C. Felmeden (2004). Antiplatelet agents and anticoagulants for hypertension. *Cochrane Database of Systematic Reviews*, Issue 3. Art. No.: CD003186. DOI: 10.1002/14651858.CD003186.pub2.

28. J.P. Baguet, B. Legallicier, P. Auquier and S. Robitail (2007). Updated meta-analytical approach to the efficacy of antihypertensive drugs in reducing blood pressure. *Clinical Drug Investigation* **27**: 735–53.

29. E. Boersma and the PCAT-2 trialist collaborative group (2006). Does time matter? A pooled analysis of randomized clinical trials comparing primary percutaneous coronary intervention and in-hospital fibrinolysis in acute myocardial infarction patients. *European Heart Journal* **27**: 779–88.

30. M.I. Aguilar and R. Hart (2005) Oral anticoagulants for preventing stroke in patients with non-valvular atrial fibrillation and no previous history of stroke or transient ischemic attacks. *Cochrane Database of Systematic Reviews*, Issue 3. Art. No.: CD001927. DOI: 10.1002/14651858.CD001927.pub2.

31. V. Fuster, L.E. Ryden, D.S. Cannom, H.J. Crijns, A.B. Curtis, K.A. Ellenbogen et al. (2006). ACC/AHA/ESC 2006 guidelines for the management of patients with atrial fibrillation. *Circulation* **114**: e257-e354.

32. S.H. Little and D.R. Massel (2003). Antiplatelet and anticoagulation for patients with prosthetic heart valves. *Cochrane Database of Systematic Reviews*, Issue 4. Art. No.: CD003464. DOI: 10.1002/14651858.CD003464.

33. R.O. Bonow, B.A. Carabello, K. Chatterjee, A.C. De Leon, D.P. Faxon, M.D. Freed et al. (2006). ACC/AHA 2006 guidelines for the management of patients with valvular heart disease. *Journal of the American College of Cardiology* **48**: e1-e148.

34. S. Yusuf, D. Zucker, P. Peduzzi, L.D. Fisher, T. Takaro, J.W. Kennedy et al. (1994). Effect of coronary artery bypass graft surgery on survival: Overview of 10-year results from randomised trials by the Coronary Artery Bypass Graft Surgery Trialists Collaboration. *Lancet* **344**: 563–70.

35. E.O. McFalls, H.B. Ward, T.E. Moritz, S. Goldman, W.C. Krupski, F. Littooy et al. (2004). Coronary-artery revascularization before major vascular surgery. *New England Journal of Medicine* **351**: 2795–804.

36. D. Poldermans, O. Schouten, R. Vidakovic, J.J. Bax, I.R. Thomson, S.E. Hoeks et al. (2007). A clinical randomized trial to evaluate the safety of a noninvasive approach in high-risk patients undergoing major vascular surgery: The DECREASE-V Pilot Study. *Journal of the American College of Cardiology* **49**: 1763–9.

37. D.M. Bravata, A.L. Glenger, K.M. McDonald, V. Sundaram, M.V. Perez, R. Varghese et al. (2007). Systematic review: the comparative effectiveness of percutaneous coronary interventions and coronary artery bypass graft surgery. *Annals of Internal Medicine* **147**: 703–16.

38. E.L. Hannan, M.J. Racz, G. Walford, R.H. Jones, T.J. Ryan, E. Bennett et al. (2005). Long-term outcomes of coronary artery bypass grafting versus stent implantation. *New England Journal of Medicine* **352**: 2174–83.

39. E.L. Hannan, C. Wu, G. Walford, A.T. Culliford, J.P. Gold, C.R. Smith et al. (2008). Drug-eluting stents vs. coronary-artery bypass grafting in multivessel coronary disease. *New England Journal of Medicine* **358**: 331–41.

40. W.E. Boden, R.A. O'Rourke, K.K. Teo, P.M. Hartigan, D.J. Maron, W.J. Kostuk et al. (2007). Optimal medical therapy with or without PCI for stable coronary disease. *New England Journal of Medicine* **356**: 1503–16.

41. D.G. Katritsis and J.P.A. Ioannidis (2005). Percutaneous coronary intervention versus conservative therapy in nonacute coronary artery disease: a meta-analysis. *Circulation* **111**: 2906–12.

42. H.K. Win, A.E. Caldera, K. Maresh, J. Lopez, C.S. Rihal, M.A. Parikh et al. (2007). Clinical outcomes and stent thrombosis following off-label use of drug-eluting stents. *Journal of the American College of Cardiology* **297**: 2001–9.

43. O.C. Marroquin, F. Selzer, S.R. Mulukutla, D.O. Williams, H.A. Vlachos, R.L. Wilensky et al. (2008). A comparison of bare-metal and drug-eluting stents for off-label indications. *New England Journal of Medicine* **358**: 342–52.

44. G.W. Stone, S.G. Ellis, L. Cannon, J.T. Mann, J.D. Greenberg and D. Spriggs (2005). Comparison of a polymer-based paclitaxel-eluting stent with a bare metal stent in patients with complex coronary artery disease. *Journal of the Americal Medical Association* **294**: 1215–23.

45. G. Weisz, M.B. Leon, D.R. Holmes, D.J. Kereiakes, M.R. Clark, B.M. Cohen et al. (2006). Two-year outcomes after sirolimus-eluting stent implantation. *Journal of the American College of Cardiology* **47**: 1350–5.

46. M-C. Morice, P.W. Serruys, J.E. Sousa, J. Fajadet, E.B. Hayashi, M. Perin et al. (2002). A randomized comparison of a sirolimus-eluting stent with a standard stent for coronary revascularization. *New England Journal of Medicine* **346**: 1773–80.

47. J.W. Moses, M.B. Leon, J.J. Popma, P.J. Fitzgerald, D.R. Holmes, C. O'Shaughnessy et al. (2003). Sirolimus-eluting stents versus standard stents in patients with stenosis in a native coronary artery. *New England Journal of Medicine* **349**: 1315–23.

48. G.W. Stone, S.G. Ellis, D.A. Cox, J. Hermiller, C. O'Shaughnessy, J.T. Mann et al. (2004). A polymer-based, paclitaxel-eluting stent in patients with coronary artery disease. *New England Journal of Medicine* **350**: 221–31.

49. C. Spaulding, J. Daemen, E. Boersma, D.E. Cutlip and P.W. Serruys (2007). A pooled analysis of data comparing sirolimus-eluting stents with bare-metal stents. *New England Journal of Medicine* **356**: 989-97.

50. A. Kastrati, A. Dibra, C. Spaulding, G.J. Laarman, M. Menichelli, M. Valgimigli et al. (2007). Meta-analysis of randomized trials on drug-eluting stents vs. bare-metal stents in patients with acute myocardial infarction. *European Heart Journal* **28**: 2706–13.

51. B. Lagerqvist, S.K. James, U. Stenestrand, J. Lindbäck, T. Nilsson and L. Wallentin (2007). Long-term outcomes with drug-eluting versus bare-metal stents in Sweden. *New England Journal of Medicine* **356**: 1009–19.

52. M. Pfisterer, H.P. Brunner-La Rocca, P.T. Buser, P. Rickenbacher, P. Hunziker, C. Mueller et al. (2006). Late clinical events after clopidogrel discontinuation may limit the benefit of drug-eluting stents. *Journal of the American College of Cardiology* **48**: 2584–91.

53. E.L. Eisenstein, K.J. Anstrom, D.F. Kong, L.K. Shaw, R.H. Tuttle, D.B. Mark et al. (2007). Clopidogrel use and long-term clinical outcomes after drug-eluting stent implantation. *Journal of the Americal Medical Association* **297**: 159–68.

54. J.A. Spertus, R. Kettelkamp, C. Vance, C. Decker, P.G. Jones, J.S. Rumsfield et al. (2006). Prevalence, predictors, and outcomes of premature discontinuation of thienopyridine therapy after drug-eluting stent placement: results from the PREMIER registry. *Circulation* **113**: 2803–9.

55. I. Iakovou, T. Schmidt, E. Bonizzoni, L. Ge, G.M. Sangiorgi, G. Stankovic et al. (2005). Incidence, predictors and outcome of thrombosis after successful implantation of drug-eluting stents. *Journal of the Americal Medical Association* **293**: 2126–30.

56. P.K. Kuchulakanti, W.W. Chu, R. Torguson, P. Ohlmann, S-W. Rha, L.C. Clavijo et al. (2006). Correlates and long-term outcomes of angiographically proven stent thrombosis with sirolimus- and paclitaxel-eluting stents. *Circulation* **113**: 1108–13.

57. J. Machecourt, N. Danchin, J.M. Lablanche, J.M. Fauvel, J.L. Bonnet, S. Marliere et al. (2007). Risk factors for stent thrombosis after implantation of sirolimus-eluting stents in diabetic and nondiabetic patients. *Journal of the American College of Cardiology* **50**: 501–8.

58. P.J. Scanlon, D.P. Faxon, A-M Audet, B. Carabello, G.J. Dehmer, K.A. Eagle et al. (1999). ACC/AHA Guidelines for Coronary Angiography: Executive summary and recommendations. *Circulation* **99**: 2345–57.

59. D.B. Mark, L. Shaw, F.E. Harrell Jr, M.A. Hlatky, K.L. Lee and J.R. Bengtson (1991). Prognostic value of a treadmill exercise score in outpatients with suspected coronary artery disease. *New England Journal of Medicine* **325**: 849–53.

6 Respiratory assessment and disease

David Lynes

SUMMARY

This chapter will describe:

- **basic anatomy and physiology of the respiratory system**
- **applied physiology of common respiratory disease**
- **blood gas analysis and implication for perioperative optimisation**
- **non-pharma and pharmacological approach to respiratory optimisation.**

INTRODUCTION

Patients with chronic respiratory problems frequently have co-morbidities that may increase the likelihood of their needing surgery. Moreover, due to the prevalence of respiratory disorders such as COPD it is often necessary to anaesthetise patients with respiratory problems and this involves a high risk of intra- and postoperative respiratory complications.[1] The perioperative clinician should be aware that, although the effects of general anaesthesia may be minor, they may nevertheless tip a patient with a respiratory condition and hence limited respiratory reserve into respiratory failure. Problems might include laryngeal or bronchial spasm due to intubation and a reduction in the ability to clear secretions due to anaesthetic agents. Excess intravenous fluids can cause pulmonary oedema in patients with cardiac failure, and some anaesthetics and drugs may depress respiratory drive.[2]

Care of the patient with respiratory conditions is therefore an essential aspect of perioperative care and this chapter describes common respiratory diseases such as COPD and asthma and discusses salient aspects of current management regimes. Pivotal aspects of perioperative management, including preoperative assessment and postoperative care, are also considered.

Respiratory anatomy and physiology: an introduction

The respiratory system can be divided into a number of sections. These include the upper respiratory tract and the lower respiratory tract; the chest wall and respiratory muscles such as intercostal and diaphragm, and the cardiopulmonary circulation. A succinct description of respiratory anatomy and physiology is provided here and in other parts of this chapter.

Figure 6.1 The respiratory system

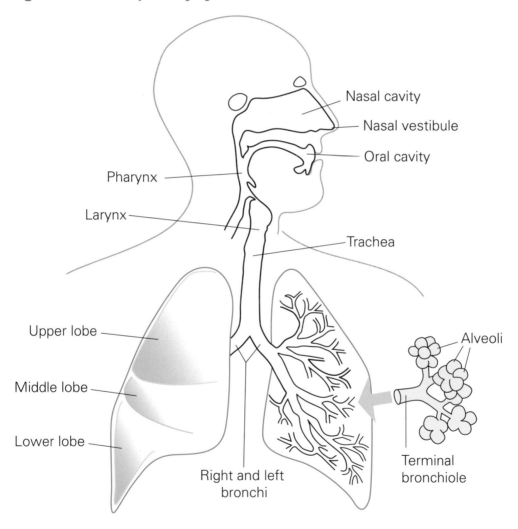

The upper respiratory tract comprises the nose, the pharynx and the larynx. Its functions include warming, filtering and moistening inhaled air.

The lower respiratory tract comprises conducting airways such as the larger trachea and bronchi, and smaller bronchioles. It also includes respiratory airways such as alveolar ducts, and the alveoli. Gaseous exchange, which involves oxygen passing from the lungs into the blood and carbon dioxide passing from the blood to the lungs, occurs at the respiratory airways and the alveoli (see Figure 6.1).

The conducting airways are made from smooth muscle and cartilage and they are lined with ciliated epithelium. Ciliated epithelium is a layer of cells with a brush border of cilia which are microscopic hair-like structures. These are interspersed with goblet cells which secrete mucus. If particles of dust or other airborne pollutants get past the upper respiratory tract into the lower respiratory tract, the conducting airways can constrict, which means that airflow through the airways becomes spiral rather than laminar and the dust is deposited onto the ciliated epithelium. Mucus traps the particles, and movement of the cilia ensures that trapped particles are removed from the lungs via the 'muco-ciliary escalator'. The airways therefore play an important role in preventing particles reaching the respiratory airways and alveoli, which do not have goblet cells or cilia. If particles do reach the alveoli, cells called macrophages detect them. Macrophages engulf and destroy micro-organisms, and can also trigger a reaction in the immune system which helps protect the lungs from future invasions of micro-organisms.

The smaller respiratory airways do not have cartilage and therefore rely on attachments to the alveoli to keep them open. This is a bit like having guy ropes on a tent to keep it up; the attachments create a radial traction on the smaller airways that keep them open. Loss of attachments, such as that which occurs in emphysema, leads to the collapse of the small airways.

The alveoli are composed primarily of a single layer of cells called type 1 pneumocytes. Type 2 pneumocytes also form part of the alveolar walls. These produce a substance called surfactant which reduces the risk of alveolar collapse during expiration. The function of the alveoli is to enable gas exchange between the air and pulmonary circulation. There are a large number of microscopic spherical alveoli, which means that there is a total surface area of between 50 and 100 square metres of membrane available for gaseous exchange in normal adults. Pulmonary venules are wrapped around the alveoli, which permit transfer of gas to and from the blood.

The chest wall is composed of twelve pairs of ribs separated by intercostal muscles, and the diaphragm below. A layer of membrane called the parietal pleura lines the chest wall inner surface, and the outer surface of the lung is lined by the visceral pleura. These membranes are in contact with each other but are not attached. There is a thin layer of pleural fluid between the two membranes.

Inspiration of air is achieved by contraction of the diaphragm, which increases the size of the thoracic cavity. Contraction of intercostal muscles also increases thoracic volume by moving the ribs upwards and outwards. This causes a fall in pressure within the lungs, and this means that air travels from the mouth to the alveoli.

Expiration is largely a passive process. It usually occurs when the intercostal muscles and the diaphragm are relaxed, although expiration can be forced with the help of muscles such as abdominal muscles.

Common respiratory disorders: asthma and COPD

Both asthma and COPD are 'obstructive' disorders, which means that the diameters of airways become smaller so that it becomes difficult or even impossible to breathe. A simple analogy is that of breathing through a drinking straw rather than a hosepipe; it takes longer to breathe in and out. This may mean that it is possible to sit comfortably, but when walking a distance or up stairs it may be necessary to stop to catch one's breath because it is not possible to breathe in sufficient oxygen to meet the additional demand due to exercise. If a smaller diameter drinking straw is used, it is possible that one may be extremely uncomfortable at rest; indeed it may take so long to breathe out that there may not be enough time for the lungs to empty before it is time to breathe in, leading to 'dynamic pulmonary hyperinflation'.

Obstructive disorders are just one category of respiratory diseases; another is 'restrictive'. In restrictive disorders the diameter of airways may not be affected, but the volume of the lungs is reduced because the patient cannot breathe in completely. Restrictive disorders include fibrosing disorders such as silicosis and fibrosing alveolitis, and bony disorders such as kyphosis. They can also include muscular weakness.

The respiratory investigation 'spirometry' is essential when diagnosing an obstructive or restrictive disorder and it is also an important preoperative investigation. An understanding of spirometry is therefore prerequisite to understanding asthma, COPD, and perioperative care of the patient with a respiratory condition.

Spirometry involves a patient breathing in as deeply as they can, blowing into a spirometer via a mouthpiece as forcibly as they can, and exhaling completely. Spirometry measures a number of variables, but perhaps the most important of these are the Forced Vital Capacity (FVC), which is the volume of air that can be exhaled from the lungs following full inspiration during a forced manoeuvre, and the Forced Expiratory Volume at one second (FEV_1), which is the volume of air expired in the first second of the FVC manoeuvre.

Results from spirometry can be displayed in a number of ways, but one of the most useful methods of displaying results is graphically on a Volume Time Curve (see Figure 6.2).

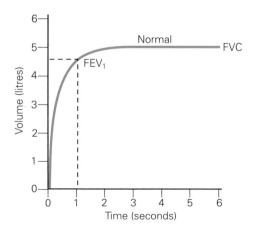

Figure 6.2
Volume Time Curve demonstrating a normal pattern

As the patient begins to exhale rapidly the graph rises sharply upwards and then curves smoothly and flattens as the exhalation slows until all air is exhaled from the lungs. FVC and the FEV_1 can be read directly from the graph.

Clearly if an individual has an obstructive disorder it will take them longer to exhale during the FVC manoeuvre (imagine trying to exhale rapidly through a narrow drinking straw). Whilst the FVC may not be affected, the FEV_1 will certainly be reduced. In order to diagnose an obstructive disorder, the FEV_1 is considered as a percentage of the FVC. This FEV_1/FVC ratio is sometimes referred to as the 'forced expiratory ratio' or FEV_1 %. This ratio defines the presence or absence of obstruction in the airways. A ratio of less than 70% is deemed to indicate obstructive lung disease.[3]

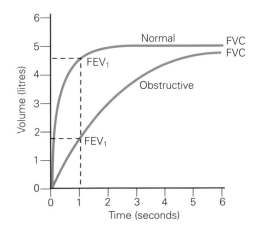

Figure 6.3
Volume Time Curve demonstrating an obstructive pattern in comparison to a normal curve

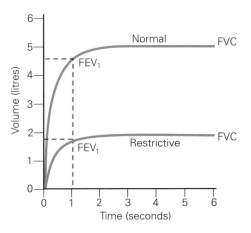

Figure 6.4
Volume Time Curve demonstrating a restrictive pattern in comparison to a normal curve

Figure 6.3 shows a typical trace of an obstructive pattern, which one might expect with either asthma or COPD. This presents as a reduction in FEV_1 from normal. Clearly the ratio of the FEV_1 to FVC is also reduced, demonstrating airflow obstruction.

Spirometry will also detect restrictive lung disorders, as shown by Figure 6.4. Restrictive disorders prevent full expansion of the lungs and may be due to changes in the chest wall, lung tissue and pleura. It is important to note that, unlike obstructive disorders, restrictive lung disorders will not necessarily reduce the diameter of airways, and the shape of the curve is therefore similar to a 'normal' curve.

The reduction in lung volume caused by restrictive disorders will mean that the FVC and FEV_1 are reduced compared to normal (see Figure 6.4). The forced expiratory ratio, however, is normal (above 70%) or high. This is because, although the vital capacity is low, the airflow is not reduced because the size of the airways remains normal. Clearly it is important to calculate the FEV$_1$/FVC ratio when diagnosing an obstructive disorder, and not simply rely on an FEV$_1$ measurement.

An example of the interpretation of spirometry: COPD

COPD involves progressive airflow obstruction. The NICE guidelines[3] indicate that COPD disease is characterised by airflow obstruction and that the airflow obstruction is usually progressive, not fully reversible and does not change markedly over several months. Unlike asthma, once COPD is established, the changes are irreversible and the disease continues to progress so long as the patient continues to smoke. In healthy non-smoking adults, FEV$_1$ will decline by an average of 30ml per year. However, in the subgroup of smokers who develop COPD, FEV$_1$ decline is an average of 70ml per year. Some smokers will decline faster than this.[4]

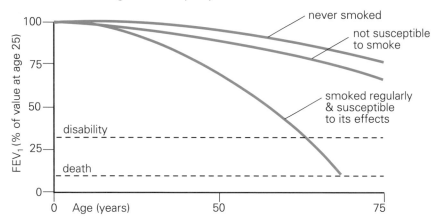

Fig 6.5 FEV$_1$ decline Based on the work of Fletcher and Peto *et al* (1976)

It is vital to ensure that the spirometry recording is accurate prior to interpretation of results. There must be a minimum of three technically acceptable recordings. The curve should be smooth, convex and free from irregularities that may, for example, be caused by coughing during the forced manoeuvre. It should rise steeply upwards and plateau for at least 2 seconds. Reproducibility is demonstrated by comparing each FVC attempt. At least two should be within 100ml and 5% of each other.

Spirometry interpretation
Step I: is obstruction present?
As discussed, this information is acquired from the FEV1/FVC ratio, which is less than 70% in obstructive lung diseases, such as COPD. If the ratio is greater than 70%, no obstruction has been demonstrated and the individual may not have COPD.

The calculation for this ratio is as follows: $\dfrac{\textbf{Measured FEV}_1}{\textbf{Measured FVC}} \textbf{ x 100}$

Step 2: What is the level of FVC and FEV_1?

The values obtained from spirometry can be compared to predicted values for the individual. These are based on the patient's height, age, gender and ethnicity. Some spirometers will do this following input of appropriate data prior to the test. The measured values are compared to the predicted value and are expressed as a percentage.

According to NICE guidelines,[3] a normal FVC is defined as being greater than 80% of the predicted value. If the FVC is low, that is less than 80% of the predicted value, this indicates small lung volumes which may be due to a restrictive lung disease. If detected, this would indicate the need for further investigation.

The calculation for percentage of predicted for FVC is as follows: $\dfrac{\textbf{Measured FVC}}{\textbf{Predicted FVC}} \times \textbf{100}$

Once it has been established that a patient has an obstructive curve, defined as an FEV_1/FVC ratio below 70%, FEV_1 can be compared to predicted values in order to calculate the severity of COPD. A normal FEV_1, is defined as being greater than 80% of the predicted value[3] although some guidelines suggest that a patient can still have COPD if FEV_1 is above 80% predicted, if the FEV_1/FVC ratio is also reduced.[5]

The calculation for percentage of predicted for FEV_1 is: $\dfrac{\textbf{Measured FEV}_1}{\textbf{Predicted FEV}_1} \times \textbf{100}$

For patients with COPD, the severity of the disease is determined by comparing the FEV_1 to the predicted value. Guidelines for the diagnosis and classification of COPD exist and vary; for example, severity classified by NICE[3] is outlined in Table 6.1.

Table 6.1 Classification of severity of COPD according to NICE (2004)

MILD COPD	FEV_1 50–80%
MODERATE COPD	FEV_1 30–49%
SEVERE COPD	FEV_1 <30%

It can be seen that spirometry is a pivotal investigation, and it will be discussed in relation to perioperative care later in this section.

Asthma and COPD have many similarities, including the fact that both diseases are obstructive and therefore limit expiratory flow; indeed asthma and COPD can coexist or overlap. However, it is important to understand that they are different disorders, and whilst they can coexist, their treatment, including aspects of pharmacological management, is different.

Whilst airway inflammation plays the central role in the pathogenesis of both diseases, the inflammation in COPD is different to that seen in asthma; in COPD it is driven by neutrophils whereas inflammation in asthma is driven by eosinophils.[6] This has important implications for pharmacological management and prognosis, which are clearly different in asthma and COPD, not least in that COPD inevitably leads to death and no current treatment can halt disease progression, whereas deterioration in asthma can be prevented and the condition can be managed for life.

The asthma inflammatory process involves the airways becoming infiltrated with inflammatory cells, and these cells are activated, meaning that they produce and contain chemicals that cause inflammation. The airflow obstruction seen in asthma is usually at least partially and often fully reversible, but if a patient ignores the symptoms or does not treat the inflammation the airways may become damaged and some changes in airway structure and function may become irreversible. For example, the basement membrane, which is the layer of tissue immediately below the lining layer of the airway wall, can become thickened. This results in the airways becoming narrowed and stiff, which can mean that the airways become less responsive to bronchodilator drugs.

Most people with asthma develop inflamed airways due to an allergic response. This means that their airways become inflamed due to an external stimulus which triggers the asthmatic response, and indeed asthmatic attacks. These triggers include allergens such grass pollen, food and drink, dust, and animal fur. However, other triggers may not be allergens. For example, exercise, respiratory viruses, psychological stress and pollution may cause asthma attacks in some people.

The inflammatory process and pathological changes in COPD are quite different from those in asthma. A pollutant, usually smoking, irritates the bronchiolar wall. The body responds by producing additional mucus, and the patient can develop chronic bronchitis. Smoke can also damage the respiratory bronchioles and the alveoli by attracting neutrophils which release enzymes called proteases. These enzymes can damage respiratory bronchioles and alveoli in susceptible individuals, which in the long term can result in the destruction of alveoli seen in emphysema. However, some smokers will not develop COPD, and it is probable that this is because they have an efficient protective mechanism against the enzymes released by white cells. Alpha 1 antitrypsin is an 'antiprotease' which is an example of a protective mechanism. A deficiency in alpha 1 antitrypsin will result in the early development of COPD, and may result in the development of COPD in a non-smoker. Alpha 1 antitrypsin deficiency is a rare condition which is probably responsible for about 1% of cases of COPD.

COPD affects different people in different ways, but there are some pathological processes that are common to most patients. In the large airways the mucous glands increase in size and number, which results in increased mucus production. The epithelium becomes chronically inflamed, and breakdown of the integrity of the epithelium is often seen. The viscosity of mucus increases and the cilia that line the airways become destroyed. Because of this the lungs' ability to remove mucus is impaired, as the mucociliary escalator becomes inefficient. This is called chronic bronchitis.

In the medium airways the airway smooth muscle becomes thickened and excessively contracted, which reduces the diameter of the airway. The small airways can become inflamed, oedematous, and infiltrated with cells such as macrophages and neutrophils. Smoking causes the neutrophils to release various enzymes such as proteases, and these digest and damage the alveoli. Inflammation also occurs within the walls of the distal bronchi and bronchioles, and this, together with the impact of repeated infections, leads to irreversible structural damage to the walls and sub-mucosa of the small airways.

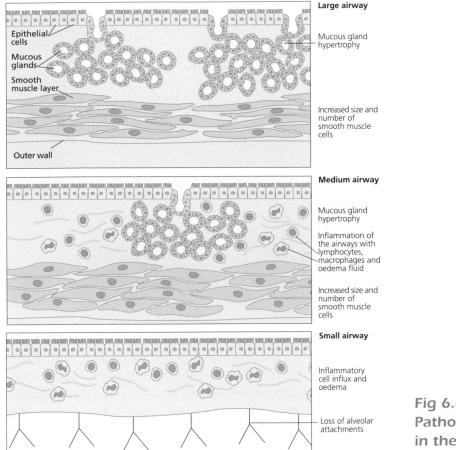

Large airway

Epithelial cells

Mucous glands

Smooth muscle layer

Outer wall

Mucous gland hypertrophy

Increased size and number of smooth muscle cells

Medium airway

Mucous gland hypertrophy

Inflammation of the airways with lymphocytes, macrophages and oedema fluid

Increased size and number of smooth muscle cells

Small airway

Inflammatory cell influx and oedema

Loss of alveolar attachments

Fig 6.6
Pathological changes in the airways

This process can result in the destruction of alveoli and when alveolar walls are damaged they can coalesce; this means that some of the smaller alveolar sacs merge to become larger ones. Instead of small alveolar sacs that are highly elastic, the alveoli coalesce into large inelastic sacs. This is called emphysema and is seen in Figure 6.7 (page 110).

If alveoli continue to merge they can form sacs that are larger than 1cm in diameter. These larger sacs are called bullae. This coalescence results in a reduction of the surface area of alveolar membrane, which results in impaired gaseous exchange. The smaller airways that supply air to alveoli have microscopically thin walls, and their shape and patency is maintained by attachments which act like guy ropes applying radial traction. Emphysema also causes a reduction in radial traction, which means that the small airways are not supported so they tend to close and collapse, especially during expiration. This will lead to air trapping, to increased work of breathing that is less efficient, and to areas of the lung not being ventilated. Hence gas exchange is further impaired. This can cause a disturbance in the matching of ventilation to perfusion.

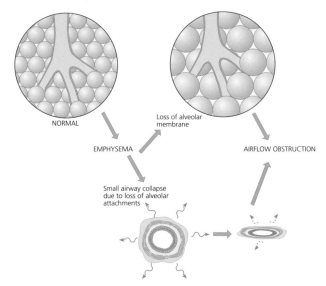

Fig 6.7
Pathological changes in the alveoli and small airways

COPD is a disorder that affects the whole body including the heart, kidneys and muscles. It also has cognitive and emotional aspects such as panic and anxiety which may directly contribute to the sensation of dyspnoea.

Importantly, as far as perioperative management is concerned, significant airflow obstruction may have developed before the COPD patient is aware of it. Indeed a substantial degree of lung damage can take place before any clinical symptoms become apparent. Many patients with COPD may have a 50% reduction in FEV_1 before they present to a doctor. This is probably because we have more alveoli than are needed for gas exchange; therefore we can afford to lose a substantial percentage before dyspnoea becomes apparent.

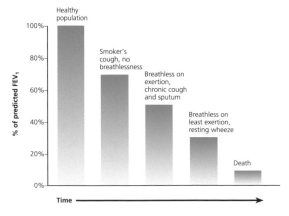

Fig 6.8
Lung damage can occur before symptoms become obvious

This means that a patient may present 'normally' and may not believe that they have a respiratory disease, but their FEV_1 may be significantly reduced, which has implications for surgery.

With increased disease severity, alveoli become hypoventilated and the patient becomes hypoxic. The patient will develop respiratory failure, and will need long-term oxygen therapy (LTOT). LTOT can double survival if given appropriately.[7,8]

Pharmacological management of asthma and COPD

The evidence base for the pharmacological management of asthma and COPD is rapidly changing, and today's good practice soon becomes dated. Up-to-date guidelines can be downloaded from the British Thoracic Society (http://www.brit-thoracic.org.uk).

Drug therapy for asthma includes inhaled bronchodilators and anti-inflammatory agents. Bronchodilators relieve the symptoms of asthma, thus patients sometimes call them relievers. Inhaled bronchodilators can be short or long acting; short acting typically lasting from 4 to 6 hours, and long acting 12 hours. Anti-inflammatory drugs do not directly cause bronchodilation so do not give immediate relief, but they can modify the underlying inflammation. Patients sometimes call anti-inflammatory drugs 'preventers' or 'controllers'. Anti-inflammatory drugs include inhaled and oral corticosteroids, and other drugs such as leukotriene receptor antagonists.

Asthma is variable, and an asthmatic can have severe symptoms at times, yet at other times can have normal respiratory function. Pharmacological therapy in asthma is therefore 'stepped up' or 'stepped down' depending on the severity of the patient's asthma, which can change. Asthmatic patients therefore need regular review, the aim being to control the disorder and prevent deterioration. Pharmacological therapy is adjunct to other aspects of management, such as allergen avoidance.

The management of COPD is different. Unfortunately treatment does not slow the underlying disease progression or slow decline in lung function. Bronchodilators can help increase exercise capacity and reduce breathlessness. The classes of bronchodilators used for COPD include inhaled beta-2 agonists, inhaled anti-muscarinics, and oral xanthine derivatives. These can be taken in short or long acting forms, they can be combined with each other, and in some circumstances can be combined with other drugs such as inhaled corticosteroids. Generally patients start off with the 'weaker' and less expensive bronchodilators, and progress to the stronger drugs in isolation and in combination with others as their disease progresses.

Pharmacological therapy can also reduce the frequency of exacerbations that a patient is likely to experience. Inhaled corticosteroids are particularly effective in this respect,[9,10,11] and exacerbation frequency can be reduced even further if these are combined with long-acting bronchodilators.[12,13,14] Systematic reviews suggest that mucolytics can also reduce exacerbations in patients with chronic bronchitis and COPD.[15] NICE[3] therefore recommend mucolytic therapy be considered in patients with a chronic cough productive of sputum.

Management of exacerbations

A patient with asthma may occasionally exacerbate, and patients with COPD exacerbate with increasing frequency and severity as their condition deteriorates.

When the asthmatic patient is in hospital, the treatment of an uncontrolled attack usually involves the use of a beta-2 agonist given by nebuliser, and if the peak flow reading is less than 75% of the predicted value then a course of oral corticosteroids is usually prescribed for at least one week. High flow oxygen is administered (usually 40% via a facemask).

The features of an acute severe attack of asthma include the inability to complete a sentence without having to draw a second breath, a pulse rate greater than 110 per minute, a respiratory rate of greater than 25 breaths per minute, and a peak flow of less than 50% predicted or best value. Thus if a patient has a silent chest, cyanosis, bradycardia and an FEV_1 of less than 33% predicted the attack is deemed to be life threatening and management should be in a critical care or specialised respiratory unit. The use of high flow oxygen therapy and intravenous hydrocortisone may be required along with other treatments including intravenous magnesium and intravenous aminophylline along with local guidelines in discussion with senior medical staff.

Acute exacerbations of COPD which require hospitalisation can be difficult to treat, and require a skilled and knowledgeable practitioner. For example, it is not sufficient to give a fixed percentage of oxygen; the patient needs enough to correct hypoxia, yet too much can cause death by respiratory failure so careful titration of oxygen is necessary.

The signs of an exacerbation of COPD include a high respiratory rate, shallow breathing, use of accessory muscles and tachycardia. The patient may be centrally cyanosed, and may show signs of carbon dioxide retention such as confusion and agitation, a bounding pulse, vasodilation (warm, flushed peripheries) and a flapping tremor of the hands.

The treatment of an exacerbation of COPD includes antibiotics, oral corticosteroids, bronchodilators and oxygen therapy. It may also include non-invasive ventilation. The use of antibiotics is contentious, as many exacerbations have viral or non-infective causes. Ram *et al*.[16] concluded that antibiotics should be used for those who have increased cough and sputum purulence and are moderately or severely ill. Oral corticosteroids can shorten the duration of an exacerbation and NICE[3] advise giving 30mg prednisolone for 7 to 14 days.

Perhaps the most difficult aspect of managing an exacerbation of COPD is oxygen therapy. If a COPD patient is hypoxic it is important that they are given sufficient oxygen to correct their hypoxia. Yet giving too little oxygen will not correct hypoxia whilst giving oxygen in excessive concentrations can be dangerous because it can result in some patients retaining carbon dioxide leading to the development of respiratory acidosis, which can be fatal. Careful monitoring of pulse oximetry and arterial blood gas analysis is therefore essential.

If it is not possible to maintain an acceptable arterial oxygen level without causing an increase in carbon dioxide and a drop in arterial pH, non-invasive ventilation (NIV) should be considered. NIV is safer than invasive ventilation, and patients do not need to be managed in an intensive care setting.[17] Indeed NICE3 recommend that NIV should be used as treatment of choice for chronic hypercapnic patients during acute respiratory failure despite optimal medical therapy.

Bi-level Positive Airway Pressure or BiPAP is probably the most important mode where management of acute on chronic hypercapnic respiratory failure in COPD is concerned. This Bi-level ventilation delivers a set pressure of air as the patient breathes in, called Inspiratory Positive Airways Pressure (IPAP) and on expiration a lower volume of pressure is delivered called Expiratory Positive Airways Pressure (EPAP). Bi-level therefore alternates between IPAP and EPAP and in doing so it provides assistance during the inspiratory phase of respiration in the form of pressure support, but why would a patient also need EPAP, which effectively means that they breathe out against a pressure that is generated by the ventilator? The answer is that a COPD patient's airways can collapse, and the delivery of EPAP effectively means that a positive pressure is maintained within the airways during the expiratory phase, helping to inflate them and keep them and the alveoli open.

NIV has transformed the management of an exacerbation of COPD, but it requires specialist knowledge and skills, and it is important that practitioners are competent and appropriately educated.

Blood gas analysis

Blood gas analysis is an essential aspect of the management of an exacerbation of a respiratory condition, and it is an important aspect of preoperative screening, preparation, and perioperative care. A discussion is merited at this juncture.

Arterial blood gases are the most sensitive indicator of respiratory function, particularly the levels of oxygen and carbon dioxide, and can be used to initiate effective treatment. In order to interpret blood gases it is important to understand acid–base balance and the role the lungs and kidneys play in maintaining that balance.

Acids and bases

The pH is a measure of a solution's acidity or alkalinity and can have a value from 0 to 14. Pure water has a pH of 7 which is neutral, whereas a solution below 7 is acidic, the lower pH value being more acidic. Likewise, a pH of over 7 is alkali with higher pH value being more alkaline.

An acid is a chemical that can release hydrogen ions (H^+). The more H^+ is in a solution, the more acidic it becomes. A base or alkali can receive or absorb H^+. Bicarbonate (HCO_3^-) is an example of a base and the more that is present in a solution, the more alkaline it becomes.

When carbon dioxide is carried in the blood, some of it combines with water to produce carbonic acid. Carbon dioxide + water = carbonic acid. Expressed as an equation this is:

$$CO_2 + H_2O = H_2CO_3$$

The carbonic acid then dissociates (releases its hydrogen ion into the blood) which causes blood pH to drop. It follows that the more carbon dioxide, in the blood, the more acidic the blood is. If a patient has respiratory problems and retains carbon dioxide they can develop respiratory acidosis. The pH of blood is normally between 7.35 and 7.45 so if a patient has too much carbon dioxide in the blood and the pH is below 7.35 they have developed respiratory acidosis.

It also follows that the less carbon dioxide is in the blood, the less acidic the blood is. So if a patient hyperventilates and there is too little carbon dioxide and therefore too little carbonic acid in the blood the patient will have developed respiratory alkalosis (pH above 7.45).

If a patient has too much carbon dioxide in the blood and therefore too much acid, the body will respond by increasing the respiratory rate and will exhale the carbon dioxide. However, if the patient has a respiratory or other problem, such as a head injury, they may not be able to do this. If this persists over hours or days the kidneys can produce bicarbonate (HCO_3^-).The bicarbonate stabilises the carbonic acid in the blood; in other words it stops the carbonic acid dissociating and releasing its hydrogen ion. This means that although the patient has too much carbon dioxide in the blood and therefore too much carbonic acid the kidneys have produced bicarbonate which will ensure that the pH will be within normal limits (7.35–7.45) but will not be as high as the upper limit. This situation is called 'compensated' respiratory acidosis, because the kidneys have compensated by producing bicarbonate. It takes a number of days for the kidneys to compensate in this way.

Acute respiratory acidosis is characterised by arterial blood gas analysis showing a high $PaCO_2$, a low pH and normal bicarbonate. On the other hand in chronic hypercapnic respiratory failure the arterial blood gas analysis will show a high $PaCO_2$, and unlike acute failure the pH will be within normal limits and the bicarbonate will be high. The pH of blood will have returned to normal limits due to this 'renal compensation'. Therefore a high bicarbonate level will be evident on blood gas analysis. This is sometimes called 'compensated respiratory acidosis'. Patients with compensated respiratory acidosis can be clinically stable but will have significant lung disease. Their arterial blood gases will always be abnormal.

Sometimes patients with chronic type II respiratory failure can deteriorate, perhaps due to an exacerbation. When this happens it is called 'acute on chronic respiratory failure'. This indicates an acute deterioration of a pre-existing chronic hypercapnic respiratory failure. Arterial blood gases show a high $PaCO_2$, low pH and high bicarbonate. In this situation the pH is low despite the high bicarbonate levels. Whilst this may be due to an exacerbation of COPD, it may also be due to injudicious use of oxygen therapy.

Acidosis and alkalosis can also be caused by non-respiratory problems, such as diabetic keto-acidosis. In situations such as this, alterations in pH are not explained by levels of carbon dioxide. For example, in diabetic acidosis the pH will be low but this is not explained by a high carbon dioxide.

Interpretation of blood gases

Investigations only make sense in the context of clinical examination and blood gases may be misleading if relied upon in isolation. It is important to label the sample and complete any forms correctly. Details regarding the patient's condition should be recorded, especially if they are receiving oxygen therapy. The percentage of oxygen being given needs to be stated, as this will have an effect on the results and subsequent treatment.

Normal values of blood gases vary from hospital to hospital, so it is important to familiarise yourself with the values used in your unit. The table below gives the values used in this chapter.

Table 6.2 Normal values of blood gases

	kPa (kilopascals)	mm Hg
pH	7.35–7.45	
PaCO$_2$	4.7–6.0	35–45
PaO$_2$	11.3–14.0	80–100
HCO$_3^-$	22–28 mEq/L	22–28 mEq/L
Base excess	+/- 2.5 mEq/L	+/- 2.5 mEq/L

In order to analyse and interpret blood gas results it is preferable to follow a systematic process which involves five steps.

1) Look at the PaO$_2$ (oxygen). This indicates whether the patient is being oxygenated adequately. If below 8.0 kPa the patient is in respiratory failure, and if below 6.7 kPa the patient is dangerously hypoxic.

2) Look at the pH. Is it acid or alkali?

3) Look at the PaCO$_2$ (carbon dioxide). Could this explain a low or raised pH? CO$_2$ combines with H$_2$O to form carbonic acid, so a high CO$_2$ would explain a low pH, and a low CO$_2$ would explain a high pH. If the PaCO$_2$ explains why the pH is high or low, then the problem is likely to be respiratory in origin. If it does not, then the problem is likely to be 'metabolic', or non-respiratory.

4) Look at the HCO$_3^-$ (bicarbonate). Could this explain a change in pH? A high bicarbonate may explain a high pH, and a low bicarbonate may explain a low pH. If changes in bicarbonate levels explain pH the problem is likely to be metabolic, or non-respiratory.

5) Assess for compensation. For example, the kidneys can compensate for respiratory acidosis by producing bicarbonate, which would mean that pH may be within normal limits despite a high PaCO$_2$. Similarly, the lungs can compensate for metabolic acidosis by 'blowing off' CO$_2$ resulting in a low PaCO$_2$.

A COPD patient with compensated respiratory acidosis might have blood gas results similar to the example below.

pH	7.37
PaCO$_2$	8.29 kPa
PaO$_2$	7.9 kPa
HCO$_3^-$	34 mEq/L

Using the steps to analyse the sample:

1. Look at the PaO_2: it is low, but is there adequate oxygenation for a person with COPD?
2. Look at the pH: it is in the lower range of normal.
3. Look at the $PaCO_2$: it is high, indicating a respiratory acidosis.
4. Look at the HCO_3: it is high, so the acidosis is not due to metabolic problems.
5. Assess for compensation: the HCO_3^- is high and the pH is within normal range; therefore a compensated respiratory acidosis is indicated.

Obstructive sleep apnoea

Obstructive sleep apnoea is thought to result from decreased upper airway patency in sleep compared to wakefulness. The airway partially occludes; arousals from sleep can restore airway patency but this is followed by a repetitive cycle of airway collapse and arousal. Patients may be at risk of complications related to anaesthesia and postoperative analgesia. Indeed it may be a risk factor for anaesthetic morbidity and mortality.[18] This may be because anaesthetic and narcotic agents can increase the tendency for airway collapse and they may also impair normal arousal, thus worsening apnoea severity.[19]

There is a positive correlation between obstructive sleep apnoea severity and complication rate, but even sleep apnoea which may not be otherwise significant may become dangerous under the influence of anaesthetic or analgesia, or with oedema of the airway from intubation.[20]

Unfortunately patients may not have a diagnosis of obstructive sleep apnoea prior to surgery, and clinical presentation alone may be a poor predictor. Nevertheless preoperative evaluation should include assessment of the likelihood of obstructive sleep apnoea. If suspected, preoperative consultation with a sleep specialist is appropriate but if surgery cannot be postponed patients may require CPAP postoperatively when the endotracheal tube is removed.[20] The first 24 postoperative hours are probably the most critical time, but deaths can occur later. This should be considered when prescribing analgesia[21] and consideration should be given to the potential synergistic effects of medications with regard to central nervous system depression.

The necessity of identifying patients with respiratory problems

Patients with respiratory disease have an increased chance of developing complications postoperatively.[2] This may be due to specific respiratory disorders, or problems may be caused by shallow breathing, poor lung expansion, and infection.

To minimise the risk of complications, respiratory patients should be identified preoperatively, and their lung function should be improved as much as possible by providing optimum treatment for their disorder, and interventions such as physiotherapy can help teach patients in the preoperative period to participate with techniques in the postoperative phase. This can help to mobilise secretions and increase lung volumes in the postoperative period, which can reduce pulmonary complications.[2] Postoperative complications can be minimised by treating respiratory conditions prior to surgery. Respiratory infection should be treated and resolved, and asthma should be well controlled. Before surgery, patients should be free of wheeze and ideally have a peak flow reading of above 80% or the patient's personal best value. Inhaled steroid dose may have to be increased or oral steroids commenced one week prior to surgery.[2,22] Elective surgery should be postponed until the patient is ready.

Smoking cessation is also an important aspect of preoperative preparation. According to Sharma,[22] patients who smoke have a two-fold increase in risk of postoperative complications even in the absence of a diagnosed disease; however, patients who quit smoking for 6 months have a risk similar to those who do not smoke. The risk of pulmonary complications following major surgery in smokers is estimated to be six times higher than that in the non-smoking population.[23]

The airways of smokers have poor muco-ciliary clearance of secretions, and they are at increased risk of postoperative complications such as pneumonia. Even abstinence for the 12 hours before anaesthesia will allow time for clearance of nicotine, a coronary vasoconstrictor, and a fall in the levels of carboxyhaemoglobin, thus improving oxygen carriage in the blood.[2]

Preoperative assessment is therefore essential, and full pulmonary function tests are sometimes warranted. Clearly this is very much dependent on the patient's condition and the nature of the surgery, and there is no definitive guide that will give reliable 'cut off' points which would prevent patients from receiving surgery. This is definitely depends on the clinical judgement of the surgeon, anaesthetist and other specialists.

Lung cancer is an illustrative example. Clearly if a patient is to receive surgery which will remove part of their lungs and reduce their FEV_1, preoperative FEV_1 is important because if it is already low, any further reduction due to surgery could be significant. Because of this it is important to calculate an 'Estimated Post Operative FEV_1' (EPOFEV$_1$). Techniques to calculate this vary considerably, and include simply counting the number of lung segments to be removed, or inserting the number of lung segments that are obstructed (a) and the number of unobstructed segments (b) into a formula. The $EPOFEV_1 = $ pre FEV_1 x $[(19 - a) - b]/19 - c$ where c = the total number of segments in the lung. The right upper lobe has three segments, middle has two, right lower has five, left upper three, lingual two and left lower has four.

For general surgery, a low FEV_1 might result in low postoperative survival. An FEV_1 of FVC less than 70% predicted, or a ratio of less than 65%, is associated with an increased risk of pulmonary complications[2] and COPD patients with an FEV_1 of less than 40% predicted are six times more likely to have a major postoperative complication. Yet it is not possible to state that there is a prohibitive level of pulmonary function for an absolute contradiction to surgery, and the clinical decision will depend on a range of factors.[22]

Spirometry alone is not a good prognostic factor[1,24] and other things are important, such as age, nutrition, hypoxia, general condition – therefore full assessment is needed. The procedure itself is of course important. For example, preoperative hypoxia or carbon dioxide retention indicates the possibility of postoperative respiratory failure which may require a period of assisted ventilation postoperatively[2] and chest X-rays may identify collapse, consolidation, infection, pulmonary oedema, or hyperinflated lungs. With some respiratory conditions, such as COPD, pre-op arterial blood gas analysis is recommended to show severity of hypoxia and hypercapnia.[23]

Postoperative care is complicated, and much of this chapter can be applied to the post-operative management of any patient with a respiratory condition. Clearly it should be tailored to the individual patient and their situation; some patients may require high flow oxygen, but other patients may require carefully controlled, titrated oxygen which is adjusted depending on blood gas analysis. Patients should be closely monitored, and COPD patients will require postoperative oxygen therapy that should aim to maintain arterial oxygen level without inhibiting respiration, thereby preventing respiratory acidosis.[23]

Postoperatively the patient may develop bronchospasm. The patient may be breathless, have a rapid respiratory rate, and may be using their accessory muscles. An expiratory wheeze may be audible on auscultation, but a quiet chest may be ominous as it may mean that very little airflow is taking place. Treatment may be similar to that discussed in this chapter, including nebulised bronchodilators, titrated oxygen and intravenous steroids.

Above all it is important to appreciate that there are no rigid rules that can be applied to the management of all respiratory patients perioperatively. Each patient's situation is unique and perioperative management should be agreed in consultation with the anaesthetist and the specialist team.

REFERENCES

1. R. Larsen (2003). *Anestezjojogia.* Wroclaw: Urban and Partner. MRC (1981). Long term domiciliary oxygen therapy in chronic hypoxic cor pulmonale complicating chronic bronchitis and emphysema.

2. M. Mercer (2000). Anaesthesia for the patient with respiratory disease. *Practical Procedures* **12**: 1–17.

3. NICE (2004). Chronic Obstructive Pulmonary Disease. National clinical guideline on management of chronic obstructive pulmonary disease in adults in primary and secondary care. *Thorax* **59** (Suppl 1): 1–232.

4. C.M. Fletcher and R. Peto (1976). The natural history of chronic airflow obstruction. *British Medical Journal* **1**: 1645–8.

5. GOLD (2004). Global Initiative for Chronic Obstructive Pulmonary Disease. http://www.goldcopd.com/ (last accessed February 2010).

6. P.J. Barnes (2000). Mechanisms in COPD: differences from asthma. *Chest* **117**: 10S–14S.

7. MRC (1981). Long term domiciliary oxygen therapy in chronic hypoxic cor pulmonale complicating chronic bronchitis and emphysema. *Lancet* **1**: 681–6.

8. NOTT (1980). Continuous or nocturnal oxygen therapy in hypoxaemic chronic obstructive lung disease. *Annals of Internal Medicine* **93**: 391–8.

9. P.S. Burge, P.M.A. Calverley and P.W. Jones (2000). Randomised, double-blind, placebo controlled study of fluticasone propionate in patients with moderate to severe chronic obstructive pulmonary disease: the ISOLDE trial. *British Medical Journal* **320**: 1297–1303.

10. P.M.A. Calverley, R. Pauwels, J. Vestbo, P. Jones, N. Pride and A. Gulsvik (2003). Combined salmeterol and fluticasone in the treatment of chronic obstructive pulmonary disease: a randomised controlled trial. *Lancet* **361**: 449–56.

11. D.D. Sin, F.A. McAlister, P. Man and N.R. Anthonisen (2003). Contemporary management of chronic obstructive pulmonary disease: Scientific review. *Journal of the American Medical Association* **290**: 2301–12.

12. W. Szafranski, A. Cukier, A. Ramirez, G. Menga, R. Sansores, S. Nahabedian, S. Peterson and H. Olsson (2003). Efficacy and safety of budesonide/formoterol in the management of chronic obstructive pulmonary disease. *European Respiratory Journal* **21**: 74–81.

13. P. Kardos, M. Wencker, T. Glaab and C. Vogelmeier (2007). Impact of salmeterol/fluticasone versus salmeterol on exacerbations in severe chronic obstructive pulmonary disease. *American Journal of Critical Care Medicine* **175**: 144–9.

14. P.M.A. Calverley, J.A. Anderson, B. Celli, J. Vestbo *et al* (2007). Salmeterol and fluticasone propionate and survival in chronic obstructive pulmonary disease. *New England Journal of Medicine* **356**: 775–89.

15. P.J. Poole and P.N. Black (2006). Mucolytic agents for chronic bronchitis or chronic obstructive pulmonary disease. *Cochrane Database of Systematic Reviews*, Issue 3. Art no.: 001287. DOI: 10.1002/14651858.CD001287.pub2.

16. F.S.F. Ram, P.W. Jones, A.A. Castro, J.R. De Brito Jardim, A.N. Atallah, Y. Lacasse, R. Mazzini, R. Goldstein and S. Cendon (2002). Oral theophylline for chronic obstructive pulmonary disease. *Cochrane Database of Systematic Reviews*, Issue 3. Art. No.: CD003902. DOI: 10.1002/14651858.CD003902.

17. British Thoracic Society (2001). Guidelines on the selection of patients with lung cancer for surgery. *Thorax* **56**: 89–108.

18. J.A. Loadsman and D.R. Hillman (2001). Anaesthesia and sleep apnoea. *British Journal of Anaesthesia* **86**: 254–66.

19. R.W. Robinson, C.W. Zwillich, E.O. Bixler, R.J. Cadieux, A. Kales and D.P. Whide (1987). Effects of oral narcotics on sleep disordered breathing in healthy adults. *Chest* **91**: 197–203.

20. A.M. Meoli, C.L. Rosen, D. Kristo, M. Kohrman, N. Gooneratne, R. Aguillard, R. Fayle, R. Troell, R. Kramer, K. Casey and J. Coleman (2003). Upper airway management of the adult patient with obstructive sleep apnea in the perioperative period – avoiding complications. *Sleep* **26**(8): 1060–5.

21. D.J. Cullen (2001). Obstructive sleep apnea and postoperative analgesia – a potentially dangerous combination. *Journal of Clinical Analgesia* **13**: 83–5.

22. S. Sharma (2006). Perioperative pulmonary management. www.emedicine.com/med/topic3169.htm (last accessed February 2010).

23. K. Rutkowska, H. Misiolek, H. Kucia and P. Knapic (2006). Perioperative management of COPD patients undergoing nonpulmonary surgery. *Anaesthesiology Intensive Therapy* **38**: 153–7.

24. D.H. Wong, E.C. Weber, M.J. Schell and A.B. Wong (1995). Factors associated with postoperative pulmonary complications in patients with severe COPD. *Anesthesia and Analgesia* **80**: 276–84.

7 Assessment of the airway

Cheng Ong
Adrian Pearce

SUMMARY

This chapter will describe:

- **why all patients require a preoperative assessment of the airway**
- **how assessment determines the airway management strategy of the anaesthetist**
- **the importance of predicting difficulty with intubation or ventilation**
- **important predictive factors: a history of problems in previous anaesthetics, a disease process affecting the head, neck or mediastinum, signs or symptoms of difficulty with breathing, limitation in mouth opening or in head and neck mobility**
- **a structured approach involving taking a history, looking at the patient and doing a few tests**
- **how linking findings at preoperative evaluation to clinical practice in an individual patient requires professional judgement.**

INTRODUCTION

Failure to adequately protect and maintain the airway throughout anaesthesia leads rapidly to impaired oxygenation and ventilation or complications of aspiration. The airway is managed during anaesthesia by either the facemask, supraglottic airway such as the laryngeal mask or tracheal intubation and these 'devices' offer differing levels of protection and maintenance of the airway. Tracheal intubation offers the highest level of airway protection and maintenance and plays a central role in both planned and emergency airway management. An assessment of the airway should be made in all patients.

Basic Science

Anatomy

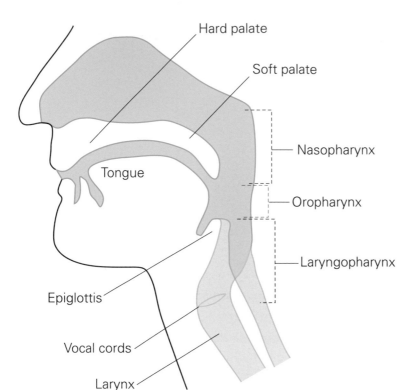

Hard palate

Soft palate

Nasopharynx

Tongue

Oropharynx

Laryngopharynx

Epiglottis

Vocal cords

Larynx

**Figure 7.1
Anatomy of the airway**

The airway consists of the passage air takes as it is conducted between the external atmosphere and alveolus (Figure 7.1). Air is drawn in initially through the nose or mouth with the nose being used at rest or with light activity. The nasal cavity is lined with highly vascular mucous membrane and leads to the nasopharynx. The oral cavity is bounded anteriorly by the jaw and teeth, inferiorly by the tongue and superiorly by the hard or soft palate. The pharynx is bounded posteriorly by the pharyngeal wall overlying the cervical vertebrae and leads to the laryngeal inlet and upper oesophagus. The epiglottis is a 'flap' which protects the laryngeal inlet from ingress of food into the respiratory tract. The larynx is a highly complex structure involving the hyoid bone, thyroid and cricoid cartilages, numerous small muscles, ligaments and the vocal cords. The vocal cords are the instruments of speech and also guard access to the trachea. The trachea begins at the lower border of the cricoid cartilage and comprises 12–20 C-shaped cartilages. Half the length of the trachea is superficial within the neck, before it passes behind the sternum to divide into the main bronchi. The bronchial tree continues to divide into increasingly narrower passages to the alveolus, which is the functional unit where gas exchange takes place.

The anaesthetist is able to place devices (Figure 7.2) into the airway to maintain patency, but only to the level of the main bronchus. Oral or nasal airways will bypass the oral or nasal cavities, the laryngeal mask will guide external air directly to the larynx and tracheal intubation provides a secure tube to the mid or lower trachea. From the brief anatomical description it can be seen that abnormalities (particularly swelling) of the lips, jaw, tongue, palate, epiglottis or vocal cords will lead to airway narrowing. The course and diameter of the trachea will be affected by masses in the neck (particularly thyroid enlargement) or in the mediastinum.

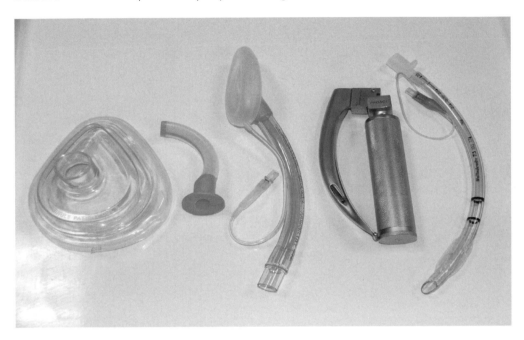

Figure 7.2 Airway devices for use during surgery

Physiology

Humans are unfortunate that their pharynx is a floppy-walled, common meeting place for anything taken in through the mouth or nose. Highly sophisticated reflexes are required to make certain that patency of the pharynx is maintained and that the contents are forwarded correctly with air to the larynx and fluid or food to the oesophagus. Anaesthesia abolishes many of these protective reflexes. In particular, in the anaesthetised supine adult, patency of the airway is abolished through the tongue and soft palate falling back to meet the posterior pharyngeal wall. Anaesthesia abolishes the protective laryngeal reflexes which guard against passage of fluid or food particles into the trachea. A particularly dangerous situation is reflux of gastro-oesophageal contents from the stomach into the pharynx and then into the lungs.

Bi-directional flow of air through the airway is normally under the control of the respiratory centre which senses blood levels of oxygen and carbon dioxide and controls the muscles of respiration. Inspiration is caused by contraction of the diaphragm and intercostal muscles, which act to increase the volume of the thoracic cage generating a negative pressure in the pleural space and alveoli. Air is drawn down the airway until the end of inspiration when relaxation of the diaphragm and intercostals reverses the gas flow in the expiratory phase. Normal negative pressures produced during inspiration are no more than -5 cm H_2O but if the airway is narrowed much greater negative pressures are required. In acute airway obstruction, respiratory muscles generate much higher negative inspiratory pressures but tire quickly. If airway obstruction develops over several weeks, the inspiratory muscles become trained and the air passage may be no more than 4–5mm wide at its narrowest point before the patient is short of breath at rest.

In normal respiration, the volume of each breath (tidal volume) in the average adult is about 500ml and the respiratory rate is normally 10–12 per minute. This gives a minute ventilation of 5–6 litres. The inspiratory gas may be air (21% oxygen) or may be controlled by the breathing circuit and gas flows to any value of inspired oxygen from 21% to 100%. The minute ventilation of 5 litres/minute replenishes the gas in the alveolus. Oxygen is being removed from the alveolus by the pulmonary blood flow and carbon dioxide delivered to it. Normal values of oxygen consumption are 250ml/min with 200ml/min of carbon dioxide being excreted during expiration. The volume of the lung at the end of a expiration (functional residual capacity, FRC) is approximately 2–2.5 litres and this provides a store of oxygen. With sudden occlusion of the airway, when breathing air, this reserve will last no more than 1–2 minutes before the patient becomes critically hypoxaemic. After breathing 100% oxygen the reserve extends the safety time to about 8–10 minutes.

Physics

Gas flow in a tube may be either laminar or turbulent and the size of the tube is an important determinant of flow. Laminar flow is more energy efficient and the factors which affect it are the pressure difference between the two ends, the length of the tube, the viscosity of the gas and the radius of the tube. The Poiseuille equation states that for laminar flow in a tube:

$$\text{Flow} = \frac{\text{Pressure difference x } \pi \text{ x radius}^4}{8 \text{ x gas viscosity x length}}$$

It can be seen that flow is proportional to the fourth power of the radius, which indicates the very great contribution that calibre and patency makes to gas flow in the airway. As the airway narrows, gas flow becomes turbulent and noisy.

Clinical practice

The first comprehensive practice guidelines for management of the airway were published in 1993 by the American Society of Anesthesiologists. It proposed a sequential five-step plan of evaluation of the airway, preparation for difficulty, airway management plan at the start and end of anaesthesia and follow-up of the patient.

Evaluation of the airway is the first of these vital steps and must be part of the preoperative assessment in all patients. The purpose of airway evaluation is to:

- decide which device will be most suitable for airway management
- judge whether there are likely to be problems with airway management
- explain the airway management plan in the explanation/consent process
- warn the patient of common or serious complications

Which airway device will be suitable?

Around the time of induction of general anaesthesia a facemask is used to preoxygenate the patient. Preoxygenation means applying a close fitting facemask to the patient whilst they are still awake and supplying 100% oxygen in the breathing circuit for a few minutes. The air in the lungs is replaced by oxygen and this provides a safety reservoir. Immediately after induction of anaesthesia the patient is ventilated initially by facemask. The factors which determine the manner in which the airway is subsequently managed are:

- risk of aspiration of gastric contents
- length of procedure
- requirement for intermittent positive pressure ventilation (IPPV)
- body mass index
- risk to the airway from proposed surgery
- ease of intubation during surgery should this be needed
- position of the patient.

Continued use of the facemask is possible for short elective procedures when there is no risk of gastric aspiration and no requirement for IPPV. One hand of the anaesthetist constantly holds the facemask in place and this makes it difficult to complete the anaesthetic record chart or respond to perioperative events.

The airway is most commonly (in the UK) managed by laryngeal mask, in approximately 70% of operations. This is because the risk of aspiration in elective surgery is low, surgery usually lasts less than 2 hours, the body mass index (BMI) is < 35, the airway will not be compromised by surgery, the anaesthetist at the head of the patient may easily intubate during surgery if the need arises and the patient is supine.

Tracheal intubation is generally required for:

- patients at risk of aspiration of gastric contents
  - preoperative food < 6hr or fluid < 2hr before surgery
  - delayed gastric emptying (including pregnancy > 16 weeks)
  - gastro-oesophageal reflux
  - acute abdomen
- surgery > 2–3 hours

- obesity
- head down or prone position
- prolonged IPPV
- head and neck surgery
- disease process affecting the airway.

Preoperative assessment and Individual devices

Difficult facemask

Difficult facemask ventilation can be defined as the inability to maintain the oxygen saturations above 90% with 100% oxygen or reverse signs of inadequate ventilation. It is rare in patients presenting for 'general' surgery. In a recent study of 22,260 patients, using a four-point scale of difficult facemask ventilation (Table 7.1), the following factors were associated with difficult facemask ventilation:

- body mass index (BMI) > or = 30kg m-2
- presence of a beard
- Mallampati class 3 or 4
- age > or = 57 years
- jaw protrusion – severely limited
- history of snoring.

Table 7.1 Grades of difficult facemask ventilation (from Han *et al.*[1])

Grade	Description	Percentage of patients
1	Ventilated by mask	77
2	Ventilated by mask with oral airway/ adjuvant with or without muscle relaxant	21
3	Difficult ventilation (inadequate, unstable, or requiring two providers) with or without muscle relaxant	1.4
4	Unable to mask ventilate with or without muscle relaxant	0.16

There are a number of severe or obvious clinical features which would suggest that the airway should be secured before induction of general anaesthesia:

- stridor (noisy breathing)
- difficulty with breathing
- severe limitation of head and neck movements

- large oropharyngeal masses or laryngo-pharyngeal disease
- grossly irregular contour of the face/jaw precluding application of the facemask.

Difficult laryngeal mask

The laryngeal mask is not designed for use in patients with a significant likelihood of gastric aspiration or those with laryngeal pathology. The seal it provides allows ventilation to a pressure of (only) 20cm H_2O which will be inadequate for patients with poor lung function or obesity. It may be difficult to insert (by the standard Brain insertion technique) in those with mouth opening < 2cm, those with large oropharyngeal masses or those with a high arched palate.

Difficult tracheal intubation

Most of the extensive literature on preoperative airway assessment is on prediction of difficult intubation. Intubation is most commonly performed by direct laryngoscopy, in which a laryngoscope is placed in the mouth and direct line-of-sight to the larynx obtained. Abnormalities of the jaw or teeth, tongue, palate, pharynx, epiglottis or larynx may cause difficulty with intubation.

Common research definitions of difficult intubation are:

- More than three attempts at laryngoscopy are required.
- It takes longer than 10 minutes to complete intubation.
- There is a poor view of the larynx – the epiglottis only or no view at all.
- Intubation can be achieved only by specialised equipment, such as a flexible fibrescope.

Prediction of difficult airway management

If difficulty with airway management is predicted preoperatively the anaesthetic team has time to consider various options and discuss these with the patient. The options are to prepare special equipment or organise more senior help, undertake intubation in the conscious sedated patient before induction of general anaesthesia, undertake the proposed surgery under local or regional anaesthesia or re-consider the need for surgery.

Prediction of the difficult airway is by:

- history
- clinical examination
- specific bedside 'predictive' tests
- special investigations.

History

The following information should be obtained from the patient and recorded:

- Previous difficult airway management during anaesthesia
- Current disease process if it affects the head, neck or mediastinum
- Any past disease, surgery or radiotherapy to the head, neck or mediastinum
- Medical diseases with some association with difficult airway management
- Difficult or noisy breathing (including snoring)
- Delayed gastric emptying or oesophageal reflux.

It is particularly important to pick up a previous problem with airway management since this is one of the most predictive factors. This may alter the scheduling of the patient and the anaesthetic department should be informed so that a consultant anaesthetist can be involved. Current diseases, such as a dental abscess, enlarged thyroid, tonsillar abscess, epiglottitis or oedema of the tongue or floor of the mouth, are relevant. Any past or current disease process which narrows or distorts the airway, limits head extension, limits mouth opening or causes difficulty with breathing is highly significant. A number of medical diseases such as rheumatoid arthritis, acromegaly and obstructive sleep apnoea have some association with difficult airway management. Rheumatoid arthritis causes limited mobility of neck movements, impaired mouth opening and jaw protrusion and may narrow the laryngeal inlet.

Table 7.2 Features of a history of previous difficult airway management

Patient knows of previous problems
Patient has written record of previous problems
Anaesthetic notes describe difficulty
After previous anaesthetics: • Front teeth displaced/chipped • Severe bruising of lips/pharynx • Unexpected admission to ICU with tear in the pharynx or larynx
MedicAlert bracelet indicating 'Difficult Airway' or 'Difficult Intubation'

Clinical examination

The patient is examined for the anatomical and pathological features listed in Table 7.3. Some of these features will be obvious on external examination (swellings, scars, receding jaw, large tongue) and others will require testing (mouth opening and movement of the head/neck). The practitioner gains an impression of whether the patient 'looks' as though airway management will be difficult. Clinical examination will also detect any noisy or laboured breathing and these are particularly important since they usually indicate narrowing or obstruction of the airway.

Table 7.3 Predictive factors on general examination

Features that suggest presence of a difficult airway
Anatomical features:
Obesity
Thick short neck
Arthritis of neck and spine – restricting flexibility or causing deformity
Receding or small mandible
Beard (this may be hiding a small lower jaw)
Limited mouth opening
Prominent 'overbite' or 'buck teeth' (maxillary incisors anterior to mandibular incisors)
Dental caps, crowns and bridges on upper front teeth
Lack of any teeth (full dentures should accompany patient to theatre)
Large and rigid hairstyles, hair extensions and wigs (especially at back of head; ponytails should not be worn)
Pathological features:
Scars and radiation changes over neck and face
Swellings on the face, neck and inside mouth
Presence of bleeding or secretions from the mouth or nose
Noisy breathing – hoarse voice, stridor, blocked nasal passages

Specific 'bedside' predictive tests

A number of tests have been suggested to improve the prediction of difficult airway management. The common ones used at the bedside during preoperative evaluation are described in Table 7.4. Where distances are measured, one common unit is the finger breadth (fb) equivalent to 1.5–2cm. The test most commonly used in preoperative assessment schemes is the Mallampati classification. Mallampati suggested that the oropharyngeal space was one determinant of difficult intubation and the test is done in the seated patient, asking them to open their mouth widely, protrude the tongue and the examiner scores the visibility of the posterior pharyngeal wall structures and fauces. Mallampati only described three classes (see Figure 7.3) in which Class 1 (the best) described a view of the whole uvula, fauces and posterior pharyngeal wall, Class 2 incomplete view of the fauces and uvula but some view of the posterior pharyngeal wall and Class 3 (the worst) the tongue against the palate with no view of the posterior pharyngeal wall. Later authors added Class 4, where the tongue lies against the hard palate, and Class 3 which indicates the tongue against the soft palate. There is great inter-observer variation in performing the test and whilst it is often performed it is not very predictive. It does, at least, force the practitioner to examine mouth opening.

Table 7.4 Commonly performed bedside predictive tests

Test	Method	Grading	Predictors of DI
Interincisor gap	Ask patient to fully open mouth and measure the distance between the upper and lower incisors.	Greater than 3-5cm (2-3 fingers' breadth) Less than 3cm	Below 3cm
Mandibular protrusion	Ask patient to protrude lower incisors (LI) anterior to upper incisors (UI). (See Figure 7.5, page 132)	Normal: Protrudes LI anterior to UI Limited: Protrudes LI to meet UI Severely limited: LI cannot be advanced to meet UI	Limited and severely limited
Atlanto-occipital joint extension (head and neck extension)	Ask the patient to fully extend the head and neck while a pencil is held vertically on the forehead. While holding the pencil firmly in position, ask the patient to fully flex their head and neck. Measure the angle of the arc of movement of the pencil.	Above 90° About 90° (+/- 10°) Below 90°	Below 90°
Mallampati (Samsoon and Young modification)	Sit the patient upright with the head in a neutral position and ask the patient to open the mouth as widely as possible and to protrude the tongue as far as possible, without phonating. The observer then classifies the airway according to the pharyngeal structures seen.	1 Soft palate, fauces, uvula, anterior & posterior tonsillar pillars 2 Soft palate, fauces, uvula 3 Soft palate, base of uvula 4 Soft palate not visible at all	Class 3 and 4
Thyromental distance	With the patient's head and neck fully extended, the measurement is taken between the thyroid notch and the tip of the jaw in centimetres. (See Figure 7.4)	Measurement in centimetres => or < 6cm	Distance < 6cm or 3 finger breadths

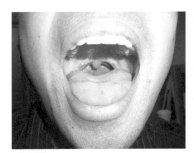

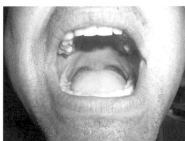

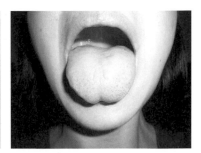

**Figure 7.3a
Mallampati 1**

**Figure 7.3b
Mallampati 2**

**Figure 7.3c
Mallampati 3**

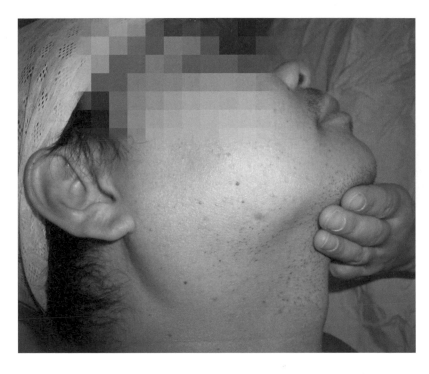

**Figure 7.4
Thyromental
distance or Patil
test. The distance
between the
chin and thyroid
notch measured
in finger breadths
with the neck fully
extended. Less than
3fb or 6cm is the
discriminant value.**

Special investigations

The following investigations are used when the disease process impinges on the airway, to provide more information. The results are particularly helpful to the anaesthetist in planning airway management.

- Chest or thoracic inlet X-ray.
- CT or MR scan from base of skull to carina.
- Flow-volume loops (respiratory function test).
- Flexible naso-endoscopy to view the supraglottis and larynx.

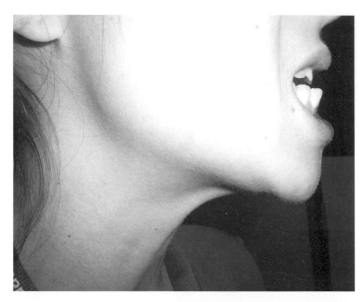

Figure 7.5
Mandibular protrusion,
or the ability to protrude the
lower teeth beyond the top
teeth. Here there is good or
normal protrusion.

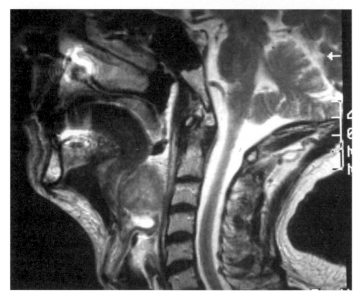

Figure 7.6
An MRI scan showing a
large tumour at the base
of the tongue. This would
make normal intubation
very difficult and the patient
was managed by a nasal
fibreoptic intubation under
sedation.

How predictive are bedside tests?

The broad answer is not very predictive. The predictive ability of a test can be understood only by mentioning a few terms. The term 'difficult patient' is used to indicate a patient with a difficult airway and to help description the Mallampati test will be used. Mallampati Class 3 or 4 would be test results indicating difficult intubation and Mallampati Class 1 or 2 would indicate a 'normal' (easy intubation) patient.

Sensitivity

Sensitivity is the ability of a test to exclude false positives or, put another way, label a difficult patient as difficult. It is the proportion of 'difficult' patients who are correctly identified. A test is 100% sensitive if it identifies all the 'difficult' patients.

Sensitivity = $\dfrac{\textbf{The number of patients tested as positive (Mallampati 3 or 4)}}{\textbf{Total number of patients who are difficult to intubate}}$

Specificity

Specificity is the ability of a test to exclude false negatives or, put another way, to label a normal patient as normal. It is the proportion of 'easy' patients who are correctly identified. A test is 100% specific if all normal patients are identified as normal/easy.

Specificity = $\dfrac{\textbf{The number of patients tested as negative (Mallampati 1 or 2)}}{\textbf{Total number of patients who are difficult to intubate}}$

Positive predictive value (PPV)

The PPV is the percentage of all patients found to be difficult out of all those predicted to be difficult by the test.

PPV = $\dfrac{\textbf{Those found to be difficult to intubate}}{\textbf{All those patients with Mallampati 3 or 4}}$

The prevalence of difficult intubation in 'general surgical' patients is no more than 1–4% and the predictive tests do not have a high enough specificity to label all normal patients as normal. The sensitivity, specificity and PPV of various tests are given in Table 7.5. A PPV of 8% means that only 8% of the patients with Mallampati Class 3/4 will be found to be difficult to intubate and such a test is of little clinical use.

Table 7.5 Sensitivity, specificity and positive predictive value

Test	Sensitivity %	Specificity %	PPV %
Mallampati	65–81	66–82	8–9
Thyromental	65–91	81–82	8–15
Wilson score (see p.135)	42–55	86–92	6–9
Mouth opening	26–47	94–95	7–25

It must be recognised that prediction of difficult intubation is not particularly accurate and patients predicted to be easy may prove difficult and those predicted to be difficult may prove to be easy intubations. Good practice requires the anaesthetist to have an airway strategy which deals with unanticipated difficult intubation and/or ventilation.

What to do if difficulty is predicted

It is easy to predict difficult intubation when there are gross abnormalities such as limited mouth opening, limited neck extension, previous difficult intubation, anatomical narrowing or distortion of the airway, small mouth, receding jaw, large tongue or previous head and neck resective surgery. Figure 7.7 shows a patient presenting for surgery with a receding jaw, limited mouth opening (Figure 7.8) and poor jaw protrusion who had a previous record of difficult intubation.

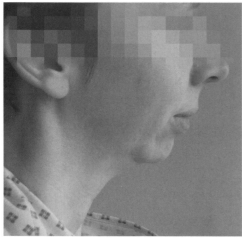

Figure 7.7
Patient with a receding jaw

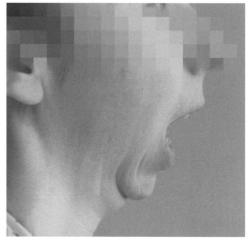

Figure 7.8
Limited mouth opening (about 1 fb)

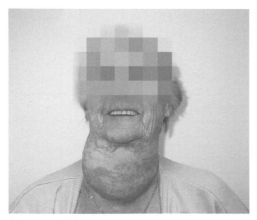

Figure 7.9
A grossly enlarged thyroid mass

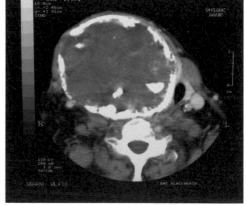

Figure 7.10
Gross deviation of the trachea from the midline

The preoperative assessment nurse contacted directly the anaesthetist scheduled for the list and the airway was managed successfully by awake fibreoptic intubation. Figure 7.9 shows a patient with a very large thyroid mass which, from the CT scan (Figure 7.10), has caused substantial deviation and narrowing of the airway. These are examples of severe problems for which the anaesthetist should be pre-warned so that they can prepare special equipment or get more senior help. Generally it is wise to contact the anaesthetic department directly and speak to the relevant anaesthetist.

Table 7.6 Wilson risk-sum score

Weight
<90kg   0
90–110kg   1
>110kg   2

Head and neck movement
> 90 degrees   0
~ 90 degrees   1
< 90 degrees   2

Jaw movement, jaw protrusion
Incisor gap > 5cm, Normal   0
Incisor gap < 5cm, Limited   1
Incisor gap < 5cm, Minimal   2

Receding mandible
Normal   0
Moderate   1
Severe   2

Buck teeth
Normal   0
Moderate   1
Severe   2

However, most patients seen preoperatively look quite normal and do not have airway narrowing. It is in these 'apparently normal' patients that the specific predictive tests are used and the results are poor. Abnormalities in several tests are more predictive than individual tests and some scoring systems incorporate up to 10 factors. One of the most well-known (but rarely used) scoring systems in the UK is the Wilson risk-sum score (Table 7.6) when a score > 2 is the discriminant value. Others used are by Arné[2] (Table 7.7) with a best-predictive score of 11 and El-Ganzouri.[3] It is worth noting that the combination of limited mouth opening and severely limited protrusion of the lower jaw usually scores highly. In patients with some findings which might indicate difficulty with airway management it is reasonable to record the findings on the preoperative assessment chart. The anaesthetist can make his or her own judgement when the patient is admitted. An illustrative flow-chart is given in Figure 7.11 (see page 138).

Table 7.7 Arné risk index

Factor	Scoring	Points
History of difficult intubation	Yes	10
Pathologies associated with DI	Yes	5
Clinical symptoms	Yes	3
Thyromental distance	< 6.5cm	4
Head/neck movement	80–100	2
	< 80	5
Mallampati	Class 2	2
	Class 3	6
	Class 4	8
Mouth opening, jaw protrusion	3.5–5.0cm, Limited	3
	< 3.5cm, Minimal	13

Patient explanation and consent

At preoperative assessment it is usual to provide an explanation, tailored to an individual, of the plans for airway management. Preoxygenation is undertaken in most patients and is performed by 'clear plastic facemask, which allows you to breathe oxygen so that your lungs are filled with oxygen before starting the anaesthetic'. Intubation is commonly described as 'placing a breathing tube in your windpipe so that your breathing is protected whilst you are asleep'. There is no UK requirement currently for written consent for anaesthesia but the national consent form does specify that the patient will have the opportunity to talk to the anaesthetist. The Association of Anaesthetists of Great Britain and Ireland (www.aagbi.org) recommends that it is not appropriate to gain consent for each specific aspect of management, such as tracheal intubation.

Patients should be warned of common or serious complications:

Teeth

The patient should be asked to detail any false, loose, capped or crowned teeth and these should be recorded on a chart. Of particular importance are the upper and lower incisors, which will bear the brunt of the biting force on an oral airway or laryngeal mask, or may be damaged during intubation. The damage may be chipping or gross displacement. It is good practice to warn the patient that loose or capped teeth are at risk and that the anaesthetist will take steps to minimise the chance of this happening. Intraoperative strategies involve placing a posterior bite-block, using nasal rather than oral tubes or airways, avoiding intubation if possible and intubation by flexible fibrescope rather than direct laryngoscopy. The most common problem reported by anaesthetists to Medical Defence organisations is dental damage.

Sore throat

Both the laryngeal mask and tracheal intubation are associated with a sore throat which usually responds to simple analgesia such as paracetamol and improves within 24 hours. The complication is common enough to be mentioned in preoperative assessment. The incidence of sore throat is about 5.8 to 34% with the laryngeal mask and 14.4 to 50% with tracheal intubation.

Voice change

Tracheal intubation may cause some degree of short-term voice change, such as huskiness. This is assumed to be due to vocal cord dysfunction secondary to the presence of a tracheal tube. Most anaesthetists would avoid intubation in a professional singer although long-term complications from perioperative intubation are exceedingly rare. Any alteration in timbre or strength of voice should have recovered in 48 hours. Prolonged alteration needs to be investigated.

CONCLUSION

Complications of difficult airway management are serious and include brain damage and death due to hypoxia. Preoperative airway assessment is the first essential step in airway management. It starts the process of planning, allows discussion with the patient of options and common complications and allows a judgement to be made as to whether there will be any problems with airway management. These judgements are easy to make if there are obvious or severe problems in the history or clinical examination. Even in patients who do not look difficult to intubate and have no history of previous problems, the practitioner must always check for adequate mouth opening and neck mobility. The seriousness of difficult airway management has led to the description of many 'predictive' tests but the rarity of the condition renders these tests poorly predictive.

Figure 7.11 Guide for airway assessment

History

Very important factors:

- Previous difficult airway management during anaesthesia
- Disease e.g. tumour, abscess, scarring ⎫
  Previous surgery ⎬ affecting head, neck
  Previous radiotherapy ⎭ or mediastinum
- Difficult or noisy breathing, e.g. snoring, stridor
- Medical disease associated with difficult airway
  e.g. morbid obesity BMI > 35 kg m^{-2}, rheumatoid arthritis, acromegaly

Important contributing factor:

- Delayed gastric emptying, difficulty swallowing

> **Report very important factors**

General examination

Very important factors:

- Mouth – difficulty opening
- Neck – rigid, deformed, e.g. fixed flexion or short and thick
- Scars, deformity or masses ⎫
  Radiation scarring and pigmentation ⎬ on face, neck
  Bleeding and secretions ⎭ inside the mouth
- Noisy breathing or stridor
- Receding or small chin – often hidden by a beard
- Prominent 'overbite' or 'buck teeth'

Important contributing factors:

- Dental caps, crowns and bridges on upper front teeth
- Beard or lack of any teeth – makes for a poor facemask fit

> **Anticipate a difficult airway**
> *Inform the anaesthetist*

Bedside tests – *with threshold for action*

- **Interincisor gap** – is *'less than 3cm'*
  – less than two fingers' breadth between top and bottom teeth
  in a fully open mouth

- **Mandibular protrusion** – is *'limited'* or *'severely limited'*
  – cannot protrude lower incisors (LI) anterior to upper incisors (UI):
  'Limited' – protrudes LI to meet UI
  'Severely limited' – LI cannot be advanced to meet UI

- **Atlanto-occipital joint extension** – is *'limited'*
  – unable to extend their head and neck beyond 90°
  (if sitting upright cannot extend to face the ceiling)

- **Modified Mallampati** – is **'Class 3 or 4'** in a fully open mouth
  with tongue protruding:
  'Class 3' – soft palate and base of uvula seen only
  'Class 4' – soft palate not visible at all

> **Report the results of all the bedside tests**

The tests, though, are commonly found in preoperative assessment schemes. Ultimately, the anaesthetist must make a judgement as to whether the factors picked up in preoperative assessment should change their normal airway management plans. This judgement remains one made commonly through experience rather than scientific tests.

REFERENCES

1. R. Han, K.K. Tremper, S. Kheterpal et al. (2004). Grading scale for mask ventilation. *Anaesthesiology* **101**: 267.

2. J. Arné, P. Descoins, J. Fusciardi et al. (1998). Preoperative assessment for difficult intubation in general and ENT surgery: Predictive value of a clinical multivariate risk index. *British Journal of Anaesthesia* **80**: 140–6.

3. A.R. El-Ganzouri, R.J. McCarthy, K.J. Tuman et al. (1996). Preoperative airway assessment: Predictive value of a multivariate risk index. *Anesthesia and Analgesia* **82**: 1197–204.

8 Preoperative testing and perioperative management of endocrine and renal disease

Sudarshan Ramachandran
David Kennedy
Munirul Haque

SUMMARY

This chapter will describe:

- **basic anatomy and physiology of the endocrine and renal systems**
- **the role of biochemical laboratory testing in the preoperative phase**
- **a clinical approach to preoperative optimisation of endocrine and renal disease**
- **therapeutic treatment of endocrine and renal disease and implications for perioperative care.**

INTRODUCTION

The purpose of this chapter is to help those carrying out preoperative assessment to use laboratory investigations in a rational manner to augment their clinical skills when faced with possible endocrine pathology. It must be clearly stated that laboratory guidelines must be applied in conjunction with clinical judgement rather than as a substitute, which would result in a deskilled process.

The role of preoperative investigations is to add diagnostic and prognostic data that could influence surgical outcome. These investigations could be either related or unrelated to the surgery planned, but may lead to alteration in clinical management. It is necessary to have some basic understanding of the endocrine system before being able to diagnose endocrine pathology or to assess current function in a preoperative setting. We therefore offer an overview of commonly encountered endocrine diseases, including the more prevalent clinical features, some of the relevant hormones and the general principles of testing.

A practical understanding of the function and regulation of hormones

Endocrine hormones can be defined as chemical agents that are secreted by specialised cells and are carried in the circulation to act on non-adjacent target tissues. This is in contrast to paracrine and autocrine actions where the effects, after secretion, are on neighbouring and secreting cells respectively. The word 'hormone' is derived from the Greek *hormao* meaning 'arouse'. Hormones are synthesised from amino acids (protein or peptide hormones), cholesterol (steroid hormones) or phospholipids (prostaglandins and related compounds). The steroid hormones include vitamin D as well as the adrenal and sex hormones secreted by the adrenal cortex and reproductive system respectively. Chemical side chains and/or changes in their tertiary structure determine the specificity of protein/peptide and steroid hormones.

Many of the hormones circulate in the body bound to binding proteins (synthesised in the liver). Thus measuring total hormone concentrations (protein bound and unbound) may be a less accurate index of biological activity, as this is generally considered to correlate with the free hormone fraction.

The actions of protein and peptide hormones are mediated by cell surface receptors, because they are less able to cross the lipid cell membrane. They mainly bind to the extracellular aspect of the receptor complex and this in turn leads to dissociation (most hormones) or activation (e.g. insulin, growth hormone, etc) of intracellular components.

Steroid and thyroid hormones can cross the cell membrane and bind to intracellular or nuclear receptors, which in turn act as transcription factors, acting on the cell's DNA. Greater mechanistic details of hormone actions are beyond the scope of this chapter and will not be described further.

It is essential to understand how control is exerted via negative and positive feedback on endocrine systems. Some endocrine systems (thyroid, adrenal cortex, sex organs etc), which are controlled by the anterior pituitary, are subject to feedback from the hormones secreted by the gland. For example, secretion of TSH by the anterior pituitary is suppressed by high concentrations of thyroid hormones (T3 and T4) and increased when concentrations are low (see Figure 8.1, page 144).

In contrast, most of the other endocrine systems are controlled by the concentration of the substances that they regulate, e.g. insulin production is controlled by glucose concentration, parathyroid hormone by calcium concentration, etc The commonly encountered human hormones are classified by system and presented in Table 8.1.

Table 8.2: Some commonly encountered hormones are classified by system and described.

Endocrine Organ	Hormone/Peptide	Endocrine Organ	Hormone/Peptide
Hypothalamus	Thyrotrophin releasing hormone (TRH)	Parathyroid	Parathyroid hormone (PTH)

Endocrine organ	Hormone/Peptide	Endocrine organ	Hormone/Peptide
Hypothalamus *(cont)*	Gonadotrophin releasing hormone (GnRH)		Calcitonin
	Growth hormone releasing hormone (GHRH)		
	Corticotrophin releasing hormone (CRH)	Adrenal cortex	Cortisol
	Prolactin releasing factor		Aldosterone
	Somatostatin		Androgens
	Dopamine		
	Arginine vasopressin (AVP)	Adrenal medulla	Adrenaline
			Noradrenaline
Anterior pituitary	Thyroid stimulating hormone (TSH)		Dopamine
	Adrenocorticotrophic hormone (ACTH)	Reproductive organs	Testosterone
	Follicular stimulating hormone (FSH)		Oestrogens
	Luteinising hormone (LH)		Progesterone
	Growth hormone (GH)		Human chorionic gonadotrophin (hCG)
	Prolactin		
	Melanocyte stimulating hormone (MSH)	Kidney	Renin
			Angiotensin
Posterior pituitary	Vasopressin		Erythropoetin
	Oxytocin		1,25 dihydroxy vitamin D

Endocrine organ	Hormone/Peptide	Endocrine Organ	Hormone/Peptide
Thyroid	Thyroxine (T4)	Skin	Vitamin D
	Tri iodothyronine (T3)		
		Heart	A type natriuretic peptide (ANP)
Pancreas	Insulin		B type natriuretic peptide (BNP)
	Glucagon		
	Somatostatin	Pineal Gland	Melatonin

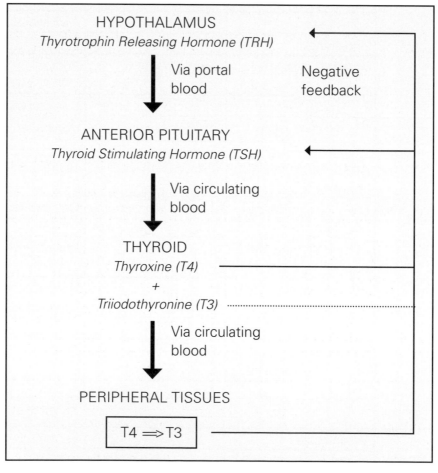

Figure 8.1 The hypothalamic-pituitary-thyroid axis illustrating negative feedback at the pituitary and hypothalamic levels

Common endocrine pathology and appropriate investigations

We briefly describe a few selected endocrine disorders that should be considered, appropriately investigated and managed prior to surgery.

Thyroid disorders

The levels of thyroid hormones (triiodothyronine – T3 and thyroxine – T4) are under the control of the hypothalamic-pituitary axis. Thyrotrophin releasing hormone (TRH) released by cells in the hypothalamus stimulates thyrotrophs in the anterior pituitary to produce thyroid stimulating hormone (TSH). TSH synthesis is inhibited by somatostatin, dopamine and various cytokines. TSH binds to specific receptors found on the surface of follicular cells in the thyroid and triggers a series of cascades leading to synthesis and release of thyroid hormones.

TSH concentration is also subject to negative feedback from thyroid hormones via alterations in the sensitivity of the pituitary thyrotrophs to TRH. This sensitivity to TRH (via TRH receptor numbers) depends on the pituitary intracellular concentration of T3 (80% of which is derived from intra-pituitary conversion of T4). TRH and TSH release is also affected by other physiological conditions (e.g. body temperature) and non-thyroidal hormone levels.

The common causes and clinical manifestations of hypothyroidism and hyperthyroidism are widespread and are described in Table 8.2.

Table 8.2:
Common causes and clinical manifestations of hypo-and hyperthyroidism.

Hypothyroidism	Hyperthyroidism
Causes	
Autoimmune thyroid disease (Hashimoto's disease)	Graves' disease (antibodies stimulating the TSH receptor)
Primary atrophic hypothyroidism	Toxic multinodular goitre
Post radioactive treatment	Thyroid adenoma
Post surgery	Thyroiditis
Thyroiditis	TSH secreting tumour
Over treatment with carbimazole/propylthiouracil	Hyperemesis gravidarum
Some forms of thyroid hormone resistance	
Secondary to hypopituitarism	

Hypothyroidism	Hyperthyroidism
Common clinical features	
Fatigue	Anxiety
Cold intolerance	Irritability
Weight gain	Heat intolerance
Constipation	Fatigue
Voice changes	Weight loss
Dryness of skin	Increased appetite
Loss of hair	Tremor
Bradycardia	Tachycardia/atrial fibrillation
Anaemia	Increased sweating
	Goitre

Disorders of the adrenal cortex

The adrenal cortex produces glucocorticoids (mainly cortisol), mineralocorticoids (mainly aldosterone) and sex hormones. Cholesterol (mainly acquired from circulating low density lipoprotein – LDL) is the precursor of all these hormones, with each group synthesised by specific enzymes differentially expressed in distinct regions of the adrenal cortex. Some of the causes of adrenocortical pathology (Cushing's syndrome, hyperadrenalism and hypoadrenalism) and associated clinical features are shown in Table 8.3. Although many of these conditions are rare, the consequences of not detecting some of these conditions (e.g. Addison's disease) in a preoperative setting can be dire.

Glucocorticoids

Cortisol, the principal glucocorticoid, is essential to a wide variety of metabolic and cellular functions, by affecting DNA transcription. The metabolic effects, inhibiting muscle and adipose tissue glucose uptake, increased insulin resistance, increasing gluconeogenesis and increasing lipolysis, all result in hyperglycaemia and hyperlipidaemia. Other effects include increased cardiac output and vascular tone resulting in hypertension and maintaining the extracellular fluid volume.

Mineralocorticoids

Aldosterone, the principal mineralocorticoid, stimulates the active reabsorption of sodium from the glomerular filtrate reaching the distal convoluted tubule in the kidney. Synthesis and release of aldosterone is under the control of the renin-angiotensin system. A decrease in renal perfusion, increased sympathetic activity or a reduction in sodium delivery to the macula densa stimulates the release of renin. Renin stimulates a cascade, culminating in the synthesis of aldosterone by the adrenal cortex. Aldosterone binds to receptors in the renal distal tubule, causing salt and water absorption with a consequent increase in extracellular volume.

Table 8.3: Causes of adrenocortical disease and associated clinical features

Hypoadrenalism	Cushing's syndrome	Hyperadrenalism
Causes		
Sudden discontinuation of steroid therapy	Iatrogenic (exogenous steroids)	*Secondary causes*
Addison's disease *(due to autoimmune destruction, infection, haemorrhage, metastases, drugs)*	Pituitary adenoma Ectopic ACTH secretion	(Physiological (pregnancy), hypovolaemia, CCF, cirrhosis, nephrotic syndrome, salt losing states, renal artery stenosis, diuretic treatment)
	Adrenal adenoma	*Primary causes*
Hypopituitarism		(adenoma, hyperplasia)
Common clinical features		
Postural hypotension, collapse	Weight gain	Hypertension
Weakness	Central obesity	Hypokalaemia
Weight loss	Moon face appearance	Alkalosis
Pigmentation	Striae/acne/bruising/ hirsuitism	
Hypoglycaemia	Hypertension	
Abdominal pain	Diabetes/impaired glucose tolerance	
	Proximal myopathy	
	Osteoporosis	

Disorders of the adrenal medulla: Phaeochromocytoma

Chromaffin cells in the adrenal medulla (which comprises 20% of the adrenal gland and part of the autonomic nervous system) secrete catecholamines. Adrenaline forms about 80% of adrenal catecholamine synthesis whereas noradrenaline is the principal catecholamine produced by the sympathetic nervous system. Dopamine is a precursor of both.

Catecholamines cause either vasoconstriction (via alpha receptors) or increases in heart rate, blood pressure, sweating and metabolic changes (via beta receptors). The released catecholamines have a very short half-life, being rapidly metabolised within minutes by the enzyme monoamine oxidase.

Phaeochromocytoma is a rare endocrine tumour, which may result in paroxysmal symptoms, due to a sudden release of catecholamines. Although rare, it is essential to diagnose the presence of phaeochromocytoma, especially preoperatively to prevent potential mortality. Palpation of the tumour and certain therapeutic agents used in anaesthesia can precipitate sudden hormone release, which may be fatal. Clinical features that lead to suspicion are presented in Table 8.4.

Table 8.4: Some of the physiological effects of catecholamines and clinical features ofphaeochromocytoma

Effects of catecholamines	Clinical features of phaeochromocytoma
Cardiovascular *(increase in heart rate, increases peripheral resistance)*	Anxiety
	Increased sweating
Visceral *(smooth muscle relaxation)*	Palpitations
	Hypertension (paroxysmal or sustained)
Endocrine *(increased secretion of glucagon, aldosterone)*	Tremor
	Headaches
Metabolic *(increased glycogenolysis and lipolysis)*	Abdominal pain
	Hyperglycaemia
Renal *(Decrease in glomerular filtration and sodium excretion)*	

Calcium regulation and parathyroid disorders

Calcium is essential for life and has an important role in many physiological functions. Thus hormone regulation of the calcium concentration in the blood is vital. The hormones act via regulation of extracellular calcium (0.1% of total calcium), but total body calcium levels also depend on the same process.

The hormones regulating calcium also control phosphate homeostasis and so both must be considered together. Phosphate has an important physiological role; including being a component of DNA, RNA, phospholipids, ATP, enzymes and second messengers (c-AMP).

In plasma, calcium is present in three forms: protein bound (mainly to albumin), complexed (with citrate and phosphate) and a free fraction. Only the free fraction is considered physiologically active and is the component maintained by homeostatic mechanisms.

Total calcium concentration is usually the measure reported by the laboratory, varying between 2.2 and 2.6mmol/L. However, measurement of the free ionised calcium fraction is often available from blood gas analysers, and is approximately half that of total calcium, i.e. 1.0–1.30mmol/L. Both the free and the bound fractions are in equilibrium. Thus, protein concentrations and alkalosis or acidosis, which affect protein binding of calcium, all affect the measured total calcium level.

Calcium and phosphate levels are dependent on absorption from the gastrointestinal tract, loss via urine and faeces and bone turnover. Hormones such as parathyroid hormone (PTH) and vitamin D play a crucial part in calcium homeostasis.

Serum calcium concentration exerts an influence on PTH secretion via negative feedback, i.e. high calcium concentrations reduce PTH release. The half-life of PTH in the serum is a few minutes. PTH acts on bone, resulting in immediate osteolysis, thus increasing serum calcium whilst a more delayed resorption process leads to increased calcium and phosphate concentrations in the extracellular fluid. PTH also acts on renal tubular cells, where it inhibits renal phosphate reabsorption and increases renal calcium reabsorption. PTH also stimulates conversion of 25 hydroxy- vitamin D to the active 1, 25 dihydroxy- vitamin D, which results in increased active calcium and phosphate absorption in the gut.

Vitamin D prohormones are obtained principally from the skin (stimulated by UVB exposure) but also from the diet. The inactive prohormones are metabolised to 25 hydroxylated forms in the liver and further converted in the kidney to the 1,25 dihydroxylated compounds, which are physiologically active. Calcium, phosphate, PTH and 1,25 dihydroxy- vitamin D concentrations regulate 1-α hydroxylase enzyme activity in the kidney, thus providing a feedback loop.

Vitamin D stimulates calcium, phosphate and magnesium absorption in the gut. Its action on bone is more complex and still unclear. The clinical features of both hyper- and hypocalcaemia which suggest a disruption of normal calcium homeostasis are described in Table 8.5 (page 150).

Pituitary gland disorders

The posterior pituitary comprises of axons and nerve terminals of neuronal cells situated in the hypothalamus, which secrete vasopressin and oxytocin. Anterior pituitary hormone secretion is controlled by hormones released into the hypophyseal portal veins by the hypothalamus. In response, the anterior pituitary lobe releases either TSH, ACTH, or gonadotrophins (LH and FSH), which in turn control hormone secretion by the thyroid, adrenal gland and sex organs.

Table 8.5: Causes and clinical features of hyper- and hypocalcaemia

Hypercalcaemia	Hypocalcaemia
Causes	
Primary hyperparathyroidism (adenoma, hyperplasia, carcinoma)	Post thyroidectomy/parathyroidectomy
	Vitamin D deficiency
Malignancies	
	Disordered vitamin D metabolism e.g. CRF
Excess vitamin D (overtreatment, sarcoidosis, tuberculosis)	Hypomagnesaemia
Familial hypercalcuric hypercalcaemia	Hypoparathyroidism/pseudohypoparathyroidism
Clinical features	
Fatigue/lethargy	Weakness
Depression/confusion	Muscular e.g. cramps/tetany
Polydipsia/polyuria	Behavioural disturbances/stupor
Musculoskeletal symptoms	Convulsions
Constipation	Cataracts (chronic)
Renal calculi/nephrocalcinosis	
Cardiac arrhythmias/hypertension	
Corneal and vascular calcification	

The anterior pituitary also secretes GH and prolactin, the former stimulates IGF-1 production by GH receptor proteins, the latter stimulating lactation. This network of hormonal control via endocrine axes is shown in Figure 8.2.

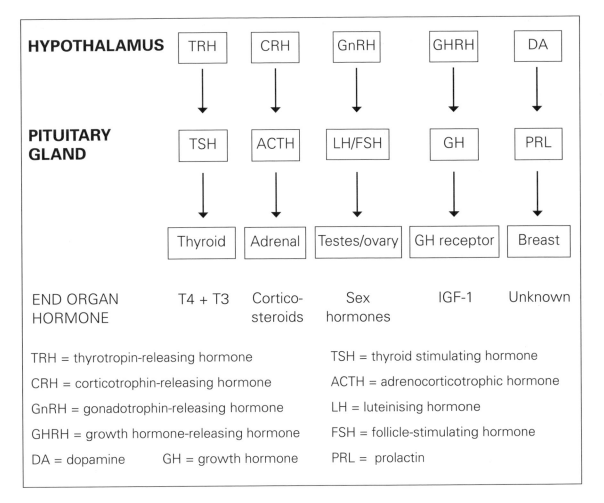

Figure 8.2 Hormonal control via endocrine axes

Diseases affecting the anterior pituitary can be divided into deficiency and hypersecretory states. The deficiency states can be either generalised or axis specific. Some of the causes of generalised or pan-hypopituitarism include non-functional pituitary adenomas, cranio-pharyngiomas, metastases, inflammatory diseases (granulomatous lesions, lymphocytic hypophysitis), haemorrhage and infarction. In a significant number of cases, hypopituitarism is evident following clinical and biochemical investigations without an underlying cause being identified and these are classified as 'idiopathic' hypopituitarism. Axis-specific deficiency states can be detected due to any of the above causes including 'idiopathic' hypopituitarism. The common clinical symptoms and signs of hypopituitarism are mainly due to deficiency of hormones produced by the end organs under its control.

Vasopressin is synthesised in the hypothalamus and thus pituitary adenomas are unlikely to lead to deficiency causing diabetes insipidus. More likely causes of vasopressin deficiency are craniopharyngiomas, inflammatory conditions and non-pituitary tumours. Familial diabetes insipidus of unknown aetiology has been described as presenting soon after birth. Biochemical investigations depending on the symptoms of deficiency states can be broken down into front-line tests such as TSH and free thyroxine (FT4), testosterone/oestrogens and LH, FSH, cortisol, prolactin and IGF-1. Should the hormone values suggest an abnormality, dynamic function tests, in addition to radiological investigations, should be performed. These are best carried out in consultation with the endocrine team and clinical biochemistry staff, as strict protocols have to be adhered to and often the interpretation of the results is not clear-cut.

Hypersecretory states are usually due to benign pituitary adenomas (rarely malignant) synthesising and secreting specific hormones. Clinical features are due to excess levels of these specific hormones and once again the relevant investigations are similar to those previously described for the deficiency states.

Diabetes mellitus

Diabetes is a disease characterised by hyperglycaemia caused by a relative deficiency of insulin secretion and/or insulin resistance. Current views on aetiology are beyond the scope of this chapter. An understanding of the actions of insulin will also not be dealt with for the same reason. It is essential that diabetes is detected in undiagnosed patients and glycaemia is controlled optimally to reduce surgery-related complications. For the purposes of this chapter we will define diabetes as Type 1 and Type 2; other types of diabetes (e.g. associated with single gene disorders, syndromes with severe insulin resistance and secondary causes) are rare. The clinical features of Type 1 and Type 2 diabetes are presented in Table 8.6. The presenting features (together with age and ketosis) often but not always differentiate Type 1 from Type 2 diabetes.

Table 8.6: Clinical features of Type I and Type 2 diabetes.

Clinical features	Type 1 diabetes	Type 2 diabetes
polyuria/thirst	++	+
fatigue/weakness	++	+
weight loss	++	-
vulvovaginitis/pruritis	+	++
peripheral neuropathy	+	++
nocturnal enuresis	++	-
asymptomatic	-	++

Type 1 diabetes is due to an autoimmune-driven process, leading to infiltration and destruction of the endocrine pancreas: the islets of Langerhans; and is associated with a loss of insulin secretion. There appear to be both genetic and environmental elements to the pathogenesis. Ketoacidosis is due to insulin deficiency and can be seen in type 1 diabetes. Insulin, an anabolic hormone, acts to inhibit lipolysis, with ketone bodies being the end products of this pathway. Thus a deficiency of insulin (or omission of exogenous insulin) promotes an increase in ketone body production and resulting acidosis. Therefore, it is essential that insulin is not completely discontinued even when the patient is 'nil by mouth' immediately prior to surgery.

Type 2 diabetes is also associated with genetic and environmental causative factors, but in contrast is thought to be due to insulin resistance causing the cells to fail as they become unable to provide adequate compensation.

Preoperative testing

Patients with endocrine disease presenting for anaesthesia and surgery can represent a significant clinical challenge. This section considers how appropriate and well targeted laboratory testing, following a detailed clinical history, can help uncover endocrine disease in patients with undiagnosed endocrine conditions, as well as aiding the management of those with established disease. Here we cover a range of endocrine conditions, highlighting information of particular relevance to perioperative care.

Patients with previously undiagnosed endocrine disease

Patients with undiagnosed endocrine disease can often have vague non-specific symptoms that can delay a positive diagnosis considerably. It is therefore a significant challenge to identify individuals at the preoperative stage with previously unknown endocrine conditions without causing unacceptable levels of inappropriate testing and delay due to the inevitably high false positive rate.

Routine, or generic, testing of asymptomatic individuals prior to surgery, even for common endocrine diseases such as diabetes mellitus, has now been clearly identified as inappropriate. However, a detailed clinical history prior to surgery should help identify key indicators that suggest endocrine disease may be present.

Clinical screening for endocrine disease

The clinical history should be detailed enough to allow identification of individuals with an increased likelihood of having an undiagnosed endocrine disease, particularly if facing major surgery. Further follow-up testing should only be requested where clinical suspicion is high and the suspected endocrine disorder is likely to impact on either response to anaesthetic agents and/or recovery. Some of the clinical features leading to the possibility of endocrine pathology are presented in Table 8.7 (page 154). As hypopituitarism is diagnosed by examining the function of all endocrine systems, we present a simplified investigation pathway in Figure 8.3.

Table 8.7
Key factors in the clinical history that may be linked to endocrine disease

General symptoms	Possible disorder(s)	Suggested initial test(s)
Recent weight loss but no loss of appetite	Hypothyroidism	TSH and FT4
Recent weight loss with severe fatigue	Hypoadrenalism (primary or secondary), diabetes mellitus	Cortisol (9am if possible), plasma glucose, TSH (Synacthen test if 9am cortisol low)
Specific symptoms		
Thirst and polyuria (± nocturia)	Diabetes mellitus, diabetes insipidus, hyperparathyroidism, hypoadrenalism	Urea and electrolytes, serum osmolality, cortisol, calcium and albumin, TSH, random plasma glucose (GTT if RPG ≥ 8.0)
Hypertension with proximal muscle weakness (especially if unexplained low potassium)	Cushing's syndrome, Conn's syndrome	Urea and electrolytes, random plasma glucose, BP
Excessive sweating (generalised)	Hyperthyroidism, diabetes, acromegaly, phaeochromocytoma, carcinoid syndrome	TSH and random plasma glucose. If other endocrine disorders suspected seek specialist advice
Hypotension	Hypoadrenalism (primary or secondary)	Urea and electrolytes, serum cortisol (9am if possible), ACTH
Recurrent fungal infection	Diabetes mellitus	Random plasma glucose
Palpitations, with headaches and anxiety attacks	Hypoglycaemia, Phaeochromocytoma (especially if paroxysmal hypertension)	Fasting plasma glucose (if symptomatic serum must be frozen within 30 minutes for insulin). If phaeochromocytoma suspected seek specialist advice
Goitre	Hypothyroidism or hyperthyroidism	TSH and FT4

Previous medical history	Possible disorder(s)	Suggested initial test(s)
Renal stones	Hyperparathyroidism	Serum calcium and albumin (PTH if calcium high)
Known hypotensive episodes or frequent dizzy spells	Hypoadrenalism (primary or secondary)	Urea and electrolytes, serum cortisol (9 am if possible), ACTH
TB with recent hypotension and/or fatigue	Hypoadrenalism (primary)	Urea and electrolytes, serum cortisol (9 am if possible)
Autoimmune disease, e.g. hypothyroidism, Addison's disease, type 1 diabetes	Another coexisting autoimmune disease, e.g. hypothyroidism, Addison's etc	Investigate selectively according to personal history and clinical signs
Family history	Possible disorder(s)	Suggested initial test(s)
Type 2 diabetes	Type 2 diabetes mellitus	Random plasma glucose if asymptomatic. If symptomatic then fasting plasma glucose (GTT if FPG $\geq$ 6)
Autoimmune disease (incl. type 1 DM)	Another coexisting autoimmune disease, e.g. hypothyroidism, Addison's etc	Investigate selectively according to personal history and clinical signs
Multiple endocrine neoplasia syndrome (MEN)	Type 1 associated with hyperparathyroidism, pituitary hormone excess and pancreatic hormone excess. Type 2 associated with hyperparathyroidism, medullary carcinoma of thyroid and phaeochromocytoma	Type 1: calcium. Type 2: calcium and 24 hour urinary catecholamines

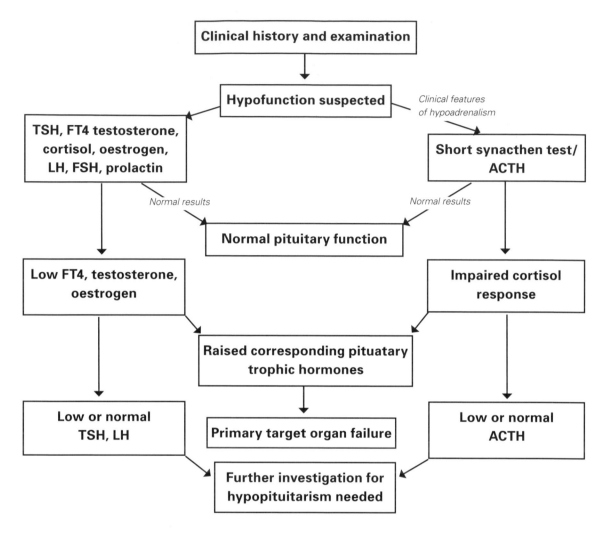

Figure 8.3: A plan of investigation when hypopituitarism is suspected

Suggested investigations for the other endocrine diseases previously described are presented below.

Diabetes mellitus

As diabetes is much more common than many other endocrine disorders, affecting up to 5% of the population, the index of suspicion can be relatively low when judging whether to screen asymptomatic individuals. Evidence-based guidelines do not support routine screening, but it is common practice in many preadmission clinic units to screen for diabetes, particularly if the population served has a high preponderance of Asian, Afro-Caribbean and/or elderly patients.

Where screening is advocated, local protocols should be agreed. However, the use of random blood glucose testing is usually preferable to urine testing, as the latter can be poorly done unless the standard of staff training is high and dipstick readers are widely available.

A random plasma glucose $\geq$ 8mmol/L should be followed up with a fasting blood glucose (FBG). If other abnormal or equivocal blood glucose results have been obtained previously then an oral glucose tolerance test (OGTT) may be appropriate. If RBG is $\geq$ 11.1mmol/L or FBG is $\geq$ 7.0mmol/L then this is diagnostic for diabetes in a symptomatic patient. In an asymptomatic patient, a further test, e.g. a repeat FBG or RBG should be performed on a subsequent day to confirm the diagnosis.

Measurement of HbA1c can be useful in a preadmission clinic for patients with previously undiagnosed diabetes, as it enables identification of those requiring intervention to improve diabetes control prior to surgery, helping to reduce postoperative complications. An HbA1c <7.5% suggests reasonable diabetic control prior to surgery whereas above 7.5% active management is indicated. Perioperative requesting of HbA1c is unnecessary if the RBG is >13 mmol/L or FBG is > 7.8mmol/L as active management is indicated anyway.

Once a patient with previously undiagnosed diabetes has been identified, other risk factors such as hypertension or peripheral vascular disease should be assessed.

Thyroid disorders

For the purpose of preoperative screening, TSH alone is recommended. Only if the TSH is above or below the reference interval is follow-up testing of free T4 and possibly free T3 required. A normal TSH confirms euthyroid status. Uncontrolled hypothyroidism or hyperthyroidism both represent significant risks for anaesthesia and surgery. Therefore, where possible, surgery should be postponed until thyroid disease is better controlled.

Hypoadrenalism

If patients are suspected of adrenal hypofunction (either primary or secondary) this can be screened for by checking a random serum cortisol. A daytime cortisol result of $\geq$ 250nmol/L in a pre-admission clinic suggests adequate adrenal reserve for minor surgery, providing the patient is not acutely ill. If clinical suspicion is high, or suspicion low but major surgery is planned, then a Synacthen test may be required to confirm adequate adrenal function.

Hyperparathyroidism

A normal serum total calcium (or corrected calcium if calculated) and phosphate is adequate for screening. Although hyperparathyroidism can exist with normocalcaemia, this is not relevant in the context of preoperative screening. However, a high normal calcium and low phosphate should raise suspicion of possible gland overactivity. A high serum calcium should be followed up by measuring parathyroid hormone (PTH). It is recommended to contact the local laboratory to check the requirements before samples for PTH are taken. PTH can be unstable if the blood is collected into certain types of sample tube and may require faster processing than other routine samples.

Cushing's syndrome

Non-iatrogenic Cushing's syndrome (i.e. patients not on steroids) is rare and therefore specific follow-up testing is only appropriate after consultation with a specialist. However, electrolytes and plasma glucose should be checked in patients suspected of Cushing's syndrome to exclude significant hypokalaemia or diabetes mellitus.

Conn's syndrome

As with Cushing's syndrome, this condition is rare and therefore does not justify specific follow-up testing during preoperative assessment other than to exclude hypokalaemia. In the event of unexplained hypokalaemia and hypertension (generally moderate, malignant hypertension is very rare) the endocrine and clinical biochemistry teams should be contacted to advise on further investigations, which include renin and aldosterone blood tests (lying and standing), suppression tests and radiology. The interpretation of these tests is often not clear cut.

Phaeochromocytoma

This is a rare disorder but poses a potentially highly significant problem for the anaesthetist and surgeon if present. Accidental palpation of an undiagnosed tumour or the use of certain therapeutic agents may precipitate a potentially fatal surge of catecholamines. Patients often present with a history of unexplained 'palpitations' or 'panic attacks' or unexplained tachyarrhythmias, with or without hypertensive episodes. Any patient for whom there is a clinical suspicion of the presence of a phaeochromocytoma should have a 24-hour urine sample collected for catecholamines (in a bottle containing acid preservative). Because of the episodic nature of catecholamine secretion by these tumours it is usual to request three separate collections to minimise the possibility of missing the secretion. However, in a preoperative setting, unless clinical suspicion is high, a single collection is probably sufficient. This test has a significant number of false positives, and certain drugs and foods can interfere. Thus any positive result will require follow-up testing and does not necessarily mean a tumour is present. Newer tests, e.g. plasma metanephrines, are not recommended for screening purposes.

Perioperative management in patients with endocrine disease

In this section we will cover the management of diabetes and thyroid disease in depth and the other endocrine disorders briefly as they are relatively rare; we would recommend that the medical endocrine team be consulted to optimise and advise on both pre- and perioperative management of these patients.

Diabetes mellitus

We will describe the management of diabetes in the perioperative setting by considering day case minor surgery separately from major surgery and Type 1 diabetes separately from Type 2 diabetes.

Day case surgery

Type 1 diabetes

Patients with Type 1 diabetes who are scheduled for surgery after 10am can be permitted to have their breakfast together with the morning insulin. A sliding scale of insulin replacement (please refer to local hospital guidelines) can be initiated an hour prior to surgery. Should the patient be scheduled first on the theatre list, the sliding scale could be started two to three hours prior to surgery.

Perioperatively the sliding scale is continued with intravenous fluids and close monitoring of blood sugar is recommended during and immediately after surgery. One strategy to avoid hypoglycaemia and hypovolaemia is to use the GKI protocol (10% dextrose, 20mL KCL and actrapid infused at 80mL per hour with an increase in infusion rate if hypoglycaemia develops).

Postoperatively if the patient is able to begin oral feeding the GKI protocol can be discontinued and the patient's subcutaneous insulin regime can be recommenced. Should oral feeding not be possible or if vomiting complicates postoperative care, then the patient should be continued on the insulin sliding scale.

Type 2 diabetes

The management of Type 2 diabetic patients varies considerably from the above. Surgery can be permitted even in the presence of significant hyperglycaemia providing there is no ketosis. Although conversion to an insulin regime is often unnecessary, the surgeon or anaesthetist may insist on tighter glycaemic control and a sliding scale can be initiated as for the Type 1 diabetic patient.

In patients presenting with Type 2 diabetes controlled with diet, regular blood glucose monitoring (pre-breakfast and two hours after main meals while an inpatient) should be the only extra precaution in addition to those carried out for a non-diabetic patient. However, should complications arise that result in hyperglycaemia and ward admission interim, conversion to insulin therapy may be necessary.

Patients on metformin and/or a thiazolidinedione, as either monotherapy or part of the oral hypoglycaemic regime, should be treated with these agents on the morning of surgery, regardless of whether breakfast is given. Neither agent is associated with resulting hypoglycaemia, unlike sulphonylureas. When a sulphonylurea is part of the regime it should be omitted. Insulin is not generally required for these patients, even if hyperglycaemia occurs, and the patient can restart the entire preoperative treatment regime once oral feeding commences.

Major surgery

Management of hyperglycaemia is more critical when major surgery is scheduled. Preferably,

Type 1 diabetic patients and insulin-treated Type 2 diabetic patients should be first on the surgical list. Oral intake is stopped from midnight and an insulin sliding scale and a GKI protocol can be initiated in the morning. However, should this not be possible or if the surgical list is scheduled in the afternoon a 'nil by mouth' restriction on intake should be placed four to six hours prior to surgery and an insulin sliding scale with fluids should be commenced. The sliding scale and fluids should be continued until oral intake is recommenced. At this point the Type 1 diabetic patient may return to the preoperative insulin regime, although the dose may have to be titrated depending on nutritional intake.

Patients with diet-controlled Type 2 diabetes need to have regular checks (every two to four hours) of blood glucose during and after major surgery. Insulin may not be needed if preoperative blood glucose remains consistently below 10mmol/L and close monitoring is essential. If the glucose concentration becomes erratic postoperatively, or the patient becomes unstable, then a sliding scale regime can be initiated. A similar management strategy applies to patients on metformin monotherapy (metformin should not be discontinued). However, if the patient is on sulphonylurea, it should be omitted with the discontinuation of oral feeding prior to surgery.

On perioperative checking if the glucose remains between 10 and 15mmol/L, then the patient must be monitored closely and the diabetes specialist nurses consulted. Should the glucose levels be persistently above 15mmol/L, insulin therapy should be initiated in the short term, again with management advice from the diabetes specialist nurses.

Thyroid disorders

When a treated thyrotoxic patient presents (clinically euthyroid) for day surgery, the carbimazole or propylthiouracil should be given as usual and continued thereafter. A similar approach is taken when preparing a patient for major surgery; however, perioperatively the patient should be monitored for signs of thyroid crisis. Intravenous propranolol can be used to control tachycardia.

If a patient presents for day surgery in a thyrotoxic state, the surgery should preferably be deferred, with the medical teams' advice sought and appropriate treatment begun. When elective major surgery is planned for a patient who is clinically thyrotoxic, the risks of surgery should be balanced against those of not carrying out the procedure. If surgery is carried out then appropriate emergency care protocols must be followed.

If hypothyroidism is diagnosed when surgery is initially planned, thyroxine should be commenced (dose depends on the thyroid function tests and the severity of the symptoms and advice should be sought from the endocrine team). TSH and Free T4 should be checked, preferably a week before surgery, allowing further titration of the thyroxine replacement dose. As absorption is rapid, thyroxine can be given even on the morning of surgery.

Perioperative steroid cover for patients on long-term steroid treatment

Many patients undergoing surgical procedures may have abnormalities of the hypothalamic-pituitary-adrenal (HPA) axis. This may be due to primary pituitary disease, e.g. hypopituitarism or following treatment for a pituitary tumour) or adrenal hypofunction (Addison's disease). However, more commonly it is due to suppression of endogenous glucocorticoid production due to the administration of high doses of steroids.

The physiological stress of surgery is a potent activator of the HPA axis in normal subjects and failure to provide adequate steroid cover may precipitate potentially fatal acute adrenal insufficiency following surgery. Normal endogenous cortisol production is approximately 15–25mg per day. Patients receiving hydrocortisone replacement for primary pituitary or adrenal failure typically receive 20–30mg daily. See Table 8.8 for equivalent doses.

Table 8.8 Approximate equivalent doses

Hydrocortisone	20mg	
= Cortisone	25mg	
= Prednisolone	5mg	i.e. 4 x potent c.f. hydrocortisone
= Methyprednisolone	4mg	i.e. 5 x
= Dexamethasone	0.5 mg	i.e. 40 x

The following categories of patients require steroid cover:

- any patient with known past history of hypopituitarism or Addison's disease who is on long-term replacement steroids
- any patients on therapeutic glucocorticoids with clinical features of Cushing's syndrome
- patients who have received > 10mg prednisolone (or equivalent, see Table 8.8) daily for > 3 weeks continuously in the last 3 months
- patients taking high dose glucocorticoids (e.g. 4mg dexamethasone t.d.s.), even for short periods, who may have significant adrenal suppression for many months
- patients taking high dose inhaled steroids long-term (i.e. fluticasone ≥1000mcg daily or >1500mcg of other inhaled steroids).

Suggested replacement doses

Traditionally, large doses of IV hydrocortisone have been suggested, which were largely empirical and based on little evidence. Overtreatment with steroids perioperatively is of concern due to its possible effects on wound healing, immune function and glucose tolerance. The likelihood of a patient having HPA axis suppression depends on the dose of steroid received and duration of therapy.

For high dose steroid regimes, HPA axis suppression may last for several months. Therefore a detailed past medical and drug history is essential. In the majority of cases, testing for HPA axis suppression is unnecessary but a Synacthen test may be helpful in a minority of cases, e.g. inhaled steroids.

Table 8.9 Suggested steroid regimes[1]

Current steroid regime	Type of surgery	Perioperative treatment
Low dose (< 10mg prednisolone or equivalent daily)	Assume normal HPA response	Additional steroid cover unnecessary
Moderate dose (> 10mg Prednisolone or equivalent daily)	Minor surgery	25mg hydrocortisone @ preop or induction. Resume normal dose postop
	Moderate surgery	Usual preop dose + 25mg hydrocortisone @ induction + 100 mg i.v. for 24 hours
	Major surgery	Usual preop dose + 25mg hydrocortisone @ induction + 100 mg i.v. for 48–72 hours
Immunosuppressive doses		Give usual doses throughout perioperative period
Steroids stopped < 3 months		Treat as if on steroids
Steroids stopped > 3 months		No perioperative steroids necessary

Renal impairment and preoperative management

As there are usually no specific symptoms, renal impairment is picked up in one of the following two ways:

1. routine biochemical testing (increased urea, creatinine and reduced estimated glomerular filtration rate (GFR))
2. patient presenting with features associated with renal dysfunction, e.g. hypertension, oedema, haematuria etc

Increasing numbers of patients are now picked up following the introduction of formula-based estimations of GFR (eGFR), which are now routinely provided by all clinical biochemistry laboratories using the abbreviated 4-variable MDRD study equation, as recommended in *The National Service Framework for Renal Services*.[2]

The initial approach should be to evaluate the cause and the severity of renal impairment. This includes:

1. estimation of disease duration (acute or chronic)
2. examination of the urine
3. estimation of the glomerular filtration rate (eGFR).

Acute renal failure (ARF) is worsening of renal function over hours/days, resulting in increasing urea and creatinine concentrations, often associated with coexisting medical or surgical conditions. The previous biochemistry is useful in making this distinction. Identification of normal urea and creatinine concentrations over the preceding weeks/months helps define acute renal failure. In the absence of previous records, the presence of anuria/oliguria, hypotension, sepsis, dehydration, and clinical evidence of fluid loss point at acute renal failure. It is important to examine all medications, as drugs can cause or exacerbate renal failure.

In contrast, chronic renal failure (CRF) results from increased loss of renal function over a longer period, a progressive rise in creatinine and a steady fall in eGFR. While anuria/oliguria is unusual, anaemia and small kidneys (on ultrasound examination) are more likely in chronic renal failure. Distinguishing acute and chronic renal failure is important for appropriate management, both immediate and long-term.

Chronic renal failure is currently graded according to the eGFR with actions dependent on the stage and progression. It must be kept in mind that eGFR will decrease with age. (see Table 8.10).

Table 8.10 Gradations of severity of renal impairement:

Grade 1	Normal GFR + proteinuria	$>90ml/min/1.73m^2$
Grade 2	Mild CKD	$90-60ml/min/1.73m^2$
Grade 3	Moderate CKD	$60-30ml/min/1.73m^2$
Grade 4	Severe CKD	$30-15ml/min/1.73m^2$
Grade 5	End stage renal disease	$<15ml/min/1.73m^2$

While patients included in grades 1–3 are asymptomatic, in grade 4 non-specific symptoms are often evident. Figure 8.4 shows a treatment algorithm for investigating patients with reduced GFR.

The cause of the renal dysfunction can be further anatomically classified as pre-renal, intrinsic and post-renal (see Table 8.11, page 164).

Table 8.11 Causes of renal failure

Acute renal failure		
Pre-renal	**Renal**	**Post-renal**
Hypovolaemia blood loss *Dehydration* diarrhoea, vomiting, etc *Medications* diuretics *Ischaemia (renal artery)* embolism, aortic dissection etc *Renal vein thrombosis*	*Sepsis* *Medications* NSAID, ACEI, ARB, contrast medium, lithium *Rhabdomyolysis* *Myeloma* *Acute glomerular nephritis* primary glomerular secondary – SLE, vasculitis, etc	*Obstructive* bladder outlet, ureter abdominal or pelvic mass prostatic pathology renal stones
Chronic renal failure		
Pre-renal	**Renal**	**Post-renal**
Acute or chronic similar causes as in ARF	*Diabetic nephropathy* *Hypertensive nephropathy* *Chronic glomerulonephritis* *Polycystic kidneys* *Reflux nephropathy* *Renal stones*	*Obstructive* similar causes as in ARF

The following points must be remembered in the preoperative management of ARF.

- The fluid status of the patient must be estimated and appropriately corrected. This is essential, as prolonged hypotension can result in irreversible renal damage.
- Careful monitoring of both input and output of fluids is essential.
- All potentially nephrotoxic drugs must be discontinued. The advice of relevant specialists must be sought if possible if a new drug is substituted.
- The critical care team must be involved early as patient care may need to be optimised preoperatively.
- In the event of the patient remaining hypotensive despite adequate fluid replacement, ionotropic support may be required.
- In severe ARF, or in the event of mild to moderate renal impairment not significantly improving, or worsening, the renal team must be consulted; interim haemofiltration/dialysis may be required prior to surgery.

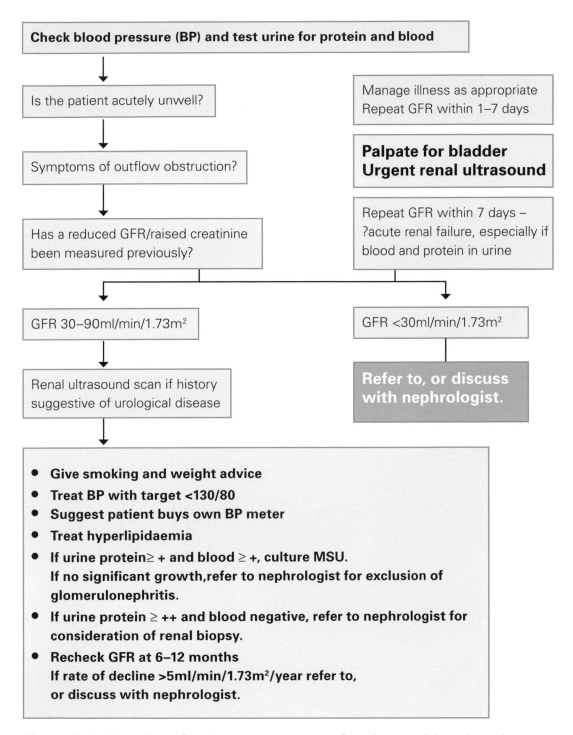

Figure 8.4: Algorithm for the management of patients with reduced glomular filtration rate (GFR)

Patients diagnosed as CKD grades 1–3 need judicious fluid and electrolyte replacement with careful assessment to avoid dehydration leading to further deterioration of renal function or fluid overload. Patients classed as grade 4 CKD need to be reviewed and managed by a nephrologist (during the entire period of admission) ahead of surgery.

REFERENCES

1. G. Nicholson, J.M. Burrin and G.M. Hall (1998). Peri-operative steroid supplementation. *Anaesthesia* **53**: 1091–104.

2. Department of Health (2004). *The National Service Framework for Renal Services.* London: HMSO.

FURTHER READING

British Association of Day Surgery Working Group (2004). Day Surgery and the Diabetic Patient: Guidelines for the assessment and management of diabetes in day case surgery patients. *British Association of Day Surgery Handbook* 2nd edn. London: BADS.

Royal College of Physicians of London (2006). Chronic Kidney Disease in Adults: UK Guidelines for Identification, Management and Referral. Available at: www.renal.org/CKDguide/full/UKCKDfullguide.pdf, accessed 08/06/08.

Chapter 9

Preoperative assessment and management of neurological disease

John Andrzejowski
Stefan Jankowski

SUMMARY

This chapter will describe:

- **basic anatomy and physiology of the neurological systems**
- **the role of testing in the preoperative phase**
- **clinical approach to preoperative optimisation of neurological conditions**
- **therapeutic treatment of neurological conditions and implications for perioperative care.**

INTRODUCTION

This chapter will address the essential background physiology and pathology that will help you undertake an evaluation of a patient presenting for neurosurgery. It will also detail how to assess patients with pre-existing neurological conditions who are due to undergo other types of surgery.

Basic science: anatomy and physiology

The brain can be considered as freely communicating fluid volumes within a fixed box (the bony skull). Intracranial pressure results from the contributions of three intracranial fluid compartments: brain tissue (parenchyma), cerebral blood vessels and cerebrospinous fluid (CSF). An increase in one of these volumes (e.g. brain tumour with surrounding oedema) increases intracranial pressure unless there is a compensatory decrease in one of the others (e.g. ventricles compress or CSF moves out).

The brain is a very greedy organ. Despite only making up 2–3% of the body's weight, (average 1.4kg), it receives 15% of the cardiac output and uses 20% of the body's resting oxygen consumption. Needless to say it needs careful looking after, so let us start by considering the five things a brain needs to keep it 'happy' (see Figure 9.1).

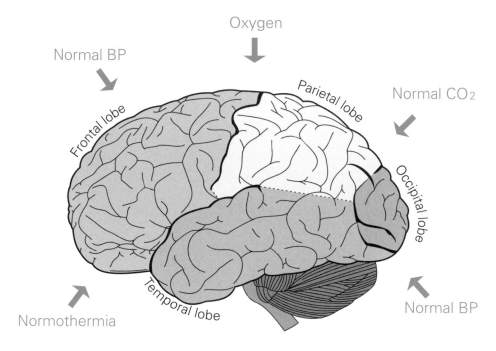

Oxygen

Normal BP

Parietal lobe

Normal CO$_2$

Frontal lobe

Occipital lobe

Temporal lobe

Normal BP

Normothermia

Fig 9.1 The brain's requirements

Maintain blood pressure and minimise ICP

The brain keeps its blood flow steady at 50mls/100gm by a process known as autoregulation. This is what stops you fainting every time you stand up. It involves the cerebral blood vessels dilating if blood pressure (BP) is low or constricting if BP is too high. However, changes in blood vessel diameter can lead to large changes in intracranial pressure (ICP). In an at-risk brain, it is therefore a good idea to maintain a decent cerebral perfusion pressure (CPP) by keeping the mean blood pressure (MAP) about 60mmHg above intracranial pressure. Normal ICP is around 10–15mmHg, so try to keep the patient's MAP about 80mmHg. This is essentially a normal BP. It may involve giving IV fluids, or raising the foot of the bed.

In certain conditions, a high BP can put the patient at risk of intracranial haemorrhage so it may need treating. Raising the head of the bed will help in such circumstances.

If raised ICP is the biggest risk, it can be minimised by raising the head of the bed, avoiding tight clothing or ties around the neck. Osmotic diuretics (mannitol) can be given if the patient is deteriorating rapidly due to raised ICP.

Oxygen

Administer oxygen to any patient suspected of having raised ICP or depressed neurological status. All cells need oxygen to survive. Oxygen saturation can be measured and should be kept >96% if possible.

Control CO_2

Figure 9.2 illustrates what can happen to cerebral blood flow with changes in carbon dioxide. A small 1kPa rise in CO_2 results in a 20% increase in blood flow to the brain due to cerebral vasodilatation. The dilated blood vessels in the brain may supply the brain with more blood, but this is at the expense of increasing ICP.

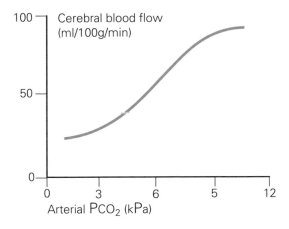

Figure 9.2 Effect of arterial carbon dioxide on cerebral blood flow

Avoid any drugs that may cause sedation or suppress respiration, since they are likely to increase CO_2 levels and/or cause oxygen desaturation. Opiates are particularly hazardous in neurology patients who have raised ICP.

Control temperature

A hot brain uses more energy and consumes more oxygen; it tolerates insults badly. Try to prevent fever in neurology patients. There is evidence that patients who are hot when they have a stroke have a worse outcome. Many hospitals now cool patients following cardiac arrest to try to prevent secondary brain damage. Use paracetamol, wet towels and ice packs. Intravenous fluids can be cooled.

Provide nutrients

Patients need to have good nutrition prior to undergoing surgery. Try to maintain oral intake. Consider nasogastric feeding particularly in patients with no gag reflex who may be at risk of aspiration. TPN may be required in certain cases. The advice of a dietician may be useful at preassessment clinic in order to optimise nutrition.

The choice of intravenous fluids in neurology patients is of paramount importance. Avoid fluids that may result in hyponatraemia, since it causes cerebral oedema. Too much normal saline however can result in a hyperchloraemic acidosis due to the high chloride content. A suitable alternative is Hartmann's (lactated Ringer's) solution. Dextrose solutions have traditionally been avoided in neurology patients since they amount to giving free water that is rapidly redistributed throughout the body potentially exacerbating cerebral oedema. In addition, neurological damage in the presence of hyperglycaemia has a worse outcome. You should start a sliding scale insulin regime early if there is concern about blood sugar levels.

Certain neurological conditions (e.g. subarachnoid haemorrhage) may result in heavy electrolyte losses, so careful management of sodium, potassium, magnesium and phosphate levels is required.

History taking in patients presenting for neurosurgery

In addition to the usual thorough preoperative assessment, you might consider the following aims:
1. Identify significant co-morbidity that may impact upon the balance of the 'happy brain' discussed above.
2. Focus on the presenting condition, consider how this might complicate the perioperative course, and predict what changes might follow surgery.

Co-morbidity may include the following aspects:

Airway

Cervical spine pathology includes rheumatoid arthritis, degenerative spondylosis, intervertebral disc prolapse or tumour. Neck movements can be limited and there may be instability of the spinal column. Severe disease may affect the function of the spinal cord (myelopathy). Anticipate airway difficulty in acromegalic patients presenting for pituitary surgery. Investigations might include lateral C/Spine X-ray in flexion and extension. The patient may require neck immobilisation, and consent for awake fibreoptic intubation by the anaesthetist. Consider an antisialagogue in these cases.

Respiratory

Chronic obstructive pulmonary disease (COPD), asthma and chest infections are common in the elderly. Patients presenting with intracranial tumours may have a primary in the lungs. Recurrent aspiration (often silent) may complicate neuro-muscular disorders, as swallowing and the cough reflex may be impaired. These conditions can cause problems with oxygenation and ventilation (removal of carbon dioxide), so consider whether optimisation is possible. Investigations might include pulmonary function tests (PFTs), chest X-ray, arterial blood gases (ABGs). Preoperative optimisation includes the use of bronchodilators, antibiotics, and physiotherapy. Surgery may need to be postponed.

Cardiovascular

Hypertension should be controlled to prevent falls in cerebral blood flow (CBF). Autoregulation maintains CBF between 60 and 100mmHg in most people. These limits may be somewhat higher, however, in chronically hypertensive patients, with the result that an intraoperative fall in blood pressure (which is not uncommon) may detrimentally decrease CBF. Resetting of these limits occurs only after hypertension has been treated for some time. Untreated hypertensives may need surgery postponing for six weeks whilst their blood pressure is controlled. Ischaemic heart disease is common in the elderly, and ideally should be stable with no evidence of heart failure. Subarachnoid haemorrhage may be complicated by ECG changes and neurogenic pulmonary oedema.

Endocrine

It is thought that hyperglycaemia may aggravate ischaemic brain injury by increasing cerebral lactic acidosis (possibly by the supply of a substrate for metabolism, glucose, when no oxygen is being delivered to the cell). Diabetes should therefore be well controlled. Steroids, used acutely for cerebral oedema, and the stress response to acute illness, may cause hyperglycaemia. Inpatients may be managed with sliding scale insulin. Blood sugars of 6–9 are acceptable.

Patients with pituitary disease may have complex endocrine disorders with excess or depletion of hormones. A specialist endocrine opinion should be sought.

Disorders of sodium balance are common in neurological patients and necessitate the checking of urine and plasma osmolalities. Diabetes insipidus manifests with a high urine output and results in hypernatraemia. Treatment often involves the administration of desmopressin. The syndrome of inappropriate antidiuretic hormone secretion (SIADH) is more common and results in hyponatraemia. It may require fluid restriction.

Examination of neurological status

It is important to be able to assess a patient's neurological condition (level of consciousness) rapidly and reproducibly. Changes in a patient's condition have to be communicated to other members of the team and to this end there are two scoring systems that are commonly used.

The Glasgow Coma Scale (GCS)

Assessment should be carried out above the level of any suspected spinal cord damage. Response to pain should be by a central stimulus. Sternal rub, nailbed pressure and trapezius pinch are all often employed, but are not central stimuli. Firm pressure on the supraorbital ridge (supraorbital nerve) is used on neurosurgical units (see Table 9.1).

Table 9.1 Glasgow Coma Scale

score	Best Motor Response	score	Best Verbal Response	score	Eyes open?
6	Obeys Commands				
5	Localises to pain	5	Orientated		
4	Withdraws to pain	4	Confused	4	Spontaneous
3	Flexes to pain	3	Inappropriate words	3	To speech
2	Extends to pain	2	Incomprehensible sounds	2	To pain
1	No response	1	None	1	None

An alert patient has a score of 15 (M6, V5, E4). Patients with a GCS of less than 9 are rarely able to protect their airway (absent gag/cough) and so are at risk of hypoxia, raised CO_2 and further deterioration by aspiration of gastric contents. A drop of two or more points on this scale, or an absolute score of less than 9, should prompt immediate medical review. The minimum score is 3 (M1, V1, E1) for a patient who has no response at all.

AVPU score

This is an easier scale that is often used for rapid assessment (see Table 9.2).

Table 9.2 AVPU score

AVPU score	Assessment	Corresponding GCS
A	Alert	14–15
V	Responds to Voice	11–14
P	Responds to Pain	7–11
U	Unconscious	3–7

The approximate GCS scores are given for comparison; it is evident that a 'P' (responds to pain) may give cause for immediate concern, since the GCS could be less than 9 as discussed above.

In addition to assessment of the level of consciousness it is important to document:

1. Pupillary size and response to light, as part of ongoing neurological observations.
2. Motor function of upper and lower limbs bilaterally, where GCS allows.
3. Findings of a full neurological examination. This is normally performed by the admitting clinician and is an important baseline.

Investigations

NICE guidelines for routine preoperative investigation are available, and are intended to avoid over-investigation of healthy patients. Neurosurgical units have their own protocols, but investigations should be prompted by findings in the history and examination.

Full blood count (FBC). Intercurrent infection associated with a raised white cell count or inflammatory markers (e.g. CRP/ESR) may delay surgery where implants are planned (metalwork, shunts).

Group and save (Screen)/**Cross match** (G&S/X-match). Craniotomy and major spinal surgery requires blood cross matching, although blood transfusion is rarely required. An agreed 'tariff' is usually available.

Urea and electrolytes (U&Es). Intravenous contrast agents are avoided in patients with renal impairment. Disorders of salt balance are common in sick and elderly patients, and those with endocrine disorders. The serum sodium may be high or low; a cause should be sought and treated.

Random blood glucose. Poor glycaemic control may worsen outcome in the brain injured; perioperative steroids may cause hyperglycaemia. Consideration should be given to the avoidance of dextrose-containing solutions in the management of diabetic patients. (Intravenous dextrose infusion is included in most intravenous insulin protocols, to protect from inadvertent hypoglycaemia. The free water given in such protocols may, however, worsen cerebral oedema.)

Coagulation screen. Intraoperative bleeding would make most neurosurgical procedures difficult, and be catastrophic in some. Coagulopathy should be investigated and corrected. Patients on long-term anticoagulants (e.g. warfarin), including anti-platelet agents (e.g. aspirin, clopidogrel) need careful management to minimise the risks of discontinuing treatment. Specialist haematology advice should be sought and local guidelines should be agreed.

Pulmonary function tests (PFTs). Problems with oxygenation and carbon dioxide retention may compromise the needs of the injured brain, or cause intraoperative brain swelling. Results of PFTs help guide preoptimisation where a reversible element is present (e.g. asthmatic component of COPD). A record of peak expiratory flow rate, where kept, should be examined to confirm stability in asthmatics.

Chest X-ray (CXR). Baseline in severe disease, exclusion of lung primary in patients with cerebral metastasis.

Arterial blood gases (ABGs). Rarely indicated as most neurosurgical interventions do not compromise lung function; history (exercise tolerance) and examination (respiratory rate, lung fields, pulse oximetry in air) are usually sufficient. Patients with severe respiratory or neuromuscular disease or those with bulbar palsies should have a baseline check.

Electrocardiogram (ECG). Neurosurgery is usually only considered in fit patients, but many are elderly, or have an exercise tolerance masked by the pain or weakness of their presenting condition. An ECG is mandatory following subarachnoid haemorrhage (SAH), since some myocardial damage can occur.

Pregnancy test. Intraoperative X-ray screening, particularly for lumbar surgery, presents some risk in pregnancy, and a pregnancy test should be performed on admission for surgery. Radiology departments may have local policies in this respect.

Premedication/Usual medication

Anxiolytics can be used where anxiety may, understandably, be a problem. Marked anxiety can contribute to hypertension and benzodiazepine premedication can be useful, but must not be administered until informed consent has been obtained.

Antisialagogue (drying) agents may be useful if an awake fibreoptic intubation is planned.

Anti-emetics should be prescribed with reference to local policy. Neurosurgery is usually considered medium risk for postoperative nausea, but the consequences of vomiting in those with swollen brains/obtunded airway reflexes would be significant.

Analgesia to treat ongoing pain must continue up to surgery. Simple analgesics, non-steroidals and opioid-based drugs may all be used. Consideration should be given to postoperative analgesia.

Patients on **chronic opioids**, and opioid abusers, need careful management; protocols exist and liaison with the acute pain team is vital.

Timely **discontinuation** of warfarin, anti-platelet agents (aspirin, clopidogrel), antihypertensive agents and oral hypoglycaemics, will prevent unnecessary cancellation of surgery. Discontinuing drugs is done on a balance of risks only after careful consideration.

Patients taking **anti-epileptics** (e.g. phenytoin) may need levels checking.

Steroid medication may need to be converted to intravenous dosing and should be continued perioperatively. Dexamethasone is often given during craniotomy.

Neurosurgical conditions

Intracranial

In general, mass lesions in the brain present with focal (localising) neurology, symptoms and signs of raised intracranial pressure (headache, vomiting, papilloedema, drowsiness), seizures, or occasionally are found incidentally during imaging for other reasons.

Scheduling of surgery tends to be more urgent than other surgical specialties; fewer elective cases mean the planning of preoperative assessment needs to be flexible. Patients admitted on-call may require surgery in a planned manner before discharge, but importantly there are some patients who require surgery as true emergencies, often admitted directly to theatre.

Examples of emergency intracranial surgery

- Intracranial haemorrhage. Bleeding can occur into different compartments in the brain, e.g. epidural/subdural/subarachnoid (see Figure 9.3).

- Cerebral abscess.

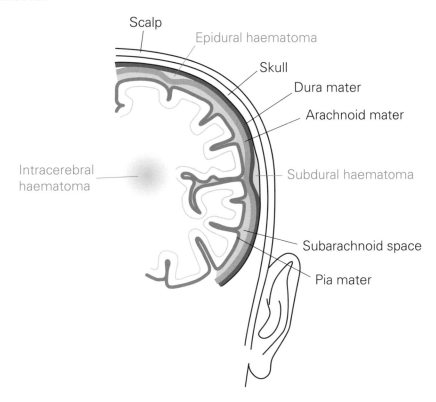

Figure 9.3
Location of epidural, subdural and intracerebral haematomas

Such neurosurgical emergencies leave little time for preoperative optimisation. If possible, a general history should be taken, with focus on neurological status and commencement of neurological observations, allowing a rapid response to any change in the patient's condition. The need for urgent surgery should not compromise acute trauma care, with attention to ABC, spinal immobilisation, secondary survey and ongoing resuscitation.

We now consider other intracranial pathologies, by specialisation.

Oncology (tumour surgery)

Supratentorial and posterior fossa mass lesions. The intracranial content is divided into compartments by dural folds. In practice two compartments are considered:

1. That above the tentorium cerebelli (supratentorial) containing the cerebral hemispheres. This compartment contains lateral and third ventricles, which contain cerebrospinous fluid (CSF) that can move from the compartment (either by circulation or absorption) and consequently compensate for expanding mass lesions.

2. That below (termed the posterior fossa) housing the cerebellum, brainstem and fourth ventricle. This is a small compartment, bound by bony structures with little room for expansion. Brainstem function can be rapidly effected by expanding lesions. Lesions here are also more likely to compress and obstruct the ventricular drainage system, causing hydrocephalus. The most common tumours are:

- Meningiomas (benign, arising from the dura and as such often vascular with risk of intraoperative bleeding). Surgery is usually intended to remove the entire tumour.
- Gliomas (malignant, arising from the cellular components of the brain, following a variable and unpredictable course).
- Metastasis. Often associated with oedema that responds to treatment with steroids. Surgery is usually intended to debulk tumour to alleviate symptoms/prolong life.

An oncology multi-disciplinary team usually plans the management of these cases. If surgery is planned, preoperative management should include continuation of steroids and anticonvulsants, and avoidance of neurological or respiratory depressants.

Stereotactic biopsy

Some intracranial lesions may require biopsy to establish/confirm a diagnosis. This is sometimes achieved by stereotactic biopsy. A frame is applied (usually under local anaesthetic) to the patient's head; the brain is imaged (e.g. CT scan) with the frame in place; the patient is transferred to theatre, where the lesion can be biopsied using co-ordinates generated by the scan, and using the frame as a fixed point of reference. Patients are understandably often very anxious.

Aneurysmal disease

Blood is supplied to the brain by the internal carotid and vertebral arteries, which join together around the base of the brain as the Circle of Willis. This arrangement is intended to protect the brain should a single vessel become blocked, as flow can be recruited from other vessels in the 'Circle'. An aneurysm occurs when there is 'outpouching' of the vessel wall. These can be associated with smoking, hypertension and a family history. The aneurysm is at increasing risk of rupture as it increases in size.

Some patients present post rupture, an emergency called subarachnoid haemorrhage (SAH). Life-threatening complications of this dangerous condition include re-bleeding, cardiovascular and respiratory problems and spasm of the intracranial blood vessels (vasospasm). Patients considered at risk need their aneurysm securing, either surgically, by placing a clip across the neck of the aneurysm, or radiologically, by packing the aneurysm sac with detachable titanium coils (coiling).

Patients will need careful preoperative assessment to exclude neurological, cardiac and respiratory complications. Nimodipine (a calcium antagonist shown to decrease severity of vasospasm post subarachnoid haemorrhage) should be continued up to surgery/coiling. An ECG is essential, chest X-ray (CXR) is useful; results and scans, including cranial CTs and angiograms, should be made available.

Arterio-venous malformations (AVMs)

Vascular malformations, which include AVMs, are a cause of intracranial bleed, or may present with seizures or neurological deficit. Preoperative management is as for aneurysmal disease, but a third option for treatment in some cases includes stereotactic gamma irradiation – see stereotactic radiosurgery below.

Endocrine

Tumours of the **pituitary** gland are quite common (8–15% of all symptomatic intracranial tumours); its complex endocrine function, and positioning within the cranial cavity, can lead to a number of different presentations. Preoperative investigation should be in conjunction with an endocrinologist. The usual surgical approach is transnasal transphenoidal resection.

Pituitary adenomas secreting growth hormone may cause **acromegaly**, which can make the airway difficult intraoperatively (macroglossia, malocclusion and upper airway lymphoid tissue excess). Diabetes is common, as are hypertension and cardiomegaly. Postoperatively the difficult airway can contribute to airway obstruction if the nose has been packed. Hormone replacement may be required.

Shunt

The ventricular drainage systems are subject to obstruction by tumours, trauma and intra-cerebral/SAH. Obstruction causes hydrocephalus (other causes include congenital abnormality) and the increase in intracranial pressure may require treatment. This can be done in a number of ways, but shunting CSF from the ventricle to the peritoneal cavity is often employed (a V-P Shunt).

Patients are often children, or have had numerous previous shunts in childhood. Signs and symptoms of raised ICP may be present.

Functional

These are highly specialised procedures for patients with movement disorders such as Parkinsonism, dystonia and tremor. One example is deep brain stimulators. Electrodes are placed, guided by neuroimaging, within the brain. The patient may be awake during the procedure (to optimise electrode placement) and intraoperative transfers for neuroimaging may be required. The electrodes are stimulated, and where benefit is seen, connected to an implanted stimulator, usually at a second operation. The surgeon might request that medical treatment is omitted preoperatively to exacerbate dystonia. However for some patients dystonia is so severe that a general anaesthetic is required for surgery.

Epilepsy

Patients with medically resistant epilepsy may be considered for neurosurgery. Operations include craniotomy to excise/disconnect the focus of seizures such as amygdalohippocamp-ectomy and corpus callosotomy. These are complex patients, often with other neurological problems; communication can often be difficult. A carer who knows the patient well can be very helpful.

An alternative procedure to craniotomy that is helpful for some patients is implantation of a **vagal nerve stimulator**. During general anaesthesia an electrode is wound around the left vagus nerve (through a small incision in the neck), and connected to a stimulator, which is implanted.

Preoperative assessment should focus on epilepsy history and medication, which should be continued, and consideration given to the social needs of these patients.

Extracranial

Vascular

Carotid endarterectomy is a surgical technique to widen the carotid artery at the neck. Patients usually present with recurrent 'mini-strokes' (TIAs) due to a stenosis (stricture) of these vessels. The procedure may be performed under local or general anaesthesia. These patients often have cardiovascular co-morbidity, and a careful cardiovascular history and examination are important.

Spinal decompression

Conditions affecting the spinal cord may present:

1. electively; e.g. unremitting sciatica
2. urgently; e.g. cervical myelopathy
3. emergently; e.g. epidural abscess, cauda equina syndrome.

Surgery, which usually entails some form of decompression, may be required at one or more levels:

- craniocervical (usually a posterior approach)
- cervical spine (usually an anterior approach)
- thoraco-lumbar spine (usually a posterior approach).

Where the spine is unstable, fixation is required with grafts or metalwork.

Patients usually have restricted mobility secondary to pain or weakness, and the cardiorespiratory system may be difficult to assess. Degenerative disease is more common in the elderly and co-morbidity should be sought. Remember that rheumatoid arthritis is a multisystem disease. Chronic pain is common, and analgesia can be a challenge.

Complex spinal surgery

More complex surgery may be required for spinal tumours or instability. As with other major surgery perioperative problems are more likely and a high dependency bed should be available.

Chronic pain/palliative

Procedures such as spinal cord stimulators and intrathecal pumps are sometimes used in the chronic pain or palliative setting. These patients may have a number of co-morbidities and a complicated drug history.

Stereotactic radiosurgery

Gamma irradiation can be focused on some intracranial pathologies using a specialised radiotherapy machine – the gamma knife. Slow-growing tumours which cannot be accessed surgically because of their proximity to vital brain structures, and vascular malformations are two examples.

The patient has a frame fixed to their head (which can be done under local anaesthetic). They are imaged with the frame in situ, and co-ordinates (fiducials) are calculated for the gamma knife to target the lesion. If a general anaesthetic is required (patients are often paediatric, or may be claustrophobic or unable to lie still/flat), the procedure may involve a number of transfers from one location to another, under prolonged anaesthesia.

Diagnostic and interventional radiology

Although minimally invasive, patients having investigations or procedures in the radiology suite are still at some risk and require the same preoperative assessment as those undergoing surgery in theatres. In particular, any allergy to radiocontrast media, evidence of renal impairment, and a negative pregnancy test (where appropriate) should be documented. Patients may require anaesthetising if procedures are very prolonged, or they are required to keep very still.

Neuromedical conditions

Concurrent disease may affect all systems of the body. Remember to fully assess the cardiovascular and respiratory systems in all patients and take a good medication history.

Autonomic dysfunction

The autonomic nervous system regulates key functions of the body including the activity of the heart muscle, the smooth muscles (e.g., the muscles of the intestinal tract), and the glands. Possible causes of a disruption in this regulation include: diabetes mellitus, Guillain Barré syndrome, Parkinson's disease and Shy-Drager syndrome.

Look for postural hypotension (decreased BP or dizziness when altering posture, e.g. changing from lying to sitting), sweating disorder, and gastrointestinal problems such as constipation. An

ECG can be done while the patient performs a Valsalva manoeuvre (involves trying to breathe out through a closed glottis) with particular attention paid to the RR variability. Sympathetic skin response and sweat tests may be requested. Optimisation may include increased salt intake, fludrocortisone and graded compression stockings or even IV fluids to increase plasma volume.

Chronic spinal cord lesions

After an initial period of flaccidity these patients suffer from spasticity and increased reflexes. Depression and phantom pain may complicate their perioperative care.

Autonomic dysreflexia can be a serious problem. Any stimulus (e.g. cutaneous, blocked bladder catheter or bowel distension) can trigger an acute sympathetic discharge. This may cause hypertension, flushing, headache and arrhythmias. If untreated it can cause myocardial ischaemia and strokes. Patients will often be aware that they have such symptoms and need to have any triggers minimised. Prevention of blocked catheters is vital. Renal problems are increased so function should be assessed with UandEs. Check PFTs. Patients with respiratory muscle weakness and difficulty coughing will require extra physiotherapy and maybe high dependancy unit (HDU) care including non-invasive ventilation. Preoperative blood gases may be required.

Spinals are frequently used in these cases to ablate visceral and peripheral stimuli. Avoid clexane within 6 hours of surgery. Incidence of latex allergy is increased.

Dementia

This may take the form of senile or presenile dementia (Alzheimer's). Impaired memory is followed by impaired thought and speech and finally complete helplessness.

Written reminders about perioperative starvation and medications are useful in the early stages. To avoid overtaxing the patient, the number of people looking after them should be kept to a minimum. A close family member or carer may provide a more accurate medical and surgical history, including past response to drugs, and a current list of medications prescribed. They should be encouraged to remain with the patient prior to surgery to ensure compliance with preoperative instructions and with medication, perioperative starvation and fluid prescription. Postoperatively they will also help reorient and reassure the person with dementia emerging from anaesthesia. They may help to protect against falls and the accidental removal of catheters and intravenous lines.

The patient should be kept warm and well hydrated perioperatively because hypothermia and dehydration can contribute to postoperative confusion.

Anaesthesia can contribute to postoperative cognitive dysfunction (POCD). Unfortunately there is no evidence that regional anaesthesia protects from this state. This group of patients may have a delayed recovery from general anaesthesia and they are at greater risk of an acute confusional state.

Acute confusional state is seen frequently in hospitalised patients of any age, but particularly in geriatric patients with dementia. Clinically there is clouding of consciousness, memory impairment, impaired cognitive function, impaired perception, disturbance of emotion, and depression of psychomotor activity, but repetitive, stereotyped activity such as plucking at bedclothes or tossing from side to side may be seen.

Epilepsy

Find out about frequency of seizures, their type and pattern and any triggering factors (e.g. flashing lights, etc). A complete drug history is vital; some drugs such as phenytoin may necessitate plasma levels and further loading. The drugs can all be given (via nasogastric tube if necessary) even when a patient is fasting preoperatively. In patients with ongoing absorbtion problems, IV phenytoin or phenobarbitone can be used. Complications such as anaemia, thrombocytopenia and hyponatraemia and deranged liver function should be excluded with the appropriate blood tests. Most patients will benefit from a benzodiazepine premed.

Guillain Barré

Patients have a progressive weakness of more than one limb. This usually ascends symmetrically and is due to peripheral nerve demyelination. They must be assessed for bulbar problems and chronic aspiration. PFTs are essential since respiratory muscles are frequently affected. Dehydration and electrolyte abnormalities should be excluded with blood tests. Excessive sweating and postural hypotension may allude to autonomic dysfunction; an ECG is indicated. Invasive cardiovascular monitoring will usually be required. HDU facilities should be available postoperatively.

Motor neurone disease (MND)

This progressive disorder is due to degeneration of motor neurones in the brain and spinal cord. Symptoms include spastic limb weakness, atrophy of muscles with fasciculation and bulbar palsies (problems swallowing with risk of aspiration). Later on respiratory muscle weakness may lead to problems breathing and coughing. Specific tests of diaphragmatic function include mouth occlusion pressures and looking for a >30% decrease in vital capacity when lying flat. Ask about dyspnoea when lying flat. Most cases that are unsuitable for regional anaesthesia (preferred technique), should be prepared as for awake intubation including acid aspiration prophylaxis.

Multiple sclerosis (MS)

Inflammation of white matter in the central nervous system leads to what can be a progressive disorder characterised by optic neuritis, limb weakness, bladder and bowel dysfunction. Symptoms may relapse and remit and could include dysarthria, dysphagia, depression or cognitive decline. Patients may be on steroid medication. Symptoms of bulbar dysfunction with aspiration as well as evidence of relapse should be noted. Poor respiratory function may require

PFTs and ABGs. There is no evidence that anaesthesia can precipitate a relapse of MS; however high concentrations of local anaesthetics, for example in epidurals, may cause a relapse. Severe demyelination of the spinal cord can lead to autonomic dysreflexia. This can result in a dangerous autonomic response (hypertension, bradycardia, flushing) to stimuli below the level of demyelination. The presence of contractures or pressure sores makes careful positioning essential. Treat pyrexia aggressively since it may cause a relapse.

Duchennes muscular dystrophy

This is a genetic condition in which patients have atrophy and weakness of muscles. Repeated aspirations and spinal deformities can restrict respiratory reserve even though PFTs may be normal. Look for tachypnoea with small Tidal Volume (Vt) and a paradoxical breathing pattern. There is an association with malignant hyperthermia so a review of previous anaesthetics is essential. They should all have PFTs, chest X-rays, blood gases, ECG and echo if there are any signs of cardiomyopathy. Risk of aspiration is attenuated by giving a proton pump inhibitor and full starvation for six hours. Make sure an HDU/ITU bed is available before undertaking surgery.

Dystrophia myotonica

This is an autosomal dominant condition which presents usually in the third decade. Involuntary continuation of muscle contractions occurs after stimulation. The condition is provoked by cold. Muscle weakness with atrophy is the main feature. Potassium supplements may make symptoms worse. Avoid hypothermia and shivering. Patients with this condition are prone to arrhythmias and aspiration.

Myaesthenia gravis (MG)

Antibodies to the acetyl choline receptor result in muscle weakness with fatigability. Take a careful drug history. Assess the gag reflex since bulbar involvement may result in chronic aspiration so preoperative physiotherapy may be helpful. PFTs and ABGs will give some idea as to the need for postoperative ITU or ventilation (e.g. VC < 2.9L). It is also increased if MG has been present for more than six years; this possibility needs to be discussed with the patient. Continue the anticholinesterase therapy (e.g. pyridostigmine) as long as possible. Some advocate a course of steroids preoperatively. MG is associated with thyroid disease as well as systemic lupus erythematosus (SLE) and pernicious anaemia. Patients may be immunosuppressed and prone to infection.

Muscle relaxants and neurological disease

With any systemic neurological disease, monitoring of the effect of muscle relaxation is mandatory. This is carried out using a Train of Four (ToF) monitor or more accurately using acceleromyography.

Table 9.3 lists a few conditions and the consequence of depolarising (e.g. suxamethonium) and non-depolarising (e.g. vecuronium) muscle relaxants.

Table 9.3 Muscle relaxants and neurological conditions

	Non-depolarising MR	**Suxamethonium**
Myaesthenia gravis	May have increased sensitivity. Wide variation in dose requirements.	Resistance has been reported. 1.5mg/kg usually enough. Cholinesterase levels correlated with recovery time
Myotonia	May not guarantee relaxation or prevent myotonia.	Can lead to prolonged paralysis/contraction. Avoid.
Muscular dystrophy	May be prolonged. Electro-myography may not reflect respiratory muscle function.	Contraindicated.
Motor neurone disease	Small initial dose and monitor.	Avoid (K+ release).

Suxamethonium may also cause potassium ion (K+) release (due to up-regulation of acetylcholine receptors) in patients after burns, those on prolonged bed rest, as well as those with spinal cord injury, major muscle denervation (e.g. Guillain Barré) or hemiparetic stroke. Some advocate caution in patients with MS and Charcot–Marie–Tooth syndrome.

Parkinson's

Parkinson's disease comprises a classical triad of resting tremor, muscle rigidity, and bradykinesia, with additional loss of postural reflexes. Parkinson's occurs as the result of a loss of dopamine-producing nerve cells in the substantia nigra. This disrupts the normal passage of messages to the basal ganglia. With the depletion of dopamine, these parts of the brain which coordinate movement are unable to function normally.

It is the commonest movement disorder and affects 3% of people over 65 years. Patients may present for other surgery but may also now be admitted for neurosurgical treatment, which involves stereotactic deep brain stimulation.

Patients may have concurrent dementia or depression. Autonomic dysfunction (see above) necessitates an ECG since they have increased incidence of arrhythmias. A baseline chest X-ray is useful to exclude atelectasis. They may have excess salivation and may have more risk of aspiration with upper airway dysfunction. Consider placing a catheter. Great care must be taken with management of antiparkinsonian drugs. Try not to allow disruption. The 'on-off' timing of the symptoms may dictate timing of surgery. Try to keep the patient warm since they have impaired thermoregulation. These patients may be at increased risk of dementia and postoperative cognitive dysfunction (POCD). Avoid anti-dopaminergic drugs such as metoclopramide and droperidol.

Psychiatric disorders

Anxiety disorders: these patients need sympathetic care. All drugs can be continued perioperatively. Premedication with benzodiazepines or beta-blockers is useful.

Depression: ECG is indicated with tricyclic antidepressants. These patients may be at increased risk of urinary retention. Patients on monoamine oxidase inhibitors (MAOIs) should avoid foods containing tyramine (e.g. cheese).

Manic disorders: Patients taking lithium should have plasma lithium levels checked since there is a narrow therapeutic window. The ECG may also be affected, and UandEs are indicated to exclude electrolyte imbalance.

Schizophrenia: Drugs can cause extrapyramidal symptoms (e.g. dyskinesis similar to Parkinsonism). Check for postural hypotension.

Recreational drugs

Various chemical substances and drugs are increasingly used recreationally in social settings. Healthcare professionals must be aware of the increasing abuse of these drugs and be able to recognise and manage serious reactions.

MDMA ('ecstasy') increases the release of neurotransmitters. The desired effects are euphoria, a feeling of intimacy, altered visual perception, enhanced libido, and increased energy. The most common adverse effects are agitation, anxiety, tachycardia, and hypertension. More serious adverse effects include arrhythmias, hyperthermia, and rhabdomyolysis.

Flunitrazepam is a potent benzodiazepine. At higher doses, the drug can cause lack of muscle control and loss of consciousness. Other adverse effects are hypotension, dizziness, confusion, and occasional aggression.

Ketamine is a dissociative anaesthetic used primarily in veterinary practice. It may be injected, swallowed, snorted, or smoked. Ketamine interacts with the N-methyl-D-aspartate channel. Analgesic effects occur at lower doses and amnesic effects at higher doses. Cardiovascular and respiratory toxicity may occur, as well as confusion and delirium.

GHB is a naturally occurring fatty acid derivative of [gamma]-aminobutyric acid that was originally used as a dietary supplement. Increasing doses progressively produce amnesia, drowsiness, dizziness, euphoria, seizures, coma, and death.

CONCLUSION

This chapter has given an overview of assessment and care for the patient undergoing neurological surgery. For more detailed understanding, the further reading list below will give the reader a wider perspective. It is important to understand in perioperative care that neurological conditions are relatively common and can present challenges in their assessment and subsequent management. Neurosurgical perioperative care is a more specialised field where expert advice and experience is required in relatively minor cases.

FURTHER READING

Arun K. Gupta and Andrew C. Summors (2001). *Notes in Neuroanaesthesia and Critical Care.* London: Greenwich Medical Media.

Joanne V. Hickey (2003). *Clinical Practice of Neurological and Neurosurgical Nursing* 5th edn. Philadelphia: Lippincott Williams.

Mary Jane Evans (1995). *Neurologic-Neurosurgical Nursing* 2nd edn. Philadelphia: Springhouse.

B. Matta, D. Menon and J. Turner (2000). *Textbook of Neuroanaesthesia and Critical Care.* London: Greenwich Medical Media.

Chapter **10** The role of haematology in preoperative assessment

Andrew Blann

SUMMARY

This chapter will outline:

- the basis of the main haematological investigations
- what these blood tests can tell us about the patient
- red blood cells and white blood cells in surgery
- the role of coagulation and anti-coagulation in surgery.

INTRODUCTION

Haematology involves the study of the form and function of the following blood components: red blood cells, white blood cells, platelets and coagulation proteins, the latter two components being important to form a clot (or thrombus). The haematology laboratory commonly provides support for preoperative assessment in the form of haematology investigations of which the most frequently requested is the full blood count and the coagulation screen. These tests will allow the preoperative assessor a view of the ability of the patient's blood to deliver oxygen to the tissues, and also an opportunity to pick up any abnormality that may affect the patient during the perioperative period, especially with respect to the patient's coagulation status.

The results of these investigations may require the practitioner to instigate changes in the patient's on-going care in an effort to avoid the potential delay or cancellation of this surgery. Common issues identified relate to either anaemia or a coagulopathy but may identify previously unidentified disease states such as leukaemia or aplastic anaemia. The haematology laboratory will therefore offer additional support to the practitioner in providing the expertise to advise and to agree to these changes in consultation with other members of the multi-disciplinary team such as the surgeon and the anaesthetist as well as providing information for the patient. These changes should be instigated well in advance of planned surgery but may need expediting if required in the emergency setting, such as reversal of anti-coagulation prior to emergency surgery.

The origin of blood cells

There are three types of cells found in blood – red blood cells (erythrocytes), white blood cells (leucocytes) and platelets (thrombocytes). These are produced in the bone marrow from differentiation of stem cells in response to stimuli such as hormones, whose production can be increased in response to pathological processes such as infection and sepsis. An outline diagram (Figure 10.1) shows the differentiation of the stem cells into the various categories of blood cells.

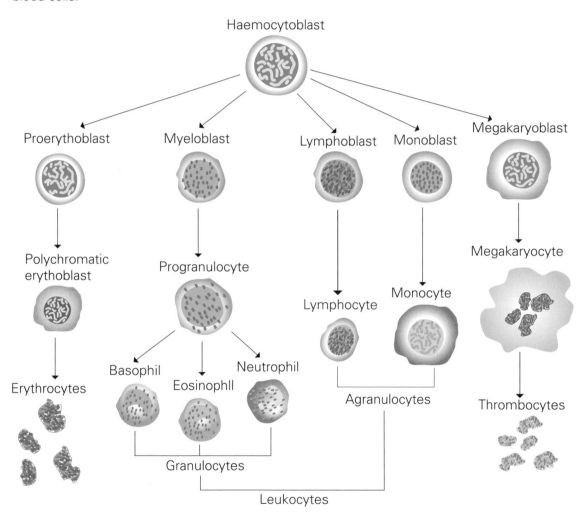

Figure 10.1 The development of blood cell types from the undifferentiated stem cells in the bone marrow. The white blood cells (leucocytes) can be divided into granulocytes and agranulocytes, the former consisting of basophils, eosinophils and neutrophils and the latter consisting of lymphocytes and monocytes.

Further information about the differentiation of the blood cell types and the pathological diseases such as leukaemia can be found in specific haematology textbooks.

The production of these blood cells can be affected by pathological processes and this may lead to failure to produce sufficient red blood cells, which will lead to anaemia, failure to produce sufficient white blood cells (leukopenia), which will lead to infections, whilst insufficient platelets (thrombocytopenia) will lead to bruising and bleeding. Each of these low levels may be present by themselves, though low levels of all three types occur simultaneously – this is known as pancytopenia. This is often seen in patients undergoing chemotherapy and radiotherapy associated with cancer, as the bone marrow is very sensitive to these toxic drugs. Routine monitoring is required to evaluate the impact of these drugs on the bone marrow of such patients.

The most common serious bone marrow disease is leukaemia, which is caused by a failure to correctly regulate the number of white blood cells being produced. Not only are there increased numbers of white blood cells generated, but also those that are produced are immature and cannot fulfil their function of defending us from infections. As the tumour of immature white blood cells grows inside the bone marrow, the production of the two other types of blood cells, red blood cells and platelets, is also affected, and levels fall, leading to anaemia and thrombocytopenia.

Haematological investigations

The two commonest requested haematological investigations from the preoperative assessment clinic are the full blood count (FBC) and the coagulation screen. Historically an allied test – the ESR or erythrocyte sedimentation rate – was requested as a measure of the physical property of the blood. Its use has reduced significantly over the last two decades as it shares common ground with the 'gold standard' serum marker of inflammation – C reactive protein (CRP). It is now rarely requested within the preoperative assessment environment.

Full blood count and coagulation screen require blood to be collected into specific blood collection bottles, each requiring a specific anticoagulant prior to processing. FBC requires the anticoagulant ethylene diamine tetra-acetic acid (EDTA), while the coagulation screen requires the anticoagulant sodium citrate. Practitioners must check with the laboratory of their specific healthcare organisation as to the particular specifications of their organisation's blood collection tubes as this may vary with geography and supplier. Collection into the incorrect tubes will require duplication of the investigation, much to the annoyance of the patient, and may delay the eventual surgical procedure.

Full blood count (FBC)

The FBC provides numerous results: those of red blood cells, of white blood cells, and of the number of platelets. An example of the results of a full blood count is displayed in Figure 10.2.

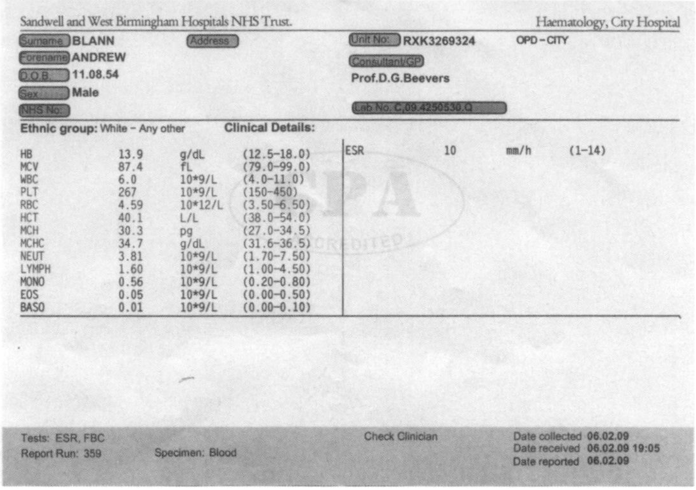

Sandwell and West Birmingham Hospitals NHS Trust. Haematology, City Hospital

Surname BLANN | Address | Unit No: RXK3269324 | OPD - CITY

Forename ANDREW | Consultant/GP Prof.D.G.Beevers

D.O.B. 11.08.54

Sex Male

NHS No: | Lab No. C,09.4250530.Q

Ethnic group: White - Any other | Clinical Details:

HB	13.9	g/dL	(12.5-18.0)	ESR	10	mm/h	(1-14)
MCV	87.4	fL	(79.0-99.0)				
WBC	6.0	10*9/L	(4.0-11.0)				
PLT	267	10*9/L	(150-450)				
RBC	4.59	10*12/L	(3.50-6.50)				
HCT	40.1	L/L	(38.0-54.0)				
MCH	30.3	pg	(27.0-34.5)				
MCHC	34.7	g/dL	(31.6-36.5)				
NEUT	3.81	10*9/L	(1.70-7.50)				
LYMPH	1.60	10*9/L	(1.00-4.50)				
MONO	0.56	10*9/L	(0.20-0.80)				
EOS	0.05	10*9/L	(0.00-0.50)				
BASO	0.01	10*9/L	(0.00-0.10)				

Tests: ESR, FBC | Check Clinician | Date collected 06.02.09

Report Run: 359 | Specimen: Blood | Date received 06.02.09 19:05

Date reported 06.02.09

Figure 10.2 Full blood count result of a middle-aged healthy male patient, showing information relating to the three cellular components, red blood cells, white blood cells and platelets

Red blood cells

The important red blood cell measurements are haemoglobin (Hb), the red blood cell count (RBC in Figure 10.2) and haematocrit (Hct). There are also three other red cell indices: mean cell volume (MCV), mean cell haemoglobin (MCH) and mean cell haemoglobin concentration (MCHC) – the MCV being the most useful.

Haemoglobin is undoubtedly the index most frequently referred to in clinical haematology. It is a protein designed to carry oxygen from the lungs to the tissues, where the oxygen is given up to participate in respiration. The normal range varies between the sexes. Lower levels in menstruating women seem obvious, but in post-menopausal women levels are still lower than age-matched men as the latter produce testosterone to stimulate red cell production. Haemoglobin is carried in the blood in red blood cells, the number of which is provided as the red blood cell count (RBC). Red cells are unusual as they lack a nucleus, which gives additional flexibility, allowing the cells to penetrate the smallest capillaries. They are the most abundant cell in the blood, are often called erythrocytes, and numbers can also vary between the sexes, being lower in women.

The haematocrit (Hct) expresses that proportion, as a decimal or as a percentage, of whole blood that is taken up by all the blood cells. Since there are approximately a thousand more red blood cells than both white blood cells and (tiny) platelets, the red cells make up the major proportion of the haematocrit. Consequently, at the practical level, it provides an idea of the proportion of red blood cells that makes up the whole blood pool.

The other red blood cell indices are the mean cell volume (MCV), which is the size of the average (mean) red blood cell. Note the stress is on 'average', as each index is the mean of millions of individual cells. The mean cell haemoglobin (MCH), as the name implies, simply reports the average amount (mass) of haemoglobin in the average cell. It does not take into account the size of the cell. Mean cell haemoglobin concentration (MCHC) is the average concentration of haemoglobin inside the average size cell. These indices are useful in diagnosing causes of anaemia, such as a microcytic anaemia which occurs with iron deficiency or a macrocytic anaemia with folate deficiency.

White blood cells
The white blood cell indices reported include the white cell count (WCC) and the differential. The latter is actually five different results – it tells us of the different proportions of the various types of white cells. These are (in order of frequency) neutrophils, lymphocytes, monocytes, eosinophils and basophils (see Figure 10.2). All these cells perform different tasks in defending us from attack by micro-organisms, and additionally take part in processes such as hypersensitivity reactions, e.g. hay fever. There may also be some unusual cells called blasts or atypical cells, and in high numbers these are likely to have considerable adverse consequences.

Platelets
These tiny bodies are fragments of a much larger cell found only in the bone marrow (the megakaryocyte). With no nucleus, they consist only of cytoplasm, but this extremely potent cytoplasm is packed full of chemicals. Platelets form a clot, or thrombus, when aggregated together with the help of the blood protein fibrin, and so minimise haemorrhage.

Coagulation screen

This generally consists of a plasma protein (fibrinogen), two clotting times (PT and APTT), and two ratios (INR and PTT ratio). Fibrinogen is one of the more important blood proteins involved in clotting and is made in the liver. It is converted into fibrin by an enzyme, thrombin (itself derived from prothrombin, and also a product of the liver), and is crucial in clot formation.

Prothrombin time (PT) and partial thromboplastin time (PTT) are measures of the ability of blood plasma to form an artificial clot in the laboratory. Some labs place an 'A' for 'activated' in front of the PTT, thus APTT. The difference between PT and PTT is that they measure different parts of the clotting pathway, can investigate different bleeding disorders, and can also be used to monitor the effects of different drugs that interfere with different parts of the coagulation system.

The PT is commonly used to assess the efficacy of the use of the oral anticoagulant warfarin which works on (some would say poisons!) the liver to prolong the PT and so make a clot less likely to happen. We use a ratio between the normal PT (i.e. when not on warfarin) and the PT whilst the patient is on warfarin to generate the international normalised ratio (INR). Similarly, the effectiveness of the injectable anticoagulant unfractionated heparin is monitored by its effect on prolonging the PTT, which also delays clot formation. Hence someone on this heparin will have a prolonged PTT, and we use a ratio between these two versions of the PTT to ensure the correct dose of the drug: hence the PTT ratio. However, unfractioned heparin is slowly giving way to an improved preparation called low molecular weight heparin (LMWH), which does not generally need laboratory monitoring. The importance of these times, the INR, and the PTT ratio will be explained in a later section.

What tests and when?

The question of what preoperative tests are required in the preoperative assessment clinic has been raised for several years. The past practice of requesting all investigations for all patients, regardless of their medical fitness or the surgical procedure that is being performed, is legendary in the teachings among many junior medical staff who historically performed the patient's 'clerking in' on admission or in an outpatient clinic. Thankfully this approach has been challenged both from a cost perspective and from an evidence-based point of view. The National Institute for Clinical Excellence released Clinical Guidance 3 in June 2003 titled 'Preoperative tests: The use of routine preoperative tests for elective surgery'.[1] The guidelines were based upon the best available evidence, which is very limited, being only level IV evidence (that is, expert opinion derived from a consensus development process and the clinical experience of the Guideline Development Group). The NICE guidelines, however, can be used as a framework, firstly for developing local guidance and secondly to improve the evidence base in forthcoming research.

In evaluating the indices of blood tests requested, the provision of a reference range (sometimes called the normal range, or the target range) helps the practitioner in deciding if further investigations are required. There is a hope that all results will be within the reference ranges, though there are three important points to remember:

- A result in the reference range does not necessarily make the patient well, but it certainly does reduce your level of anxiety!
- And in reverse, just because a result is outside the reference range does not necessarily mean the patient is at death's door. However, the further the result is away from the reference range, then the more concerned you must be.
- References ranges are not carved in granite: they change with time and between healthcare organisations.

Broadly speaking, we need to consider results which are above or below the reference range.

Red blood cells

A full blood count can indicate two possible major abnormalities with red blood cells:

1. Not enough red blood cells – anaemia
2. Too many red blood cells – erythrocytosis or polycythaemia.

Polycythaemia is rare, though uncontrolled it has been implicated as the only abnormality of circulating blood cells that has a positive impact on perioperative morbidity. The condition may cause a possible fatal stress on the heart and cardiovascular system and may precipitate a stroke. The use of elective venesection is used to control the disease, though thorough investigation of the underlying conditin will be required as a matter of urgency.

Table 10.1 Anaemia and its causes

Type of anaemia	Hb	MCV	MCH	Possible causes
Hypochromic microcytic	Low	Low	Low	Chronic blood loss (ulcers, tumours, menorrhagia) Failure to absorb iron (post-gastrectomy) Failure to utilise iron in haemoglobin production
Normochromic normocytic	Low	Normal	Normal	'Anaemia of chronic disease' • Renal disease • Severe connective tissue disease, such as rheumatoid arthritis • Carcinoma • Bone marrow failure in chemotherapy, poisoning, leukaemia or infiltration
Macrocytic anaemia	Low	High	Normal	B_{12} or folate deficiency due to: • Diet or malabsorption • Increased demand (e.g. pregnancy)

Anaemia is a far more common diagnosis that is demonstrated with the full blood count. Anaemia may be defined as the clinical (symptomatic) consequence of the failure of the blood to deliver enough oxygen to the tissues so they can adequately perform their physiological function. In contrast, other authorities will define anaemia as a level of haemoglobin below a certain level. However, a haemoglobin level of, say, 11.5g/dL may well be perfectly adequate for an elderly woman with few physiological requirements and a relatively quiet life, while the same haemoglobin level in a younger person with a very active lifestyle, perhaps including sports, will be inadequate. Thus the medical state of the individual as a whole person should be considered, not merely an arbitrary number at which one acts. An alternative view of anaemia may be the level at which concern arises, and at which further investigations are considered. Certainly, anaemia should not be seen merely as that level that automatically requires a blood transfusion, a therapy that many consider should be reserved only for life-saving situations.

The cause of anaemia should be elucidated prior to elective surgery as much as possible.

The use of all the indices reported with a full blood count will assist with this diagnosis by determining the size and haemoglobin content of the circulating red blood cells. Table 10.1 (page 193) outlines common findings.

White blood cells

White blood cells, or leukocytes, are collectively responsible for defending us from attack by micro-organisms such as viruses, bacteria and parasites. Accordingly, raised levels of these cells (which is described as leukocytosis) can be expected in the face of infections with these microbes. However, increased numbers may also be present in a number of conditions such as rheumatoid arthritis and cancer, and also after surgery and in leukaemia. It follows, in reverse, that low levels of white blood cells (leucopenia) may be a sign that the patient could be susceptible to infections. However, the causes of unexplained low white blood cells are very rare, and of these the most common is aplastic anaemia, and if present, there is also a low red blood cell count. The most common reason for leucopenia is the effect of cytotoxic drugs on the bone marrow, a therapy only undertaken in severe disease such as cancer. In this case, the patient is most likely to be aware of this problem.

The most common white blood cells are neutrophils and lymphocytes. Low levels of neutrophils and lymphocytes are, respectively, described as neutropenia and lymphopenia. Similarly, an increased number of neutrophils is called neutrophilia, or perhaps a neutrophil leukocytosis. High numbers of lymphocytes are referred to as lymphocytosis. Neutrophils and lymphocytes have different functions.

The fundamental purpose of the neutrophils is to protect the body from bacterial infections, such as may be caused by staphylococcal and streptococcal organisms. One mechanism by which neutrophils perform this function is to engulf the bacteria, and then kill and digest them with the help of intracellular enzymes and chemicals (phagocytosis). Another of the white blood cells, the monocyte, is also able to digest bacteria. Hence both neutrophils and monocytes may be described as phagocytes. Consequently, high numbers of neutrophils are often associated with bacterial infections, but may also be found in autoimmune diseases such as rheumatoid arthritis. This is because in arthritis the immune and inflammatory systems attack the body's own tissues (such as the skin and joints) instead of bacteria. Increased levels of neutrophils in the absence of an infection, such as after surgery or severe exercise, are referred to as the 'acute phase response'.

The acute phase response is a collection of physiological actions that are generated by a shock to the body, often microbiological or traumatic, including iatrogenic trauma of surgery. The body is programmed to perceive this shock as a potential threat, and so initiates steps to protect itself. A typical shock is that of surgery; another is a severe infection. The actual changes of the acute phase response include a rise in blood pressure, in white blood cells (to defend against presumed microbial attack), and increase in platelet count and coagulation proteins (to defend against potential haemorrhage). An important feature of the acute phase response is that raised levels are to be expected to fall back to normal as the cause of the stress subsides.

There are two major types of lymphocytes: B lymphocytes make immunoglobulins (antibodies – proteins designed to recognise, attack, and help destroy invading pathogens – Figure 10.1, page 188) whilst T lymphocytes cooperate in antibody production and also attack cells that are infected with viruses. Whilst many lymphocytes are present in the blood, they are also to be found in lymph nodes, the bone marrow, the liver and the spleen. These organs are collectively called 'lymphoid tissue'. Mildly increased numbers of lymphocytes in the blood may be expected in conditions that also cause a raised neutrophil count. However, the highest levels often encountered in health are found during attack against viral infections, such as glandular fever. In such cases these 'activated' lymphocytes may be larger than usual, and sufficiently large to be described as blasts. However, some viruses actually kill lymphocytes, so that the number in the blood will fall, HIV being such a virus.

Platelets and coagulation proteins

Haemostasis is the technical name for the balance between an increased risk of clotting (thrombosis) and an increased risk of bleeding (haemorrhage). If this balance is disturbed then clinically important disease may result. Good haemostasis, as evidenced by 'healthy' clot formation, requires the correct activation and numbers of platelets with the correct assembly of coagulation proteins.

An increased risk for thrombosis follows from increased numbers of platelets (called thrombocytosis) and high levels of the coagulation proteins such as fibrinogen. However, platelets and fibrinogen do not normally come together to form a clot; the process of thrombosis generally requires a trigger. A good example of such a stimulus is orthopaedic surgery, which is why patients undergoing these operations are at risk of thrombosis and so need protection with anticoagulants. Thrombocytosis is often present in infections and in autoimmune diseases such as rheumatoid arthritis.

An increased risk of haemorrhage may result from low numbers of platelets (known as thrombocytopenia) and/or low levels of coagulation proteins. Drugs such as quinine and sulphonamides may cause a low platelet count, as well as poor production from the bone marrow, or excessive consumption. Low levels of coagulation proteins will be demonstrated by prolonged prothrombin and partial thromboplastin times. However, in the absence of established drug therapies such as warfarin and heparin, excess clotting times are hardly ever encountered in a routine setting. Perhaps the best-known such disease is haemophilia, caused by the lack of coagulation Factor VIII, but if present, it will have been present from childhood and very obvious to the patient and his family.

The whole topic of coagulation is very important in surgery and will be developed in great detail in a later section. Figure 10.3 (page 196) shows how the coagulation system comes together to form a clot (thrombus).

Figure 10.3 Simplified diagram of the coagulation system

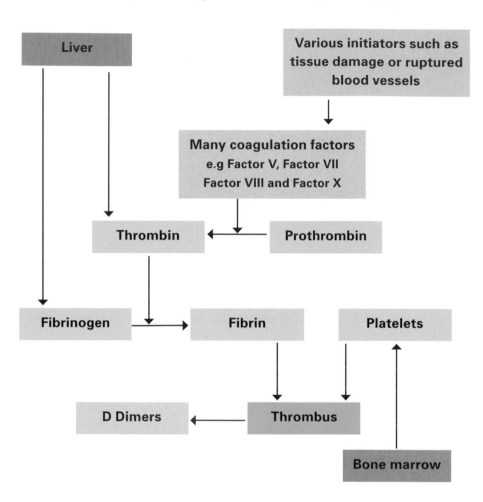

Several factors start the coagulation 'cascade', such as crush injuries, severe bacterial infections or severed blood vessels that expose collagen. Among the first coagulation factors to be activated are Factor V and Factor VII.

Later, Factor X becomes activated and so is referred to as Factor Xa. The activity of this molecule is inhibited by low molecular weight heparin (LMWH), and Factor Xa is a major contributor to the complex of Factors and other molecules whose function is to convert prothrombin into thrombin. Once formed, thrombin acts on fibrinogen to turn it into fibrin. Fibrin forms a mesh that, with platelets and other blood cells, generates a thrombus (clot) to reduce blood flow.

Table 10.2 briefly summarises the value of the full blood count and coagulation screening tests in preoperative assessment.

Table 10.2
Interpretation of major haematological tests in preoperative assessment

---

Red blood cells

- Is the patient anaemic?
- Can red blood cells provide enough oxygen to the tissues to allow them to perform their functions whilst the patient is being operated upon?
- If borderline anaemic, can the patient withstand any loss of blood during surgery?
- If so, should a number of units of packed red cells be prepared by the Blood Bank?

White blood cells

- If mildly or moderately raised: is the patient experiencing a current infection? If so, there is also likely to be a raised CRP.
- If markedly raised: does the patient have a serious disease such as leukaemia or lymphoma?
- If profoundly low: the patient may be at risk of an infection. It follows that you may well ask 'why is the patient's white blood cell count profoundly low?'

Platelets and coagulation proteins

- If thrombocytopenic (platelet count < 100): the patient may be at risk of haemorrhage, and especially so if the platelet count is < 50.
- A prolongation of PT and PTT is inevitably caused by a particular disease (such as haemophilia) or by anticoagulant drugs.

Red blood cells and white blood cells in surgery

The haematology laboratory provides the practitioner with important information not merely about the patient's general health, but also provides clues about how they may react to their surgery. As with all blood tests, the primary question in a screening setting would probably be 'Is the patient fit for surgery?'

The red blood cell, haemoglobin, and anaemia

The major concern about red blood cells before, during and after surgery, is anaemia. Although high number of red cells can be dangerous, there are few patients with this problem. However, even the textbook definition of anaemia can vary, such as a haemoglobin result of less than 12g/dL, or less than 11g/dL, or even lower values, and perhaps varying with sex. Others define anaemia as the point at which the body may suffer, or perhaps when treatment is needed. Consequently, in the light of impending surgery, a high degree of flexibility is called for.

Before surgery

The function of the red blood cell and haemoglobin is to deliver oxygen to the tissues. However, surgery increases the demand by the body for oxygen. Thus a mild or moderate anaemia may not be a problem without surgery, but under stress a smaller number of red cells may not be able to provide the amount of oxygen required. This may have severe consequences, such as a heart attack. It may also be the case that anaemia is caused by a more dangerous and hidden disease, such as pure red cell aplasia, which means that the patient may not be able to withstand the effects of the surgery.

Nevertheless, if anaemia is present, it may be treatable in the short or moderate term. If so, then this is certainly worth considering, especially if the surgery can be delayed, as in elective orthopaedic cases. If this option is taken, the patient will need to be passed to the haematologists for treatment. The time taken for anaemia to resolve depends on the basis of the disease. For example, iron-deficient anaemia may respond to oral, depot or infused iron within a month or six weeks. However, the cause of the anaemia must be investigated, as it may be related to other serious disease such as myeloma, although most common diseases can be detected by more than one sign, symptom or laboratory result. There are many possible causes of anaemia, as indicated in Table 10.3. The practitioner will be aware that few of these conditions are associated with a single abnormal result and that a broad knowledge is required to successfully confirm a diagnosis.

Table 10.3 Potential causes of anaemia

Problems with the bone marrow • Bone marrow cancer (leukaemia, lymphoma, myeloma) • Secondary cancer (originating elsewhere, e.g. breast, prostate) • Suppression (perhaps by chemotherapy)
Lack of micronutrients • Insufficient iron and vitamin B_{12} in the diet • Good diet, but malabsorption due to intestinal disease
Disease in other organs • Liver disease – this organ stores iron and synthesises crucial proteins • Renal disease – if damaged, the kidney may fail to make the growth factor erythropoietin
Destruction of mature red blood cells • Haemolytic anaemia • Infection, such as malaria • Haemoglobinopathy (sickle cell disease, thalassaemia)

Physical loss of blood
- Heavy menstrual periods
- Via a cancer in the lower intestine (colon, rectum)

If the need for the surgery is vital, perhaps acting on a life-threatening condition, then an alternative approach is to perform a short-lived but effective treatment – a blood transfusion. This is discussed in more detail in Chapter 11 of this book.

The effects of surgery

Clearly, some types of surgery can be more 'bloody' than others, especially those involving arteries. But there are several strategies to minimise blood loss, such as salvaging, followed by recycling. Despite this, surgical procedures seemingly without notable 'on table' blood loss are still associated with a fall in haemoglobin. In some cases of orthopaedic surgery, haemoglobin levels measured in the postoperative period have not reached pre-surgery levels by six weeks. Very accurate measures of blood loss indicate that the loss of a litre of blood should, in theory, lead to a fall in haemoglobin of 2.5g/dL. But in practice, this level of blood loss regularly leads to a fall of 3g/dL. This increased fall above and beyond the simple physical blood loss of surgery is well established but cannot be explained by unmeasurable blood loss (e.g. via the intestines). A healthy response to surgery sees the mobilisation of inflammatory cytokines as part of the acute phase response, and these may influence iron kinetics. For example, even simple surgery such as arthroscopy of the knee or correction of hallux valgus (with minimal blood loss) can cause a significant decrease in serum iron.

Recovery after surgery

This will be associated with a degree of reconstruction of cells and tissues and so there will be a high demand for oxygen. It is possible, therefore, that postoperative anaemia may impair recovery. However, the spleen is an effective reservoir of red blood cells, and the fact that the spleen shrinks after surgery suggests that some of these stored red cells have entered the circulation. As indicated in the previous paragraph, the red blood cell count and haemoglobin count may take months to recover.

However, red blood cell production can be actively promoted by the provision of the growth factor erythropoietin. Given subcutaneously in the perioperative period, this agent is effective in increasing levels of haemoglobin and in reducing the need for blood transfusions.

Is anaemia always bad?

It follows that the 'normal' response to surgery is to reduce the haemoglobin level. This is contrary to the clear presumption that anaemia is a disease that demands treatment. Certainly, there are numerous diseases (such as cancer, chronic heart failure and chronic renal failure) where low iron status is associated with a poor prognosis, but this may be coincidental. However, this is too simplistic since not all treatments (such as blood transfusion) are safe and beneficial. It has been argued that, in fact, some forms of anaemia are an adaptive response that may be beneficial. For example, it is established that high iron levels can promote the formation of noxious reactive oxygen species. Additionally, iron is an essential requirement of several species of pathogenic bacteria, so that minimising free iron may also restrict the growth of these organisms.

White blood cells and microbes

Leucocytes defend us from microbial attack. So whereas high levels may indicate an infection, low levels may predispose to an infection.

Before surgery
A low white blood cell count may be found in an assessment clinic. In the absence of cytotoxic chemotherapy (possibly anti-cancer, and which the surgeon and various healthcare professionals are likely to be aware of) a low white cell count is important and needs investigating. This is not merely because it may be linked with other and/or more severe diseases, but also because it may leave the patient open to attack by pathogenic microbes. Therefore, if surgery cannot be postponed, antibiotic (if neutrophils are low) or antiviral (if lymphocytes are low) prophylaxis may be necessary. However, no drug is without a side effect, and, ironically, one of the most common such side effects is suppression of the bone marrow. A compromised white cell response after surgery may lead to life-threatening septicaemia and thus a spell in intensive care.

There are a small number of reasons for a high white blood cell count (a leukocytosis). These include infection, an autoimmune disease such as lupus, and leukaemia. The latter is relatively easy to diagnose as there is also anaemia and low platelets (thrombocytopenia). It is possible that a preoperative blood sample may suggest an autoimmune disease, but if so there will be other clinical clues and a history. However, a leukocytosis is more than likely to indicate a current, possible low-grade infection. But once again, other blood tests should be informative, and there should also be an increase in CRP, the 'gold standard' marker of inflammation. If the leukocytosis does indeed suggest an infection, then postponing the surgery should be considered and the patient should be placed on antimicrobial therapy.

White blood cells do not have a great part to play during surgery. However, they are likely to be primed by the operation, as in the acute phase response.

After surgery
One of the most common and potentially life-threatening consequences of surgery is infection. As part of the acute stress response associated with surgery, the body rapidly mobilises 'dormant' white blood cells, and places them in the blood, ready in case of an infection. This is also associated with other changes, such as a rise in the CRP. Thus a modest increase in the white blood cell count after surgery does not necessarily imply an infection. However, if a leukocytosis is more marked (perhaps $12–15 \times 10^9$/L) and persistent (exceeding three to four days), then an infection will seem more and more likely.

Ideally, a leukocytosis, either as part of the acute phase response or a genuine response to an actual infection, will eventually fall. However, a persistent leukocytosis may be the consequence of an acute inflammation becoming transformed into chronic inflammation. If so, then a different class of chemotherapy may be called for.

Coagulation and surgery

The coagulation system exists to minimise blood loss and it does this by the controlled formation of a thrombus, formed from platelets and the blood protein fibrin (see Figure 10.3, page 196). Both fibrin and platelets are necessary to form a clot and an excess of either one cannot make up for a lack of the other. However, part of the normal and healthy acute phase response is an increased tendency to clot, which, if extensive, can be fatal. In such a case, prevention is essential.

Prior to surgery

It is necessary to ensure that the patient has a coagulation system that is 'capable' of functioning to minimise blood loss. A clear history of previous bleeding problems at the time of surgery, either personally for the patient or from the patient's blood relatives, needs to be elucidated, coupled with any evidence that the patient has a bleeding tendency by bruising easily or has prolonged bleeding when sustaining abrasions or cuts.

Provided that the patient is not on any antithrombotic treatment such as warfarin, the key result with such a patient initially relates to the platelet count, with further investigation of the level of fibrinogen, INR and PTT ratio. The latter two will give an indication of the workings of the two different aspects of the coagulation system. Patients with deficiencies in this pathway may be unable to form a protective thrombus and so may haemorrhage. Ideally, one would not normally operate on such patients, but life-threatening emergencies may take precedence.

Thrombocytopenia slightly below the bottom of the reference range (150×10^{12}/L) may be acceptable if the surgery is minor and blood loss is expected to be minimal. However, if the thrombocytopenia is more profound ($75–125 \times 10^{12}$/L) then a transfusion of a platelet concentrate may be appropriate, and if less than 50×10^{12}/L, transfusion would be mandatory. However, discussion between the haematologist and the surgeon and anaesthetist is important to address the risks of proceeding to surgery. The cause of the thrombocytopenia should also be determined before surgery, as this may have an impact on postoperative care. For example, in the case of immune-mediated thrombocytopenia, mediated by an autoantibody to platelets, immunosuppression with an agent such as prednisolone may be advisable.

A similar situation is present in the face of low levels of fibrinogen (possibly less than 1.0 g/L) – is the surgery really necessary, and if so, how can we improve the haemostasis of the patient? Once more, one option is a transfusion of fresh frozen plasma (FFP), which will contain fibrinogen as well as other coagulation proteins.

After surgery

A major risk of surgery is haemorrhage, and the body has its own defence system ready to cope should this occur – an increased tendency to form a clot, generally in veins. This is called venous thromboembolism, and its occurrence is a veno-thromboembolic event (therefore both abbreviated to VTE). When this happens in veins of the leg it is called a deep vein thrombosis (DVT), whereas when it happens in a vessel in the lungs it is called pulmonary embolism (PE). Not only do DVT and PE lead to considerable morbidity; clots also kill!

- A DVT leads to a swollen, painful leg such that walking can be difficult, perhaps impossible. DVTs by themselves are rarely fatal but can produce considerable long-term morbidity. There is also powerful evidence that DVT leads to PE. About two-thirds of all VTEs are DVT.

- Blockage of a crucial lung vessel (be it an artery or a vein) by a PE will lead to breathlessness and pain, can lead in the long term to congestive lung disease and heart disease, and can indeed be fatal. PEs make up about a third of all VTEs.

But how big a problem is VTE and who is likely to suffer an event? According to the House of Commons Health Committee,[2] about 10% of hospital deaths (1% of admissions) were attributable to PE. However, lower limb DVT has been documented in 50% of major orthopaedic operations performed without anti-thrombotic prophylaxis, in 25% of patients with acute myocardial infarction and in more than 50% of acute ischaemic stroke cases.

The risk of VTE after major general surgery has been extensively documented. Risk factors include abdominal or thoracic surgery requiring general anaesthesia of over 30 minutes. However, lower extremity orthopaedic operations such as total hip and knee replacement carry a particularly high risk and, without prophylaxis, about 50% develop VTE. Arthroscopy is particularly low risk, so prophylaxis is optional, depending on other risk factors. VTE is common in fracture of the pelvis, hip or long bones. Indeed, in one of the first trials of an anticoagulant, the incidence of death from PE after hip fracture fell from 10% to zero!

However, the patient may have other risk factors unrelated to surgery, such as obesity (body mass index >30), age over 60 years or cancer. Not all these risk factors and types of surgery are as dangerous as others. Depending on the risk of the different types of surgery, and on different risk factors that the patients have, they will be started on an anticoagulant. This is likely to be one of the several types of low molecular weight heparin (LMWH), such as enoxaparin, or oligosaccharide anticoagulant such as fondaparinux, and some patients may be moved on to warfarin.

Prevention and treatment of venous thromboembolism and surgery

In view of the high incidence of venous thromboembolism in the perioperative period several guidelines have been developed over the last two decades to try to reduce their incidence and also to reduce the morbidity and mortality associated with them. The guidelines identify several modalities including anticoagulant therapy as prophylaxis to be used in different clinical settings to prevent venous thromboembolism.

- Perhaps the most accessible is the British National Formulary (BNF),3 widely available in NHS hospitals and regularly updated. See http://www.bnf.org
- The British Committee on Standardisation in Haematology (BCSH) offers reasonably up-to-date guidelines for outpatient treatment of DVT with warfarin or heparin at http://www.bcshguidelines.com.
- The UK national guideline-setting body, National Institute for Health and Clinical Excellence (NICE), has released its Guideline 46, devoted to reducing the risk of thrombosis after surgery. This is available at http://www.nice.org.uk
- The National Patient Safety Agency (NPSA) has released its own guidelines on the management of the patient on warfarin, available at http://www.nrls.npsa.nhs.uk/

Local practice and management

Each healthcare organisation should have a 'thrombosis committee' to develop and issue local guidelines for the prevention of venous thromboembolism. In the UK this will be based on the NICE Guideline 46 released in April 2007, as well as the guidance from the NPSA related to the management of patients on warfarin. Each practitioner should gain access to their local guidelines for assessing the risk of each patient and ensure that the patient receives the recommended appropriate modality in their organisation in collaboration with other members of the multi-disciplinary team. Coupled with this is the need to give both verbal and written information to the patient about the risks of VTE and the effectiveness of prophylaxis.

Statement

What follows is informed comment and **NOT** guidelines.

NO responsibility is taken for their use in clinical practice.

Practitioners are expected to refer to their own Hospital Guidelines.

NB: Consider NICE Guideline 46.

Most surgical patients are likely to be at a relatively high and acute risk of thrombosis and therefore are likely to be treated with LMWH. However, it is also possible that some patients will come into hospital already taking warfarin. If so, this may need to be reduced or stopped altogether. Patients may also benefit from graduated elastic compression stockings (GECS). In many cases the risk of thrombosis will still be present after the patient is fit for discharge. If this is the case then the patient is likely to be discharged with GECS and treated with LMWH or even warfarin as an outpatient. The latter will most likely be commenced on the ward.

Risk assessment for treatment with LMWH

ALL patients (regardless of surgical indication) **MUST** be assessed prior to surgery for the risk of developing VTE to identify those at highest risk and to identify any contra-indications to thromboprophylaxis. The practitioner will identify specific risk factors and the relative score (as identified in Table 10.4) to produce a DVT risk factor score.

Table 10.4 Risk factors for VTE

Risk factors (Score 1)	Risk factors (Score 2)	Risk factors (Score 3)
Age > 60	Oestrogen-containing pill	Immobile (> 72 hours)
Obesity (BMI > 30)	Hormone replacement therapy (HRT)	History of DVT or PE
Ischaemic heart disease, congestive cardiac failure or previous stroke	Known thrombophilic conditions	
Significant chronic obstructive pulmonary disease	Malignancy	
Extensive varicose veins	Sepsis	
Inflammatory bowel disease	Known family history in two relatives (at least one first degree).	
Nephrotic syndrome	Post partum	
Myeloproliferative disorders	Pregnancy	

To this score must be added another, depending on the type of surgery (Table 10.5).

Table 10.5 Additional risk factors for surgical inpatients

Score	Surgical procedure
4	Major trauma, e.g. lower limb fractures
4	Major joint replacement
4	Surgery for fractured neck of femur

3	Thoracotomy or abdominal surgery involving mid-line laparotomy
3	Total abdominal hysterectomy, including laparoscopic assisted
2	Intraperitoneal laparoscopic surgery lasting > 30 minutes
2	Vascular surgery (not intra-abdominal)
1	Surgery lasting > 30 minutes
0	Surgery lasting < 30 minutes

The total risk score will give an initial guide to therapy, although LMWH may not be appropriate for all patients.

Contra-indications to heparin and warfarin

No drug is free of unwanted side effects, and not all patients are able to tolerate these agents. After clinical assessment has demonstrated an indication for prophylaxis with heparin or warfarin, the patient's medical and drug history must be assessed for the cautions and contra-indications to both agents. These are shown in Table 10.6.

Table 10.6 Contra-indications to heparin and warfarin

	Heparin	Warfarin
Contra-indications	Known uncorrected bleeding disorders, e.g. haemophilia	Peptic ulcer
	Severe to moderate thrombocytopenia	Severe hypertension (BP >160/100)
	Heparin allergy	Thrombocytopenia (platelet count <100)
	Heparin-induced thrombocytopenia	Bacterial endocarditis
	Heparin-induced thrombosis	Pregnancy
	Patients on existing anticoagulation therapy	Cranberry juice
	Bleeding or potentially bleeding lesions, e.g. oesophageal varices, active peptic ulcer	

Cautions	Severe hepatic and renal impairment Major trauma or surgery to the brain, eye or spinal cord	Recent surgery Alcohol abuse Previous haemorrhage Dementia Breast feeding Renal and hepatic impairment Notably, women of child-bearing age taking warfarin should be made aware of the risk of teratogenicity

Anti-platelet drugs

Aspirin is far less effective than warfarin or LMWH in reducing the risk of thrombosis. Indeed, the UK government guidelines such as NICE specifically advise against aspirin in many types of surgery. Therefore anticoagulants are preferred, saving aspirin for those who are intolerant of warfarin or LMWH, as indicated above.

Non-pharmacological treatments

All inpatients will be considered for the use of graduated elastic compression stockings (GECS). However, contra-indication and cautions apply. Contra-indications include massive oedema of the legs or pulmonary oedema from congestive cardiac failure, severe atherosclerosis of the leg, dermatitis, gangrene, and extreme deformity of the leg. Cautions include selecting the correct size, checking fitting daily for change in leg circumference, and that the top should not be folded down. GECS should be removed daily for not more than 30 minutes. Graduated elastic compression stockings may be full length, thigh length, or below knee. Most clinically important DVTs occur above the knee, which provides the rationale for using full-length stockings though knee-length may be used as a suitable alternative.

All patients, whether ambulatory or inpatient, should be mobilised as much as is practicable, and full attention should be given to adequate hydration. If the patient cannot drink, fluids should be provided intravenously.

Use of LMWH

Once (a) the patient has been assessed and found to be in need of treatment, and (b) the contra-indications or cautions to anticoagulation have been addressed, then (c) the patient must be informed and educated as to the purpose of the particular treatment, and (d) treatment can begin according to the following regimes. Depending on the risk factor score, the patients may receive none, a low dose, or a high dose of LMWH (Table 10.7). Each hospital's Thrombosis Committee should define exactly which type of LMWH is to be used.

Table 10.7 Application of risk assessment tables for the use of LMWH

Low risk: Score 0 or 1	Early ambulation, consider GECS
Moderate risk: Score 2 or 3	GECS, low dose LMWH
High risk: Score 4 or more	GECS, consider intermittent pneumatic compression in theatre, high dose LMWH
Note: For male patients <57 kg and female patients <45 kg, caution may be needed regarding the dose of LMWH prescribed. Please consult the clinician in charge of the patient's care.	

However, if LMWH is inappropriate then other anti-platelet therapy (e.g. enteric coated aspirin 75–300mg od or clopidogrel 75mg od) may be considered. Commencement on warfarin may also be considered but any of these situations should be discussed with the surgeon, anaesthetist and haematologist. However, contra-indications to aspirin exist, principally any known allergy and gastric erosions.

How much LMWH should be given?

This depends on a number of factors. First, the different varieties of LMWH all have different licences for different conditions, such as treatment of proven VTE, or the prevention of VTE that may arise from certain risky situations like orthopaedic surgery (i.e. prophylaxis). LMWHs have different potencies so the dose for one may be different from the dose for another. Some suggest doses of a certain number of milligrams, other doses are for a given number of units. Secondly, it may also be the case that doses are different for those in need of treatment foran actual DVT or PE, or in prevention of a possible VTE that may occur in the near future (i.e. prophylaxis after a high risk procedure such as hip replacement).

Prevention (prophylaxis)
A recent edition of the BNF,[3] for example, recommends the dose of a particular LMWH for the prophylaxis of DVT in low-risk surgical patients to be 20mg (2000 units) two hours before surgery, then 20mg every following 24 hours for seven to ten days. A high-risk patient by the same token needs 40mg (4000 units) 12 hours before surgery and additional 40mg doses every 24 hours for seven to ten days. However, for medical patients, the dose is 40mg every 24 hours for at least six days and until ambulant, to a maximum of 14 days. Practitioners must consult the latest edition of the BNF, as recommendations and licensed applications are subject to change.

Treatment (i.e. the patient has suffered a DVT/PE)
However, the same BNF recommends a dose of 1.5mg/kg (150 units/kg) of the same LMWH

every 24 hours for the treatment of a proven DVT/PE for at least five days and until adequate oral anticoagulation has been established. So an 80kg patient may receive 20mg for prevention, but six times as much (80 x 1.5 = 120mg) for treatment. At the practical level, this degree of treatment is likely to be of a newly acquired VTE, often in hospital and therefore as an inpatient. Other LMWHs may have a different dosing regime.

Pregnancy

Here there is a recommendation (although unlicensed) to weight-adjust the dose of LMWH used for treatment of VTE: for weight under 50kg use 40mg (4000 units) twice daily, for 50–70kg use 60mg (6000 units), for 70–90kg use 80mg (8000 units) and for over 90kg, use 100mg (10,000 units) – all twice daily.

General points

Also note that doses of some LMWHs may need to be adjusted according to factors such as the weight, body mass index, and renal function (e.g. increased serum creatinine or reduced glomerular filtration rate). Some guidelines may recommend that the dose of LMWH should be that which inhibits Factor Xa to a certain level (i.e. anti-Factor Xa activity). However, other LMWHs may not need to be dosed to this level of precision, and may be given at a standard dose.

In the United Kingdom, all hospitals should have a thrombosis committee, whose roles include producing guidance for all local practitioners on which LMWH best suits their individual requirements. These documents will inevitably refer heavily to national and international guidelines. Therefore the practitioner is likely to consult their local guidelines, and recall that these may change from workplace to workplace.

At what time should LMWH be administered?

Almost all patients will qualify for prophylaxis with a low dose of LMWH once daily at 1800 hrs the evening before surgery unless prophylaxis is contra-indicated and the patient has been identified as at highest risk of developing VTE. In this case a dose of high dose LMWH once daily at 1800 hrs should be prescribed. Aspirin is not recommended as anti-thrombotic therapy for surgical patients. However, if the patient is intolerant of LMWH then anti-platelets or warfarin are the remaining options.

A) Patients admitted the day(s) before surgery

All patients identified to require any treatment modality should commence it immediately they arrive in the hospital. For LMWH, whether with a low or high dose this should be commenced at 1800 hrs on the evening before surgery. This will achieve effective prophylaxis combined with minimal additional risk of bleeding complications at the time of regional anaesthesia (e.g. epidural or spinal) and surgery. Therefore the LMWH should be continued at 1800 hrs daily at the same time until the risk of thromboembolism is considered to be minimal or until anticoagulation with warfarin has reached its target international normalised ratio (INR).

B) Patients admitted on the day of surgery

According to the BNF,[3] patients eligible for prophylaxis should ideally receive a low dose of LMWH two hours preoperatively, unless this is contra-indicated. One of the main contra-indications is that the patient is due to be receiving regional anaesthesia (spinal or epidural).

Therefore, if a general anaesthetic only is to be administered, the anaesthetist following the assessment should prescribe the preoperative dose. Patients should then receive a further low dose of LMWH at 1800 hrs on the evening following the surgery – ideally this should have already been prescribed when they attended preoperative assessment. Thereafter a daily dose of LMWH at 1800 hrs should be prescribed at the appropriate dose depending on the patient's risk score.

C) Emergency patients

Patients admitted, who are eligible for prophylaxis and who are likely to have their operation within 12 hrs, should be treated as elective patients admitted on the day of surgery. Patients who are admitted after 0900 hrs but who are not expected to be operated on until the following day should receive the recommended dose at 1800 hrs on the evening of admission.

In all cases

For the purposes of these notes, for surgical patients it is recommended that:

- LMWH prophylaxis should be continued at the same times daily until discharge or until the risk of thromboembolism is considered minimal (the latter most unlikely).
- Consideration should be given to extending prophylaxis when the hospital stay is prolonged or the risk continues. Such prophylaxis could be either an outpatient LMWH self-administration programme or treatment with warfarin.
- Continued use of GECS on discharge from hospital to reduce the risk of late VTE may be beneficial in patients with poor mobility.
- NICE guidelines[4] recommend that LMWH or fondaparinux therapy should be continued for four weeks after hip fracture surgery.

D) Regional anaesthesia

A major caution is that when epidural/spinal anaesthesia or spinal puncture is employed, patients anticoagulated or scheduled to be anticoagulated with heparin for the prevention of VTE are at risk of developing an epidural or spinal haematoma, which can result in long-term neurological dysfunction.

It is recommended that if LMWH has been administered preoperatively, a period of 12 hours should elapse before insertion of an epidural or spinal anaesthetic and likewise LMWH should be withheld until at least four hours after the insertion of these neural blocks. The practitioner should access the local guidelines for the definitive guidance.

A general algorithm for surgical patients admitted the day before their operation can be seen in Figure 10.4 (page 210).

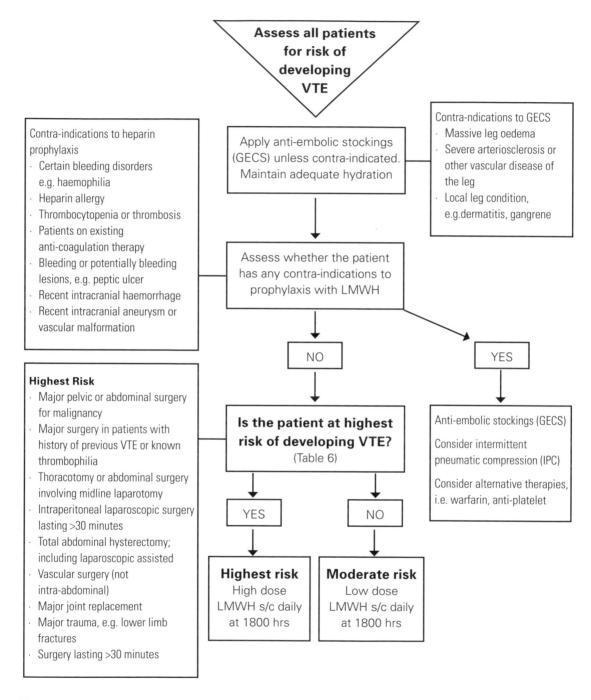

Figure 10.4

General algorithm for surgical patients admitted the day before their operation

Obstetric surgery (in cases of caesarean section)

Elective caesarean sections admitted the night before surgery
In the case of planned caesarean sections that are admitted the night before, low dose LMWH should be started at 1800 hrs the evening before surgery, or if the woman is considered to be at high risk, a high dose of LMWH should be considered following discussion with the consultant responsible for her care. Thereafter, a dose of LMWH (dose dependent on risk) at 1800 hrs should be prescribed. Where epidural or spinal anaesthetic has been administered the postop day dose should be given no sooner than four hours after spinal/epidural puncture.

Elective caesarean sections admitted on the day of surgery
Administer low dose LMWH postoperatively on the day of surgery, provided that this is not within four hours if spinal or epidural anaesthesia has been administered (see D above). Thereafter, administer low dose LMWH od at 1800 hrs commencing the next day.

For the purposes of this chapter, for surgical patients it is recommended that:

- Heparin prophylaxis should be continued at the same times daily until discharge or until the risk of thromboembolism is considered minimal.

- Consideration should be given to extending prophylaxis when the hospital stay is prolonged or the risk continues. Such prophylaxis is likely to be with warfarin.

- Continued use of GECS on discharge from hospital to reduce the risk of late VTE may be beneficial in patients with poor mobility.

Oral contraceptives and hormone replacement therapy (HRT)
As highlighted earlier, the oral contraceptive pill and HRT are risk factors for VTE, as is surgery. It follows that women taking these synthetic hormones may be at additional risk of VTE should they continue this therapy during surgery. Certainly, such women must be assessed for their risk of thrombosis, but there is no evidence in favour of routinely stopping HRT so long as there is appropriate thromboprophylaxis with LMWH or unfractionated heparin (UFH).

Similarly, there is no evidence that the progesterone-only pill is associated with increased risk of VTE, or that such preparations should be stopped prior to surgery. However, whether or not to stop the combined (oestrogen plus progesterone) pill before major surgery is a controversial issue. The risk of unwanted pregnancy, the effects of anaesthesia on pregnancy and the risks of subsequent termination are high, and therefore, rather than stopping the oral contraceptive pill, these women should receive thromboprophylaxis with LMWH as per standard guidelines.

Monitoring the effectiveness of LMWH in the laboratory
Unlike the old-style fractionated heparin previously used for VTE prevention, which required monitoring with activated partial thromboplastin time (APTT) testing, LMWH administration does not require regular monitoring, as it is so stable and its activity is relatively predictable. However, if LMWH does indeed need to be checked for efficacy, the relevant test is inhibition of Factor Xa.

Long-term anticoagulation

As the patient recovers from their surgery, the next question is the duration of anticoagulation. Once more, the thrombosis committee will provide the organisation's definitive guidance, generally based on formal recommendations such as NICE Guideline 46 – this suggested either LMWH or fondaparinux be prescribed for four weeks after most cases of 'major' surgery. This can be delivered either with the role of a 'DVT nurse' who will support the administration of the injectables in the community in collaboration with community teams or with an educated and appropriate patient self-administering the anticoagulation.

In situations where the risk of thrombosis is long-term, or the patient has other risk factors such as cancer, then injectables are not convenient and oral agents are preferable. The principal agent at present is the coumarin-based drug, warfarin, though others are currently being tested to be considered as an alternative or replacement in the future to reduce the need for long-term monitoring.

The use of warfarin for long-term anticoagulation

The commencement of warfarin for long-term anticoagulation requires a clear understanding of the benefits for the patient of this therapy weighed against its risks. The decision should involve all members of the multi-disciplinary team along with the patient and their carers (if necessary). Guidance will be available to the practitioner for its administration and monitoring within each healthcare organisation as well as from national bodies such as the British Committee for Standards in Haematology and the National Patient Safety Agency. Local guidelines will have been developed by a multi-disciplinary team to ensure a safe, effective and consistent approach to the management of adult patients in primary and secondary care receiving warfarin.

Each hospital or family doctor must give advice to prescribers and other healthcare professionals on managing patients on warfarin, e.g. prescribing considerations, monitoring requirements and factors affecting warfarin therapy. The user is reminded of the importance of the patient's handheld record in the form of the Yellow Book, an anticoagulant therapy record booklet. Due to the inherent complexity associated with warfarin use, communication between teams involved in patient care is of the utmost importance, particularly since very often patients are initiated in secondary care and managed in primary care.

Pathophysiology

Warfarin is in fact a slow-acting specific liver poison and as such attention must be paid to adequate liver function (therefore LFTs are necessary). This is pertinent as this organ is also the site of production of many coagulation proteins. In practice this means that the full effect of a fixed dose of warfarin will not be evident for several days, possibly a week or more. Conversely, the liver will be slow to recover once the drug has been withdrawn. However, vitamin K can be given to promote the return of coagulation protein synthesis.

Warfarin is available in 0.5mg, 1mg, 3mg and 5mg tablets. Patients take a combination daily, aiming to maintain an INR either between 2 and 3 (hence target 2.5), or between 3 and 4 (hence target 3.5). In practice the average dose is 4–6mg daily. The INR is monitored with venous blood or by fingerprick. Management is by simple up or down titration followed by re-testing. In case of low INR (at either target), the patient is advised to increase their daily dose of warfarin, and vice versa for an INR above the desired range. Precise algorithms for these dose changes and return visits for rechecking are available with readily accessible documents such as the British National Formulary (BNF).[3]

Rapid induction of warfarin is usually indicated for patients at high risk and/or acute risk of VTE and it should achieve the target INR within five days. LMWH should continue being administered despite the commencement of warfarin until the INR has been within range for two consecutive days. A normogram for rapid induction is available in the BNF. Care should be taken with patients with a low body weight (less than 50kg), elderly patients, those with a low albumin, liver or heart disease, or multiple interacting medications. In such cases a lower loading dose, e.g. 5mg on day one should be used, rather than the usual 10mg starting dose, or a slow induction plan should be considered.

Patients who have recently commenced oral anticoagulant therapy as inpatients will need their INR to be checked regularly, usually by venepuncture on alternate days within the first week. Once stabilised, intervals between INR checks can lengthen but changes in interacting medications must be accompanied by more frequent checks.

Most patients are likely to be fit for discharge by the time their target INR (generally 2–3) has been reached, perhaps in five to seven days, although this may take as long as a fortnight. Once again, the DVT nurse may be prominent in caring for the patient as their INR slowly rises. As an outpatient, management will most likely transfer to an oral anticoagulant team, which may also include scientists and pharmacists. But whatever route is followed, the healthcare professional will need to educate the patient, in line with National Patient Safety Agency (NPSA) guidelines.

The Yellow Book

In the UK perhaps 500,000 people are taking warfarin. An invaluable record of their treatment dose and INR is in the form of a Yellow Book that will be issued to each patient when they start on warfarin. It contains not only a record of warfarin use, but also helpful tips as to how the patients can help themselves, and possible problems to be aware of. Patients are to be strongly encouraged to take care of this book and bring it with them each time they attend hospital or their GP. It is a useful source of information for the practitioner at the preoperative assessment to assess the variability of warfarin control prior to surgery and the planning of cessation of warfarin preoperatively.

Patients to be admitted for surgery already on warfarin

Patients on long-term anticoagulation with warfarin require some careful planning prior to admission for elective surgery. Unlike other anti-thrombotic prophylaxis, such as aspirin, the effects of warfarin cannot easily be controlled in the acute setting. Withdrawal of the warfarin needs to occur before surgery to allow the INR to decrease to a level that the surgeon is happy to operate on, yet at a level to prevent recurrence of thrombosis for the patient. Invariably the warfarin will be withdrawn for four to five days preoperatively and depending on the indication for warfarin may need to be covered with alternative anti-thrombotic prophylaxis such as LMWH preoperatively as well as postoperatively. The re-commencement of warfarin will occur in the postoperative period once the risk of haemorrhage from the surgical perspective has become negative. LMWH will continue to be administered until the target INR has been reached for at least two days.

The following should be considered:

- The individual's risk of bleeding will vary both with the type of surgery, and with the presence of other risk factors for bleeding. Most surgery can be safely performed when the INR falls to 1.5.

- Period of time for INR to fall: for patients in a therapeutic range of INR 2–3, it takes approximately four days after stopping warfarin for INR to reach 1.5; for patients with a therapeutic range INR 3–4 and the elderly this may be longer.

- Once the decision is made to stop warfarin therapy preoperatively and perform the procedure when the INR has returned to safe levels, there is a need for other methods of anti-coagulation – either full-dose anticoagulation or prophylactic doses of LMWH.

The patient is admitted for elective surgery

(i) Minor risk of VTE

For minor surgery an INR of <2 should be achieved. For very minor procedures, some surgeons may operate at INR 2.5. For an INR range 2–3, omit warfarin for two days. For INR range 3–4, omit warfarin for 3–4 days. Restart warfarin postoperatively on the day of surgery at the maintenance dose (occasionally a boost in the dose of warfarin will be required).

(ii) Medium risk of VTE

These will be patients on long-term anticoagulants for atrial fibrillation, cardiomyopathy, previous single episode of VTE more than three months ago, mural thrombus, rheumatic mitral valve disease, new model prosthetic aortic valves, tissue valves.

- Before surgery: Stop warfarin four days prior to surgery. If INR is still high, a small dose of vitamin K (0.5–1mg orally) may be given if necessary. Consider stopping anti-platelet drugs (aspirin, clopidogrel) 5–7 days before surgery. Give high dose LMWH sc at 18:00, at least 12 hours before operation. On the morning of surgery check that the INR is <1.5.

- After surgery: Continue high dose LMWH od postoperatively as above. Restart warfarin as soon as patient is able to take oral fluids. When INR >2 for 48 hours stop LMWH.

(iii) High risk of VTE

These may be patients on long-term anticoagulants for prosthetic mitral valve, old model aortic prosthetic valves, recurrent VTE, antiphospholipid syndrome, recent (3/12) VTE. Patients who have had VTE (especially PE within the last month) are considered very high risk. If surgery is urgent and there are risk factors for bleeding, an inferior vena cava (IVC) filter should be considered.

- Before surgery: Recall that the risk of haemorrhage is greater than the risk of recurrent VTE providing sub-therapeutic INRs are limited to one to two days only. Generally, stop warfarin four to five days before surgery, and consider stopping anti-platelets five to seven days before surgery. Admit two days prior to surgery, check INR on admission and daily. In some cases low dose LMWH can be used when the INR is <2.0, with a prophylactic dose given the night prior to surgery. The interval between full dose LMWH and surgery should be 24 hours; and 12 hours between prophylactic LMWH and surgery.

- Day of surgery: Check INR and APTT. If INR <1.8, proceed with operation, if >1.8; delay operation. A small dose of vitamin K, e.g. 0.5–1mg IV will lower the INR. The onset of action of IV vitamin K is 6–8 hours and it may take three to four days for warfarin to work when restarted. LMWH will need to be continued postop.

- After surgery: Restart therapeutic low dose of LMWH 12 hours postop. Restart warfarin at the usual dose on the evening of the operation or as soon as the patient is able to take oral fluids and provided there is no undue bleeding. Continue LMWH and warfarin until INR >2.5 (this is usually five to seven days). Monitor INR daily. For patients who are at a higher risk of bleeding IV unfractionated heparin is preferable as it has a shorter duration of action than warfarin or LMWH, and is more rapidly reversible, although monitoring by APTT is required.

Patients admitted for emergency surgery

Again, consider is it minor or major surgery – does the INR need to be lowered? (See above.) If INR is >2.0 and urgent reversal is required, stop anticoagulant therapy, take blood samples (INR, FBC, crossmatch, other tests if indicated). If there is sufficient time before surgery, give vitamin K 0.5mg IV slowly. This will lower the INR in roughly **six to eight hours**.

The patient may be refractory to warfarin for three to four days after but this can be covered with LMWH. Larger doses of IV vitamin K 5–10mg can be given if continued anticoagulation is not needed again. Check INR prior to surgery: if > 2.0 and surgery is urgent and there is no time for vitamin K to work, give FFP 10–15ml/kg or prothrombin complex concentrates. Repeat INR after FFP and before surgery. When INR < 2.0, proceed with operation.

Note that separate guidelines exist for management of inpatients who are over-anticoagulated. Restart warfarin in the postop period as above with regard to risks of thrombosis/haemorrhage. Ensure the patient is fully educated as to the purpose of therapy.

Restarting patients on warfarin therapy.

Patients who have stopped warfarin therapy due to surgery will need re-induction on warfarin depending on their reasons for anticoagulation. Usually, patients just need to restart their warfarin on their usual dose (taking into consideration any changes in medication or general well -being). The risks of over-anticoagulation and bleeding associated with rapid induction should be considered. Patients with prosthetic valves may need anticoagulation cover with LMWH until INR is within range, depending on the age and valve type. Patients with a history of or recent VTE should receive LMWH until INR is back within range. In both cases warfarin should be inducted rapidly. Consideration needs to be given postoperatively to increased risks of bleeding.

CONCLUSION

The pathology laboratory is an essential resource, providing crucial information about the patient's blood. It helps determine whether or not the patient is fit for surgery, and answers the following questions:

- Can the patient's red blood cells provide sufficient oxygen to meet the extra demands of the surgery?
- Are the patient's white blood cells able to provide protection from attack by microbial pathogens?
- Are there any signs that the patient is suffering a sub-clinical infection?
- Does the patient have enough platelets and clotting factors to provide sufficient haemostasis?
- Are there any other reasons why surgery should not proceed (such as evidence of haematological disease)?

Once surgery has been completed, the patient is likely to need anticoagulation. The laboratory can provide the following assessment of the three major anticoagulants:

- The effectiveness of unfractionated heparin is assessed by the APTT assay (in the form of the APTT ratio).
- The effectiveness of LMWH is assessed by an anti-Factor Xa assay.
- The effectiveness of warfarin is assessed by the PT assay (in the form of the INR).

REFERENCES

1. National Institute for Clinical Excellence (2003). *Clinical Guidance 3: Preoperative tests: The use of routine preoperative tests for elective surgery.* London: NICE.

2. House of Commons Health Committee (2005). *The Prevention of Venous Thromboembolism in Hospitalized Patients.* London: Stationery Office.

3. British National Formulary (BNF) (2010). British National Formulary 59. London: BMJ.

4. National Institute for Health and Clinical Excellence (NICE) (2007). *Guideline 46. Venous Thromboembolism: Reducing the risk of VTE (DVT and PE) in inpatients undergoing surgery.* London: NICE. www.nice.org.uk

FURTHER READING

T.P. Baglin, P.E. Rose, I.D. Walker, S. Machin et al. (1998). Guidelines on oral anticoagulation: Third edition. *British Journal of Haematology* **101**: 374–87.

T.P. Baglin, D.M. Keeling and H.G. Watson (2006). British Committee for Standards in Haematology. Guidelines on oral anticoagulation (warfarin): 3rd edn. – 2005 update. *British Journal of Haematology* **132**: 277–85.

T.P. Baglin, T.W. Barrowcliffe, A. Cohen and M. Greaves (2006). The British Committee for Standards in Haematology. Guidelines on the use and monitoring of heparin. *British Journal of Haematology* **133**: 19–34.

T.P. Baglin, D. Cousins, D.M. Keeling, D.J. Perry and H.G. Watson (2007). Safety indicators for inpatient and outpatient oral anticoagulant care: [corrected] Recommendations from the British Committee for Standards in Haematology and National Patient Safety Agency. *British Journal of Haematology* **136**: 26–9. Erratum in: *British Journal of Haematology* **136**: 681.

A.D. Blann (2007). *Routine Blood Results Explained* 2nd edn. Keswick: M&K Update.

British Committee on Standardisation in Haematology (BCSH) offers reasonably up to date guidelines for outpatient treatment of DVT with warfarin or heparin at www.bschguidelines.com.

British Thoracic Society Standards of Care Committee (2003). Pulmonary embolism guideline. *Thorax* **58**: 470–83. (www.brit-thoracic.org.uk)

Y.L. Chee, J.C. Crawford, H.G. Watson and M. Greaves (2008). Guidelines on the assessment of bleeding risk prior to surgery or invasive procedures. *British Journal of Haematology* **140**: 496–504.

Department of Health (2007). Report of the Independent Expert Working Group on the prevention of venous thromboembolism in hospitalized patients. March. www.doh.gov.uk

J. Hirsch, G. Guyatt, G. Albers, H.J. Schunemann, H. Munger, S. Brower et al. (2004). The Seventh ACCP Conference on Antithrombotic and Thrombolytic Therapy: Evidence based guidelines. *Chest* **126** (3 Suppl): 174S–696S.

The National Patient Safety Agency (NPSA). (2007). Patient Safety Alert 18. Actions that can make anticoagulant therapy safer (release date 28 March). Available at: www.npsa.nhs.uk/health/alerts

Royal College of Obstetrics and Gynaecology. Guideline 28. *Thromboembolic disease in pregnancy and the puerperium: Acute Management.* RCOG, London, 2001. (www.rcog.org.uk)

The Scottish Intercollegiate Guidelines Network (SIGN) (2002) 'Guideline No 62: Prophylaxis of venous thromboembolism(released October). Available at: www.sign.ac.uk/guidelines/fulltext/62/index.html

11 The role of blood transfusion in preoperative assessment

Andrew Blann

SUMMARY

This chapter will outline:

- **the basics of blood grouping and variety of transfusion products**
- **clinical assessment and management of patients requiring transfusion**
- **the risks associated with blood transfusions**
- **strategies to reduce the use of blood products perioperatively.**

INTRODUCTION

The objective of blood transfusion has changed markedly over the decades, from being a crude instrument to maintain the haemoglobin level, to a targeted therapy to save lives. Additional changes have occurred following the realisation that blood transfusion is far from a simple and trouble-free treatment to one that can damage, possibly permanently, the health of the recipient. There are currently over two million packs of blood transfused each year in the UK, although changes in practice have brought this number down from nearly three million a decade ago.

This decrease in usage is largely due to the reduced use of blood in surgical patients, with the widespread adoption of lower thresholds for transfusion than the haemoglobin level of 10g/dl that was traditionally quoted. It is often perceived that the majority of donated blood is transfused into patients undergoing surgery but recent studies show less than 40% of blood units are transfused into surgical patients.

A further development has been the move from transfusing 'whole' blood, which therefore included plasma (with all its proteins, antibodies and other molecules), white blood cells and platelets, to transfusing only specific components, usually just the red blood cells. The latter, called 'packed cells', is not only more efficient, but also, without the white blood cells and plasma antibodies, produces fewer adverse reactions. The remaining plasma, once the red blood cells have been harvested, can provide other useful blood products (such as clotting proteins, although these can also be produced by genetic engineering). Laboratory staff can also help with albumin, fresh frozen plasma and transfusions of platelets (often needed by those at risk of, or with actual, haemorrhage) and, of course, a wealth of experience and advice.

Why is blood transfusion needed? What do I need to do? Many possible reasons exist, but before we embark on the answers to these (and other) questions, a better understanding of the topic will be helpful.

Blood groups

The major human blood groups are defined by the ABO system and the Rhesus (Rh) system. A patient's blood group consists of two parts. First the blood group of a patient is determined by the presence or absence of specific 'antigens', molecules that are present at the surface of the cell. The presence or absence of an antigen is genetically determined, with the ABO locus being identified on chromosome 9, and these genomes code for specific glycoprotein, which is displayed on the cell surface. The second part relates to the presence or absence of specific antibodies. These are specialised proteins produced by lymphocytes and are thought to develop during the first year of life. The presence of these antibodies means that transfusion of blood containing specific blood antigens will lead to complement-mediated lysis of the red blood cell.

The ABO system

Table 11.1 Determinants of ABO blood group

Blood group	Frequency (%)	Antigen structures on the red blood cell surface	Antibodies in the plasma
A	42	A	Anti-B
B	9	B	Anti-A
AB	3	A and B	None
O	46	None	Anti-A and anti-B

Antigens A and B are protein structures with 'sugars' at the end that can be present on the surface of all body cells, including red blood cells. If you have only the blood group A structure on your red blood cells, you are blood group A. Similarly, if you have only group B molecules on your red cells then you are group B. People with both A molecules and B molecules on their red blood cells are group AB, and if you have neither of these structures on your red cells, you are group O.

We also have plasma antibodies that recognise blood group structures A and B, but in the healthy individual, these are the reverse of your blood group. So if you are group A, you will have antibodies that will recognise group B red cells (i.e. Anti-B). Likewise, group B people have antibodies that recognise group A red cells (i.e. Anti-A). Group AB people have no antibodies, but group O people have both anti-A and anti-B antibodies. Most people are blood group O, followed by group A. This is summarised in Table 11.1.

The Rhesus (Rh) system

The Rhesus system is more complicated, being composed of perhaps 48 recognised antigens, although practically, five different structures on the surface of the blood cell are commonly dealt with in the blood bank. A full explanation of this is beyond the scope of this chapter. However, in practice, focus is placed on the molecule known as D (i.e. Rhesus D), as it is this structure, and the antibodies that, if not correctly treated, give rise to haemolytic disease of the newborn (HDN). About 85% of white Europeans are Rhesus D positive. Other members of the Rhesus family of antigens are C, c, E and e.

The main distinction between the ABO and Rhesus systems is that in the normal person, there are always ABO antibodies to absent antigens. Anti-D antibodies are not normally found in blood, but these can easily be provoked by an incompatible transfusion or during childbirth. However, the fact that many of us naturally have anti-A and anti-B antibodies makes an ABO incompatibility potentially fatal.

Why order a blood transfusion?

Historically blood transfusions were requested to either maintain a patient's haemoglobin at a specific level, commonly at greater than 10g/dl or in response to a volume of blood that was lost or envisaged to have been lost. Over the last two decades, this approach has been challenged and now the practitioner should consider the following questions:

- Does the patient really need it?
- What exactly is the clinical problem that requires resolution?
- Are there alternatives to resolve the problem rather than blood transfusion?
- Is iron therapy worth considering?
- Will erythropoietin be a possibililty?
- Would autologous transfusion be worth considering?

Common UK practice suggests that an otherwise seemingly healthy postoperative patient who has no particular symptoms, but has haemoglobin of 9g/dL, probably does not require a transfusion. As mentioned, historically a transfusion was often ordered simply because a physician considered it a good thing to do, with the belief that it would probably do the patient some good. This could, of course, be fine but this approach can lead to a number of problems.

- While the ABO/Rh systems are the most important blood groups, there are a host of other less frequent and (initially) less dangerous blood group antigens (with names such as Kidd,

Duffy and Kell) that can cause a problem. The more transfused a person becomes, then the greater the likelihood that these problems will build up to become a real clinical and laboratory issue.

- We are programmed by evolution to collect and save iron in stores all over the body. People who are hyper-transfused often have problems in various organs as the build-up of this iron can cause damage to the tissues (a process called haemosiderosis). Since one unit of blood contains some 250mg of iron, 15 units can more than double the body iron stores.

- Transfused blood can contain pathogenic organisms (viruses, bacteria, parasites, nvCJD) although, through screening, this is becoming less of a problem.

- Infection can also occur via the site of the transfusion.

- Transfusion practice is not without errors as will be highlighted later.

Therefore, the present view is that transfusion should be reserved only for those in danger of losing their life, or for those who will show a measurable improvement not achievable by other means. It follows that the requirement for a transfusion can only be made clinically, not in the laboratory (by a particular haemoglobin result). The haematology laboratory provides the physician with this haemoglobin result, and the physician will then decide, after consideration of the patient's state, whether or not the patient will benefit from a transfusion. However, much experience is available within the blood bank laboratory service and advice should be sought if cases fall outside established practice or guidelines.

Indications for blood transfusion

Reasons for ordering a transfusion can be many and varied, but major life-threatening indications include:

- chronic and serious anaemia unresponsive to other treatment, such as, severe cases of the haemoglobinopathies, sickle cell disease or thalassaemia

- life-threatening emergencies, such as rupture of an aortic abdominal aneurysm or massive blood loss after a road traffic accident

- haemorrhage, such as in haemophilia or because of overdoses of warfarin or heparin.

In surgery, there are other indications that need to be addressed.

- A curious response to many types of surgery is a fall in haemoglobin that cannot be accounted for by simple blood loss alone. This is presumed to have evolved to protect the body.

- Of course, if the operation is a 'bloody' affair, perhaps involving arteries or major organs, there may be significant blood loss, which needs to be replaced. However, blood volume can initially be replaced by an infusion of crystalloid or colloid intravenous fluids to maintain normal perfusion of organs.

However, transfusion should not be considered just because the haemoglobin result is less than a certain number. Various randomised controlled trials have failed to demonstrate any advantage of transfusing patients using an Hb trigger of 10g/dl compared to using lower triggers of between 7 and 8g/dl.

The mechanics of blood transfusion

Assuming the patient may need a transfusion, what are the next steps to be taken? Even before blood is taken, there must be an explanation of the process, and the patient's consent must be obtained. We can view these in separate steps, although several may take place at the same time.

Explanation and consent

All patients undergoing operations, where there is a likelihood of receiving blood, must receive written information about blood transfusion. Information leaflets are available from the UK Transfusion Services (UKTS), though these should be tailored to provide local hospital-specific information depending on availability of services such as autologous transfusion (transfusion of patient's own blood – see page 230). Information about blood transfusion is best given to patients at the time of preoperative assessment rather than on admission to hospital immediately prior to the operation.

Specific written consent is not currently required for blood transfusion in the UK but it is good practice to include mention of the possibility of transfusion in the consent for operation where there is a reasonable possibility of transfusion. These operations would be best defined as any operation where a 'Group and Save' or a 'cross-match' is routinely ordered. In addition, specific mention should be made on the consent form of any information leaflet given to the patient.

Once the requirement for a blood transfusion has been clarified, and the patient has received information and given consent, two allied blood tests are called for.

Group and Save

This is usually the first test that is done on the patient's blood and allows the laboratory to identify the blood group of that particular patient, ideally in advance of their planned procedure. This is achieved with the request 'Group and Save' (GandS) – this instruction identifies the patient's ABO blood group and often their Rhesus status (the 'Group' part of the process). The blood is then stored (the 'Save' part of the process, generally in a refrigerator) as this will be needed in the future to allow the laboratory to perform a 'cross-match'. The 'Save' process may be time-limited and therefore, when planning a service, this time limit needs to be clarified to decide on the optimal time for taking blood from the patient.

Cross-match

Although the 'Group and Save' process identifies the patient's ABO group and often their Rh status, administration of group-specific blood to a patient still puts that patient at risk of harm due to blood incompatibility. It is important therefore to match the blood group of the person needing the transfusion (the recipient) with the group of the blood that is to be transfused (the donor). This process is called a 'cross-match', and is done in the blood bank on a sample of the patient's (recipient) anticoagulated or clotted blood – in the elective situation this sample will come from the specimen submitted for 'Group and Save'.

The essential steps are:

(a) The patient must be ABO and Rh (D) typed – first part of the 'Group and Save' process.

(b) There must be screening for other clinically significant antibodies (this is as important as the cross-match).

(c) The actual 'cross-match' is where the patient's plasma or serum is tested against a panel of potential blood from several different donors.

In practice, laboratory staff in the blood bank will mix red blood cells from the patient (recipient) with a series of plasma samples from stored bloods of five or six different donors, to see if there are any matches. Prior 'Group and Save' process allows the blood bank to identify the best possible matches and identify any other problems that may frustrate a good transfusion. Sometimes the laboratory may request a fresh blood sample from the patient, especially if the cross-match process is proving complicated due to the presence of numerous antibodies (common in patients who have received numerous blood transfusions).

A good match is where the red blood cells are unaltered by this mixing, and therefore should not react when in the patient. However, blood that does not match will aggregate, forming small clots, which indicates an incompatibility due to a cross-reaction with the red blood cell antigens and antibodies in the plasma. It is presumed that, if this mismatch blood is transfused, the same reaction may happen in the blood vessels of the recipient, which may kill them.

An example of this would be transfusing blood from someone of blood group A with some blood from someone of blood group B. The group A person has group A molecules on their red cells but also antibodies against B in the plasma (i.e. Anti-B). The group B person has the reverse – group B molecules on their red cells and anti-A antibodies in their plasma. So, when mixed, the group A red cells will be recognised by the anti-A antibodies, and so will react together. Similarly, the group B red blood cells will be recognised by the anti-B, and will also react. In an incompatible transfusion, the body has no way of knowing that the 'foreign' red bloods are actually being introduced to help the recipient.

Thus incompatibility is when the mismatched antibodies and red cells are mixed. One way of avoiding this is to always transfuse red blood cells which are group O and Rh negative – these cells lack antigens that the antibodies are designed to react towards, so there cannot be this kind of a problem with mismatching. Consequently, this 'O-neg' blood can be given to any patient in an emergency if cross-matching is not possible – hence it is a very valuable commodity. People who donate this kind of blood are called universal donors.

It follows that people who are Group AB do not have anti-A or anti-B antibodies in their plasma, so can receive A-neg, B-neg, O-neg or their own group (AB), and so are called universal recipients. However, they may still be susceptible to Rhesus and minor antigen reactions.

How much blood should be ordered?

Each healthcare organisation has developed a system, often called the Maximum Surgical Blood Ordering Schedule (MS-BOS), which determines the number of units of blood that will be needed for a particular operation. This is calculated from a review of average blood usage per type of operation over a reasonable period of time – this gives a figure which will determine the number of units required to be cross-matched for a given operation, usually cross-matching between one and two times the average number of units used per operation. For example, if an average of 1.4 units were used for a particular type of operation then two units would routinely be cross-matched. If an average of less than 0.5 units of blood were used for any type of operation, with only a minority of patients requiring blood, then a group and antibody screen (GandS) would usually be performed without any blood being routinely cross-matched preoperatively.

This MS-BOS system should be regularly reviewed and adjusted to allow for changes in surgical practice, which should be endeavouring to reduce perioperative blood loss if at all possible. The MS-BOS system, however, is only applicable to patients without any unusual red cell antibodies or increased risk of bleeding. If a patient has unusual antibodies, which may attack the incoming blood (normally fewer than 5% of routine surgical patients), then extra units are usually cross-matched, depending on the type of antibody. Similarly, in patients with increased risk of bleeding, cross-matching extra units of blood should be considered. Both of these situations require discussion between the surgical, anaesthetic and blood bank staff.

Risks of blood transfusions

The risk of blood transfusion in terms of morbidity and mortality is not clear, as invariably blood and its components are administered to patients with complex medical problems and in complex clinical situations. Patients may receive blood in a relatively stable situation and this transfusion may provide little or no clinical benefit, while when blood is administered during a life-saving operation the benefits are likely to far outweigh the risks.

The use of information from national reports of serious complications and transfusion-related deaths allows the practitioner to develop good practice to ensure that the risks to a patient are minimised. In the UK the Serious Hazard of Transfusion (SHOT) group (www.shotuk.org) produces annual reports of this information. The 2008 report found that of 1040 reported cases, with the issuing of 2,845,459 units of blood components in 2007–8 in the United Kingdom, there was one death reported as a direct consequence of the blood transfusion. There were 262 cases of incorrect blood transfused, in which 10 cases were due to ABO-incompatible red cell transfusion. Four of these cases were due to bedside administration errors, three due to 'wrong blood in tube' and three due to laboratory errors. The report also identifies 76 cases of inappropriate or unnecessary transfusion and 139 cases of handling or storage errors.

Clinical and laboratory problems in transfusion practice

Errors can and do occur at all places in the 'journey' from blood donor to blood recipient. However, it is generally recognised that most errors happen in the laboratory and/or once the blood has left the blood bank for its destination.

Laboratory error

The packs of donor blood arrive from the National Blood Transfusion Service (NBTS) in good shape, having been typed for ABO and Rhesus, and screened also for major infective agents (hepatitis virus, HIV). However, the blood sample from the recipient may be labelled incorrectly. The next source of error may be the incorrect labelling of the small portion of each potential donor pack that is collected to take part in the cross-match.

Next, there may be error in the cross-match itself. These are very rare because the laboratory invests heavily in the technology and reagents to ensure that if an adverse reaction happens, it is detected. However, if the cross-match goes wrong, which is a false negative, a possibly incompatible unit of blood may be issued. If several packs are identified, the lab may assign an incompatible unit to the donor.

Post-laboratory error

Post-laboratory errors are inevitably the wrong blood being given to the wrong patient. The wrong pack of blood may be collected from the blood bank issuing refrigerator, or the blood may be given in error to the wrong patient. A common confusion is that two or more patients are to be transfused at the same place at the same time, and that the bloods are switched.

Many of these are simply incorrect patient identification, generally by a misunderstood verbal recognition question, or by misreading the patient's ID strip at the wrist. Effective checking is essential at all stages.

Prevention of transfusion reactions

Naturally, there are many steps designed to prevent a transfusion reaction: generally check, check and check again. Laser bar coding is being introduced so the sample can be traced from the requesting blood sample all the way back to the patient. Many hospitals have a policy of at least two members of staff checking the blood they are about to transfuse into one of their patients. This approach has proved to reduce mistakes and serious hazards of transfusion. Indeed, SHOT itself reports that ABO incompatible transfusions have shown a 54% reduction since 2001/2002. Blood transfusion outside core hours (mostly night time) is considerably less safe – and so it is a SHOT recommendation to avoid transfusion 'out of hours'.

Many hospitals have their own formal policy, and professional bodies (e.g. the Royal College of Nursing, the Institute of Biomedical Sciences) generally offer guidelines. Checks must be made at each part of the pathway of the blood from the laboratory to the patient. These include:

- ensuring portering staff have collected the correct blood from the blood bank
- correct transfer of the blood to the requesting practitioner: the latter must take responsibility and sign the appropriate document
- if the transfusion is not immediate the blood must be placed in a blood-designated refrigerator to keep it cool – ideally blood should only be requested for immediate use
- finally, at the bedside, the details on the blood pack must be checked against the patient, not merely against the patient's wristband, but also by confirming verbally (assuming the patient is conscious). These generally include name, sex, date of birth and hospital number and often home address.

The use of laser bar coding can help reduce errors that may arise. A further recent initiative is the requirement for a 'cold chain', which calls for blood being carried from the blood bank to the ward in cool bags. This is thought to be necessary for a number of reasons, such as to keep the blood cool and so reduce the opportunity for bacterial growth, and to maintain the integrity of the red cells.

There is a mandatory requirement that all blood must be traceable from 'vein to vein'. Relevant documents include the EU Blood Safety Directive (2005/50). In the UK, the Medicines and Healthcare products Regulatory Authority (MHRA) is the EU-designated responsible authority to ensure all UK hospital blood banks are compliant.

Clinical management of transfusion problems

Adverse reactions to a blood transfusion may be classified as those happening within minutes or a few hours (that is, early reactions), and those happening perhaps after 12 hours to days later (that is, late reactions).

Early reactions

In an acute setting a transfusion reaction may not be easily diagnosed, as the patient may not recognise that there is a problem and the symptoms and signs of a transfusion reaction vary enormously (see Table 11.2).

Table 11.2 Symptoms and signs of early transfusion reaction

Symptoms (conscious patient)
Cough
Flushing/rash

Anxiety/headaches

Diarrhoea

Nausea and vomiting

Tremble/shakes/chills

Shortness of breath/chest pain

Cognitive changes/patient restless/agitated

Pain at venepuncture site

Pain in abdomen, flank or chest

Signs (patient need not be conscious)

Fever

Hypotension

Oozing from wounds

Haemoglobinaemia

Haemoglobinuria

Tachycardia

However, there can be other acute non-red blood cell reactions such as an acute urticarial reactions (e.g. hives) or anaphylaxis as a result of the recipient responding to the donor's plasma proteins and their IgA antibodies – if so, antihistamines (e.g. chlorpheniramine 10mg, 20mg if severe) are one possible treatment.

Upon suspicion of a reaction, the infusion should be immediately stopped. All hospitals will have a defined protocol that must be followed. Clearly, clinical treatment will depend on the severity of the reaction, which if mild or moderate, can be rapidly reversed. But severe reactions can be life-threatening and will be treated accordingly (e.g. admission to Critical Care for disseminated intravascular coagulation (DIC), often with ventilation, inotropic support, and steroid treatment). One 'mechanical' way of treating an acute reaction is to try to 'flush' it out – this is attempted by giving fluids, but clearly requires good renal function. If there is a massive destruction of donor red blood cells, there may well be hyperkalaemia requiring appropriate immediate treatment.

In view of this possible transfusion reaction, any donor blood packs that have been administered will need to be collected by the blood bank. These will need to be re-analysed, along with a fresh blood sample from the patient. This transfusion reaction will require further investigation, along with reporting to national bodies such as the Medicines and Healthcare Products Regulatory Authority (MHRA) reporting system, and the Serious Adverse Blood Reactions and Events (SABRE) in the UK.

Late reactions

Problems from 12 hours to three days after transfusion may involve major organs such as acute renal failure (often oliguria with or without haematuria or haemoglobinuria), jaundice, congestive heart failure due to circulatory overload, and pulmonary oedema with or without adult respiratory distress syndrome. Thus, because of the time delay, the association with the transfusion may not be recognised; this is important, especially if the patient has been discharged from hospital. It follows that patients and/or their carers must be made fully aware of the signs of a reaction, especially as the reaction could be life-threatening.

Febrile reactions (generally with a slow rising temperature peaking at over 40°C) are seen in 0.5–1% of transfusions and may be due to anti-HLA reactions. Later complications (3–14 days) after an incompatible transfusion may consist of a 'new' immunological reaction of the recipient to the donor red blood cells, causing the destruction of the latter. This time period may also see transfusion-related infections that have escaped the screening process. There may also be reactions with rare antigens too weak to be detected in the laboratory.

An ABO-incompatible transfusion may be so severe as to result in the serious coagulopathy of DIC, which will generally result in transfer to the Critical Care facility. Another coagulation problem occasionally seen is post-transfusion purpura, which is characterised by a severe thrombocytopenia (platelet count perhaps less then 50 x 109/mL), which can last from two weeks to two months. Antibodies to antigens on the surface of platelets cause this and it requires treatment with high dose steroids and intravenous immunoglobulin. In the short term a thrombocytopenia may develop in the hyper-transfused patient, as infused blood is generally platelet-free. If the patient is haemorrhaging, then platelet transfusion may be required. If there is widespread destruction of red blood cells, jaundice may develop due to the presence of high levels of bilirubin, a breakdown product of red blood cells.

Very late consequences

Humans have evolved to store iron in case of future deprivation. However, high levels of iron stores can be damaging and cause heart failure, diabetes, and other syndromes. Accordingly, patients who are regularly or hyper-transfused (as in thalassaemia) may need iron chelation therapy (such as desferroxamine) to reduce these dangerous stores.

Other untoward consequences of a transfusion

There does not need to be an incompatibility for the patient to feel unwell. Due to anticoagulants used to prevent blood clot in blood packs (such as acid citrate dextrose), patients may become hypocalcaemic due to the binding of calcium. They may also develop a degree of hyperkalaemia due to increased potassium leaching out of the donor cells. A further metabolic problem may be seen related to an alteration in acid/alkali balance: large volumes of blood products can contribute to alkalosis.

Blood for transfusion must be kept cool at 4°C. It follows that the absorption of several units of cool blood may reduce the core temperature of the patient. Fortunately, blood warmers should be available to increase the temperature of blood packs prior to transfusion and avoid hypothermia which will not help a bleeding patient.

Initiatives to make blood transfusion safer

The preceding section has underlined the danger of transfusing blood from one person to another. What can we do to make it safer? Clearly, one way is to ensure administrative errors are minimised, if not eliminated. But another is not to transfuse someone else's blood, but to transfuse the patient's own blood. There are four ways in which this 'autologous' transfusion can be achieved.

Preoperative blood donation

Sufficiently fit patients can 'donate' their own blood for their own use in advance of their surgery. A unit of whole blood can be taken weekly and stored for up to 35 days, as with standard volunteer donor blood. The donation must be tested and stored to the same standards as donor blood, with blood banks requiring 'manufacturer's' level accreditation from the government if they collect, test and store autologous blood. The patient must be well enough to donate blood and fulfil the routine volunteer donor criteria (such as having a sufficiently high haemoglobin level) and clearly the donations must not weaken the patient. Oral iron supplementation may be necessary and erythropoietin injections may be used to increase the number of units donated in the time allowed.

The advantages of preoperative autologous donation include a reduction in risk of viral infections and avoiding the induction of antibodies to other people's red blood cell antigens. The process does not, however, reduce the risks of administration error and bacterial infection of the blood packs. Despite initial support for its use in the UK, in recent years the National Blood Transfusion Service has withdrawn this service. It may be a useful strategy in certain cases.

Acute isovolaemic haemodilution

This technique requires, immediately preoperatively, the venesection of large volumes of blood from a suitable patient, replacing the blood volume with saline or similar fluids. This reduces the red cell concentration within the patient's circulation and therefore fewer red cells and less haemoglobin are lost per litre of blood shed during the operation. The collected blood is then re-infused at the end of the operation when the circulation and blood have recovered.

Perioperative cell salvage

This is the most effective and commonly employed form of autologous blood use. Blood shed during the operation and the immediate postoperative period is collected using modified suction devices into a sterile reservoir. Depending on the amount collected, it can then be 'washed' using a cell washing device, and then re-infused back into the patient in a relatively short period. Modern devices can rapidly process large volumes of blood and re-infuse blood within five to ten minutes. With separate collection and cell washing sets, blood can be collected and then only processed if significant volumes of blood are shed, thus saving expensive consumables. This procedure cannot be used when operating on potentially infected organs (such as in contaminated open bowel surgery) and in those involving cancer, due to the risk of re-infusing malignant cells. Recent trials, however, suggest that the process can safely be used in operations on some tumours such as prostate cancer.

The technique is of maximum benefit in large procedures, where large blood loss is expected, such as emergency abdominal aortic aneurysm (AAA) rupture and therefore benefits from being available outside routine working hours. This requires training of all operating department staff to provide an on-call service and to be able to provide the service across all theatres. It has recently been introduced into obstetric practice, being acceptable in obstetric fields with a machine capable of washing away potentially thrombogenic amniotic fluid. The procedure is also acceptable to most Jehovah's Witnesses as the blood collected is continuous with the patient's circulation during the procedure. Patients who may benefit from this procedure should be identified at preoperative assessment or earlier and offered information on the procedure.

Postoperative cell salvage

This technique simply re-infuses the blood shed in wound drains, particularly in joint replacement operations. Shed blood from the modified wound drains is collected postoperatively, then re-infused via an integral filter to remove blood clots and debris. Manufacturers' instructions and recommendations vary as to the maximum amount of blood that should be returned unwashed and the maximum time between commencing collection and re-infusion using this method. There may be concerns about re-infusing activated clotting factors but studies do not show any detrimental effects with this technique.

Blood products

As discussed earlier, the blood bank can provide not only red blood cells, but also a host of other items. These include platelets and coagulation proteins such as albumin, immunoglobulins, Factor VIII, Factor IX, Factor VII, prothrombin complex concentrate, fresh frozen plasma (FFP) and cryoprecipitate. While these products are essentially often 'left over' after the red blood cells have been harvested, plasma alone and/or platelets alone can be collected from a donor – this is called apheresis. While blood proteins, if frozen, have a shelf life of a year; platelets cannot be frozen and must be used within five days. The shelf life of a pack of red cells is 35 days. Platelets for transfusion, like red cells, should be ABO compatible.

Blood products can be used in a small number of highly specialist cases.

Haemorrhage

Blood products may be needed by people at risk of haemorrhage, or with actual haemorrhagic blood loss, but who do not need red blood cells, such as those with haemophilia and severe von Willebrand's disease. The proteins are kept frozen and so must be thawed before being transfused. This, of course, may prove crucial if someone needs these products urgently with a life-threatening haemorrhage. As fragments of cells, platelets will also need to be checked for blood group compatibility.

All hospitals deal with haemorrhage due to prolonged PT, PTT, decreased fibrinogen, over-anticoagulation with warfarin or heparin, severe liver disease, trauma, surgery or disseminated intravascular coagulation. Involvement of the haematologist at an early stage of any complicated case is important to prevent delay in the patient receiving the appropriate therapy to deal with the haemorrhage. Once the haemorrhaging patient has been transfused, their new coagulation status must be confirmed with a coagulation screen as well as a repeat full blood count.

Special cases

Albumin (generally as a 20% preparation) is also available for people with low levels or who have had heavy burns (although only regional centres will deal with these risky patients) or ascites.

There are groups of patients where blood products must be carefully treated, with the provision of irradiated blood, or blood proven to be negative for cytomegalovirus. Both these would not normally be problems for the 'healthy' patient who can mount a reasonably good immune response. But the immuno-compromised patient, perhaps after bone marrow transplantation, demands extra care. This is particularly pertinent as graft-versus-host disease (where the donor's white blood cells attack the recipient) is a possible consequence. This can be minimised by filters that remove white blood cells from donated blood before they pass into the patient.

CONCLUSION

The key points regarding blood transfusion can be summarised as follows:
- This therapy is generally reserved for urgent and life-threatening clinical situations such as blood loss. It is now rarely seen as a temporary 'cure' for anaemia, where an alternative such as iron may be preferable.
- The major blood groups are A, B, AB and O, but Rhesus D is also important.
- Requests are usually to 'Group and Save', and to 'cross-match'.
- The blood bank also provides platelets, albumin and coagulation factors.
- You also have access to highly specialised services in investigating reactions and providing

ultra-specialist products, e.g. HLA matched platelets, stem cells, etc.

- Incompatible blood transfusion can be fatal and can be preceded by symptoms such as rash, shortness of breath, headache and cough.

- Most incompatible reactions are due to clerical and/or identification errors. The cause(s) of these must be investigated (SHOT, SABRE, MHRA).

REFERENCES

Department of Health. www.transfusionguidelines.org.uk/index.aspx

EU Blood Safety Directive (8 November 2005). http://www.opsi.gov.uk/si/si2005/20050050.htm.

Paediatric transfusion: www.ich.ucl.ac.uk/clinical_information/clinical_guidelines/cpg_guideline

www.learnbloodtransfusion.org.uk.

Medicines and Healthcare Products Regulatory Agency www.mhra.gov.uk.

National Patient Safety Agency www.npsa.nhs.uk/nrls/alerts-and-directives/notices/blood-transfusions.

Serious Hazard of Transfusion (SHOT) group www.shotuk.org.

Taylor C (Ed.), Cohen H, Mold D, Jones H, *et al.* on behalf of the Serious Hazards of Transfusion (SHOT) Steering Group. The 2008 Annual SHOT Report (2009).

World Health Organisation www.who.int/bloodsafety/en/index.html.

FURTHER READING

M. Popovsky, P. Robillard, M. Schipperus, D. Stainsby, J.D. Tissot, J. Wiersum, (2006) *ISBT Working Party on Haemovigilance. Proposed standard definitions for surveillance of non-infectious adverse transfusion reactions.*

NHS Confederation / NPSA Briefing No. 161. Act on Reporting: Five actions to improve patient safety reporting.

http://www.nhsconfed.org/Publications/briefings/Pages/Actonreporting.aspx.

BCSH Blood Transfusion Task Force (1999). The administration of blood and blood components and the management of the transfused patient. *Transfusion Medicine*, **9**, 227–39. http://www.bcshguidelines.com.

British Committee for Standards in Haematology, Blood Transfusion Task Force (2007). The specification and use of information technology systems in blood transfusion practice. *Transfusion Medicine*, **17**, 1–21.

D. B. L. McClelland (Ed.) (2000). *Handbook of Transfusion Medicine*, 4th edn., London: TSO.

http://www.transfusionguidelines.org.uk/index.asp?Publication+HTM&Section = 98&pageid=1105.

UK Resuscitation Council Emergency treatment of anaphylactic reactions. http://www.resus.org.uk/pages/reaction.pdf.

MHRA Background and guidance on reporting serious adverse reactions and serious adverse events. http://www.mhra.gov.uk/home/groups/dts-aic/documents/websiteresources/con2022523.pdf.

A. Morris, G. Lucas, E. Massey & A. Green (2007) 'Are HLA matched platelets being used and reviewed in accordance with British Committee for Standards in Haematology, Blood Transfusion Task Force guidelines?' http://nhsbtweb/group_services/clinical/clinical_audit/audit_reports/HLA%20Report%20%202007.pdf

Guidelines for the use of platelet transfusions, *British Journal of Haematology* (2003) **122** (1), 10–23.

12 Preoperative pharmacological optimisation

Jonathan Thompson
Simon Young

SUMMARY

The chapter will describe:
- **the importance of a detailed medication history**
- **common therapeutic treatments for systemic disease and implications for preoperative optimisation.**
- **the increasing use of herbal and illicit drugs and implications for perioperative care.**

INTRODUCTION

It is important to take a detailed drug history from all patients undergoing surgery. This includes details of prescribed drugs, non-prescription medicines (for example, herbal remedies), and drugs of addiction and abuse. In general most chronic medications can be continued throughout the perioperative period, though there are some important exceptions which are detailed in this chapter.

Perioperative medication may be prescribed for several reasons:
- the management of co-existing medical conditions unrelated to the surgery
- the medical management of surgical conditions
- premedication
- anaesthetic agents (general, regional, and local) and analgesics
- organ support in critically ill patients
- drugs administered *de novo* in an attempt to improve outcome.

Alteration of drug therapy to optimise chronic medical conditions and the judicious use of certain additional drugs may help avoid some of the complications of surgery and anaesthesia, as well as improve patient satisfaction.

In addition other factors are relevant to drug therapy in the perioperative period, including:

- fasting before surgery and altered gastrointestinal function
- the effects of surgery and anaesthesia on co-existing illnesses
- the effects of anaesthesia and surgery on drug action, metabolism and elimination.

When planning drug therapy for surgical patients, a number of specific decisions should be made:

- whether to continue a drug (the usual course of action)
- whether to discontinue a drug, and for how long before surgery
- whether to replace one drug and/or route of administration with another
- whether to prescribe additional drugs that will improve patient outcome, comfort or satisfaction
- when to restart a drug following surgery (in most cases, immediately).

Some of the most commonly used 'premedications' in anaesthetic practice are anxiolytics, analgesics and gastric acid suppression medication. Pre-emptive anti-emetic drugs may also be considered in those at high risk.

Concurrent medication

Drugs acting on the respiratory system

Asthma and chronic obstructive pulmonary disease (COPD) are the chronic respiratory diseases most commonly encountered in surgical patients. General anaesthesia, pain that reduces vital capacity and the ability to cough, and surgery per se all cause worsening of respiratory function. This may be compounded by the effects of analgesic medication, e.g. respiratory depressants (opiates) or drugs which may exacerbate bronchospasm, e.g. non-steroidal anti-inflammatory drugs (NSAIDs). Postoperative respiratory tract infection may supervene and impair respiratory function further. It is therefore important that respiratory function is optimised before surgery and perioperative management of the respiratory system has two main aims:

- treatment of acute deteriorations, and possible postponement of elective surgery until treatment is effective
- assessment and optimisation of chronic respiratory disease.

In general, all regular respiratory medications should be continued and with inhaled drugs this is usually straightforward. In addition regular nebulised beta2-agonists and anticholinergics can be usefully administered for a number of days before surgery, as well as being administered immediately before the operation, and in the postoperative recovery room (Table 12.1). Patients with severe airways disease may benefit from a preoperative course of double dose inhaled steroids or daily prednisolone (20–40mg) for seven days.

Table 12.1 Bronchodilator pharmacology

	Dose	Timing
Beta2-agonists		
Salbutamol	2.5–5mg neb	Every 15 mins as required
Terbutaline	0.5mg neb	Every 15 mins as required
Anti-muscarinic		
Ipratropium bromide	0.5mg neb	6 hourly
Non-specific phosphodiesterase inhibitor		
Aminophylline	0.5mg/kg/hr	Substitute for theophylline

Patients who have severe airways disease may also be receiving drugs such as theophylline or leukotriene receptor antagonists (e.g. montelukast, zafirlukast). Again, every attempt should be made to ensure uninterrupted perioperative administration of these drugs. Intravenous aminophylline may be used as a substitute for oral theophylline (Table 12.1) in patients unable to take tablets; drug monitoring of plasma concentrations (therapeutic range 10–20µg ml^{-1}) is strongly suggested.

Drugs acting on the cardiovascular system

Cardiovascular disease is common in patients presenting for surgery. Many drugs that surgical patients receive will have effects on the cardiovascular system, either as a direct therapeutic aim or as a side effect. Perioperative cardiovascular morbidity (e.g. acute myocardial infarction) is uncommon, but carries a high risk of death, and may be decreased by certain therapies. Management of cardiovascular drugs covers two areas:

- optimisation of chronic disease
- specific drugs to reduce perioperative cardiovascular morbidity.

Beta-adrenoceptor antagonists ('beta-blockers')

Beta-blockers are commonly used in the treatment of patients with a variety of conditions including hypertension, ischaemic heart disease, cardiac dysrhythmias, congestive cardiac failure, hyperthyroidism and anxiety. Abrupt discontinuation of beta-blockers in the perioperative period can lead to rebound hypertension and tachydysrhythmias, and has been associated with perioperative cardiovascular morbidity. Exaggerated responses to anaesthetic and surgical stimuli often occur if beta-blockers have been withheld. Every effort should therefore be made to continue beta-blockers, using intravenous preparations if the oral route is not available. For example a patient normally receiving oral atenolol 25–100mg once daily could be switched to atenolol 2.5–10mg IV (administered cautiously by slow injection) once daily. Longer-acting blockers (e.g. atenolol) may confer more benefit than shorter-acting drugs (e.g. metoprolol, propranolol) in reducing perioperative cardiovascular morbidity, as the effects of mistimed or omitted doses are lessened.[1,2]

Renin angiotensin system modifying drugs

Angiotensin converting enzyme inhibitors (ACEIs) and angiotensin II receptor blockers (ARBs) are used in the management of hypertension, ischaemic heart disease, congestive cardiac failure and renal protection in diabetes mellitus. They can be associated with profound hypotension in the perioperative period, which can be unresponsive to vasoactive drugs. Various patient and anaesthetic factors can influence the degree of hypotension. The decision to continue or discontinue ACEI/ARB should therefore be made on an individual patient basis (Table 12.2). If these drugs are to be stopped this should be considered at least 24 hours before surgery. A new class of drug has recently become available – the direct renin inhibitors (DRI), e.g. aliskiren. The therapeutic and adverse effects of these drugs are most likely similar to the ACEIs/ARBs, and until more data are available they should be treated in the same way.

Table 12.2 Considerations regarding perioperative ACEIs and ARBs

Consider continuation
Critical left ventricular function
Anti-hypertensive monotherapy
Consider discontinuation
Planned central neuraxial block:
• particularly if using thoracic epidural analgesia (particularly a high thoracic epidural placement)
• particularly if combined with general anaesthesia
Anticipated large perioperative fluid shifts (major gastrointestinal, orthopaedic, thoracic surgery)
Combined ACEI and ARB therapy – consider stopping at least one
High risk of acute renal failure in the perioperative period
Orthostatic hypotension

Anticoagulation

Anticoagulants are used for the prevention of clotting in various situations:

- patients with prosthetic valves, vessels or stents
- patients with atrial fibrillation (AF) or dyskinetic ventricular segments (to prevent arterial embolic events, particularly stroke)

- patients at risk of, or suffering from venous embolic events, i.e. deep vein thrombosis (DVT) and pulmonary thromboembolism (PTE).

Therapeutic anticoagulation increases surgical bleeding but the risks of this should be balanced against the risks of thrombotic events if anticoagulant therapy is discontinued. Thus it is important to understand the indications for anticoagulation, the problems it can cause, and the alternatives available. Warfarin (oral route) and the heparins (subcutaneous or intravenous routes) are the most commonly encountered anticoagulants in the UK. A detailed discussion of this topic is covered in Chapter 10, pages 202–16.

Anti-platelet drugs

Anti-platelet drugs (aspirin, dipyridamole, clopidogrel) are widely prescribed for the prevention and treatment of ischaemic heart, cerebrovascular and peripheral vascular diseases. They are associated with a slight increase in surgical bleeding but in most cases this is minor and should be balanced against the increased risks of thrombotic events if anti-platelet therapy is discontinued. In most cases therefore treatment can be continued in the perioperative period. Spinal or epidural catheter placement is considered to be safe in patients receiving low-dose aspirin or dipyridamole therapy. However in some high-risk situations, for example intracranial and vitreo-retinal surgery, the increased risks of surgical bleeding outweigh the potential antithrombotic benefits and in these situations anti-platelet drugs should be stopped.[3] The effects of aspirin on platelet function are irreversible, and so if aspirin is to be stopped before surgery a period of seven days should be allowed before sufficient platelets are regenerated.

Clopidogrel is a highly potent anti-platelet drug. Its action is also irreversible and if it is to be stopped this should be done at least seven days before planned surgery or spinal/epidural anaesthesia.[4] Recent developments in cardiology have included the widespread introduction of intravascular stenting for coronary artery disease. In the early weeks and months after stent placement the patient is at increased risk of potentially fatal stent thrombosis,[5,6] and it is recommended that clopidogrel is continued for one year after placement of a drug-eluting stent.[7] Clearly some of these patients will present for surgery within this time. If surgery cannot be postponed, most patients with recent coronary artery stents would benefit from continuing their dual anti-platelet therapy perioperatively, accepting that surgical blood loss will be increased, and that epidural or spinal anaesthesia should be avoided.[8] This approach may be inappropriate in situations where bleeding could be catastrophic (neurosurgery, vitreo-retinal surgery, major cardiac or hepatic surgery) in which case clopidogrel therapy may be stopped but aspirin continued.

Anti-dysrhythmic drugs

Cardiac output may be compromised by tachycardia (heart rate > 90bpm) and uncoordinated cardiac contractions (e.g. atrial fibrillation or other cardiac dysrhythmias). Anaesthesia and surgery can predispose patients to new dysrhythmias, or pre-existing benign dysrhythmias may develop into malignant dysrhythmias. Mechanisms involved include perioperative electrolyte imbalances, autonomic reflexes, or the administration of certain drugs used during anaesthesia. It is therefore very important to continue any rate-controlling drugs (e.g. digoxin, beta-blockers) and rhythm-controlling drugs (e.g. amiodarone, flecainide) in the perioperative period. In patients unable to absorb oral medication intravenous preparations of these drugs are available. In patients receiving digoxin for atrial fibulation, poor heart rate control, major surgery and critical illness would be indications for therapeutic drug monitoring of serum digoxin concentrations (usual range 1.0–2.5nmol l^{-1} or 0.5–2.0ng ml^{-1}). Optimisation of serum potassium and magnesium levels is also important. Anxiolytic premedication (e.g. benzodiazepines) may also be helpful.

Diuretics

Many patients receive diuretic medication for the management of hypertension and fluid retention, caused by congestive heart failure or chronic kidney disease. If continued during the perioperative period these can cause electrolyte disturbance and dehydration. However, withholding diuretics may worsen congestive heart failure. The decision as to whether to continue with diuretics is complex, but if large fluid and electrolyte shifts are expected (e.g. major bowel surgery) it may be prudent to withhold them.

Nitrates

Nitrates are used for symptom control in angina pectoris. Abrupt discontinuation of nitrates is unwise and additional nitrates may be useful if angina is associated with preoperative anxiety. The patient's own modified-release nitrate (e.g. isosorbide mononitrate) or a topical nitrate patch can be administered perioperatively. Topical nitrate patches are available (GTN in 5mg, 10mg and 15mg preparations) which deliver their dose over 24 hours. Anxiolytic premedication can also help reduce symptoms of angina.

Calcium channel blockers

Calcium channel blockers (CCBs) are primarily used to treat hypertension, angina pectoris and tachydysrhythmias. Sudden withdrawal of CCBs may be associated with exacerbations of angina and it is therefore prudent to continue these drugs during the perioperative period.

Drugs used for hypertension

Chronic hypertension is a sustained increase in blood pressure over 140/90mmHg,[9] as measured in the clinic or general practice setting. The British Hypertension Society guidelines[9] suggest drug treatment for the following patients:

- Stage I hypertension (SBP 140–159 or DBP 90–99) if associated with organ damage, or in the elderly
- Stage II hypertension (SBP ≥ 160 or DBP ≥ 100).

Although uncontrolled hypertension has traditionally been viewed as a reason to cancel elective surgery, recent data suggest that some of the risks may have been over-emphasised.[10,11] Patients with severe hypertension are at increased risk of perioperative swings in blood pressure, dysrhythmias and myocardial ischaemia and specific additional interventions or monitoring may be required. However, there is limited evidence to prove that postponing surgery in order to control blood pressure improves overall outcome.[11] Nonetheless every effort should be made to optimise blood pressure in elective patients prior to surgery. Eight weeks is ideally required to allow stabilisation on a particular anti-hypertensive agent. Blood pressure control should be complemented by assessment of overall cardiovascular risk, with consideration given to starting anti-platelet and statin therapy as well.

Reducing perioperative cardiovascular morbidity in non-cardiac surgery

There has been much interest recently in using beta-blockers to reduce cardiovascular complications and mortality in patients undergoing major surgery. Recent guidelines[12] recommend that patients scheduled for major vascular surgery, and who have inducible myocardial ischaemia on cardiac stress testing, should receive beta-blockers before and after surgery (Table 12.3). Beta-blockers should also be considered in patients with documented coronary artery disease or multiple cardiac risk factors undergoing other high-risk surgery, though the evidence in these groups is less conclusive. There is an increased risk of perioperative bradycardia and hypotension requiring treatment in the beta-blocked patient.[13]

Table 12.3 Beta-blocker therapy recommendations[12]

- Start several days or weeks before surgery if possible.

- Aim for a resting preoperative heart rate of 50–60bpm, and an intraoperative and postoperative heart rate of less than 80bpm.

- Use cardioselective (beta1-antagonists) agents, e.g. atenolol, metoprolol, esmolol.

- Every effort should be made to continue beta-blockade uninterrupted throughout the perioperative period.

- Use long-acting agents where possible, to minimise rebound effects, if administration is interrupted.[2]

There is growing evidence that patients undergoing major vascular surgery benefit from long-term statin (HMG-CoA reductase inhibitor) therapy (e.g. simvastatin 20–40mg daily), starting as early as possible before surgery,[14,15] and continuing for life. Even in patients having non-vascular surgery, statin therapy may reduce perioperative cardiac morbidity. Certainly statins should not be withdrawn in patients already taking them, and they should be re-introduced as soon as possible postoperatively.[15]

Endocrine system

Diabetes mellitus

Diabetes mellitus (DM) can be broadly classified as Type 1 (insulin-dependent) DM and Type 2 DM (diet-controlled, tablet-controlled, or insulin-requiring). Tight control of blood glucose concentrations can improve wound healing and reduce morbidity and mortality.[16] Guidelines vary but a target blood glucose concentration of less than 10mmol l[-1] provides a compromise between practical glycaemic control and avoidance of dangerous hypoglycaemia.[17]

Oral hypoglycaemic agents either promote the release of insulin, or improve its action in the peripheral tissues. They can be safely omitted on the day of surgery, although stopping Metformin may require specialized advice before surgery or in the critically ill. Some patients with Type 2 DM who do not normally require insulin may need to be given insulin perioperatively, and patients who usually receive subcutaneous insulin may need 'tighter' glycaemic control through the use of intravenous insulin. Most hospitals have guidelines in place for the perioperative management of patients with diabetes.

Corticosteroid supplementation

The need for steroid replacement or supplementation is determined by the dose of steroid taken regularly, the extent of surgery, and the duration of perioperative fasting. Patients regularly using lower dose inhaled steroids do not require additional steroid replacement. If high inhaled doses are being taken, perioperative steroid supplementation should also be considered (Table 12.4).[18]

Table 12.4 Perioperative corticosteroid supplementation guidelines[18]

Prednisolone	Surgery	Additional steroid cover
≤ 10mg d[-1]		Usually not needed
> 10mg d[-1]	All	25mg hydrocortisone IV at induction
Plus postoperative dosing as follows:		
	Minor	No postoperative steroids
	Intermediate	Hydrocortisone 100mg d[-1] IV for 24 hrs
	Major	Hydrocortisone 100mg d[-1] IV for 48–72 hrs

'High' daily doses of inhaled corticosteroids for asthma and COPD[26]	
Fluticasone propionate	400 micrograms or over
Beclometasone dipropionate	800 micrograms or over
Budesonide	800 micrograms or over

Notes:

If patient stopped chronic steroids less than three months ago, treat as if still on steroids. Postoperative hydrocortisone should ideally be administered as a constant infusion to minimise swings in blood glucose concentrations; alternatively hydrocortisone 25mg IV qds can be given.

Thyroid disorders and the perioperative period

Patients with thyroid disease should be clinically euthyroid (i.e. displaying neither symptoms nor signs of hyper- or hypothyroidism) and free from any adverse effects of thyroid medication. Thyroid over-activity can cause tachycardias and a hypermetabolic state (a thyroid 'storm'), whereas under-activity can lead to bradycardia, hypotension and prolonged recovery. In emergency situations the effects of hyperthyroidism can be attenuated by administration of beta-blockers, potassium iodide and carbimazole. Thyroxine is available as an intravenous preparation, liothyronine, but is seldom needed as patients can usually safely omit thyroxine for a number of days. The exception is the critically ill patient who requires thyroxine to aid recovery. The dose of intravenous liothyronine is one-fifth that of oral levothyroxine, i.e. 10–40micrograms.

Neuro-psychiatric disorders

Anti-epileptic medication

Anti-epileptic medication should be continued throughout the perioperative period to reduce the risks of seizures. Particular attention should be paid to the formulations of anti-epileptic drugs. Many are available in modified release formulations, which should not be interchanged with the standard release formulations. Some (e.g. phenytoin and sodium valproate) can be administered by intravenous infusion if gastrointestinal absorption is impaired. Changing to alternative routes of administration or alternative medications should only be undertaken with specialist advice, as interactions between these drugs are complex and toxicity common.

Anti-Parkinsonian medication

Anti-Parkinsonian drugs should be continued regularly (via gastric or jejunal tube if necessary), to ensure avoidance of distressing dyskinesis. In exceptional circumstances a subcutaneous infusion of apomorphine, a short-acting dopamine agonist, may be used during waking hours as a temporary replacement of normal oral therapy.[19,20] Newly available transdermal patch formulations (e.g. rotigotine, a dopamine agonist) may provide an alternative route of administration. Expert advice should be sought when changing formulations.

Anti-depressants, anti-psychotics and anxiolytics

Most drugs in these categories should be continued in the perioperative period. The possible exceptions to this are the mono-amine oxidase inhibitors (MAOI) and lithium. MAOI may interact unpredictably with some anaesthetic drugs and for this reason some authorities recommend their discontinuation two weeks before surgery. However, these drugs are usually prescribed for severe depressive illness and discontinuation may have serious repercussions; continuation is sometimes the best course of action. Lithium should be stopped 24 hours before major surgery as electrolyte derangements can occur, but can be continued for minor surgery.

Inflammatory conditions and immunosuppressants

In general, conditions with inflammatory components (e.g. inflammatory bowel diseases, arthritis, skin conditions) can worsen if medications are withheld. Immunosuppressants and corticosteroids are the agents most commonly used, and consideration should be given to switching to intravenous preparations if the enteral route will be unavailable for any length of time. In particular, in patients with a transplanted organ where immunosuppression is vital to the preservation of organ function, medication should not be interrupted.

Premedication

This section will deal with pharmacological management of the following perioperative concerns, which can be managed, at least in part, by medication:

- anxiety
- gastric acid suppression
- pre-emptive analgesia
- management of nausea and vomiting.

Anxiety management

Many patients are anxious about forthcoming anaesthesia and surgery. Common fears include pain, nausea and vomiting, awareness under anaesthesia, and even death. Often patients will be reluctant to voice their fears directly. Much patient anxiety can be allayed by explanation of the process of anaesthesia, analgesia, surgery and the postoperative course.

Despite reassurance, some people understandably remain anxious about forthcoming anaesthesia and surgery. Apart from the psychological upset caused by anxiety, physiological manifestations can be troublesome. Tachycardia, hypertension, hyperventilation, and gastro-intestinal upset are all common in the anxious patient. Activation of the sympathetic nervous system (the 'fight or flight' response) can be harmful. For example, the patient who has chronic hypertension may develop dangerously high blood pressure, the patient with atrial fibrillation may become tachycardic, or the patient with angina may develop chest pain and shortness of breath. Anxiolytic or sedative medication can reduce both psychological stress and the associated pathophysiological effects.

The anxiolytic medications most commonly used in anaesthesia are the benzodiazepines, which also have sedative and amnesic effects. Benzodiazepines act by potentiating the action of the inhibitory neurotransmitter γ–amino-butyric acid (GABA) on neuronal GABAA receptors.

Various different types of benzodiazepine are available (Table 12.5), and the choice of drug depends mainly on the duration of anxiolysis required.

The use of benzodiazepines can lead to prolonged sedation postoperatively. This may be undesirable in certain situations, such as day case or intracranial surgery. The metabolism of many benzodiazepines can also be significantly prolonged in the elderly, and the sedative effects can last for days, leading to postoperative delirium and somnolence. Repeated doses of benzodiazepines can lead to significant accumulation of these drugs.

When using these sedative drugs, particular thought should also be given to the potential for respiratory depression and hypoxaemia. Supplemental preoperative oxygen is indicated for any patient who may be at increased risk of respiratory depression, or when the higher doses of benzodiazepine are used. Flumazenil is a benzodiazepine antagonist that can be used in emergency situations where over-sedation has occurred.

Table 12.5. Oral benzodiazepines for premedication

	Drug	Dose	Before surgery
Short-acting (30–60 mins)	Midazolam	0.5mg kg-1	30 mins
Intermediate (2–4 hrs)	Temazepam Diazepam	10–40mg 5–10mg	30–60 mins 1–2 hrs
Long-acting (4–8 hrs)	Lorazepam	1–4mg	1–2 hrs

Gastric acid suppression

In the perioperative period, gastrointestinal dysfunction and impairment of airway reflexes can increase the risk of inhaling gastric contents, leading to aspiration pneumonitis. Reduction of gastric fluid volume or acidity can lessen this risk. Drugs that suppress gastric acid fall into to two groups:

- drugs that reduce acid secretion by the gastric parietal cells
- drugs that neutralise acid already produced and present in the stomach.

Acid-secretion inhibitors are commonly used drugs with relatively few side effects. If a patient is already taking these drugs it is wise to carry on their normal prescription uninterrupted. In some institutions the H_2-antagonist ranitidine (150mg PO or 50mg IV) is routinely prescribed the night before, and the morning of surgery.[21] Other available acid-secretion inhibitors include the proton pump inhibitor (PPI) class of drugs (e.g. omeprazole 40mg PO or IV). In obstetric practice, the administration of sodium citrate (30ml 0.3m PO) is advocated immediately before general anaesthesia to neutralise residual stomach acid.

Pre-emptive analgesia

There is evidence that prevention of pain (by analgesics or local anaesthesia before surgery) can reduce both the stress response to surgery and postoperative pain. This is termed pre-emptive analgesia and can be used alone or as an adjunct to intraoperative analgesia. It often takes the form of simple oral analgesics, which can be given to the patient whilst awake prior to general anaesthesia. The type of analgesic considered depends on a number of factors:

- routes of administration available
- allergies to, or intolerance of, a particular drug
- perceived severity of pain to be encountered
- presence of co-morbid disease (respiratory, cardiac, renal, hepatic).

The continuation of analgesics already being taken by the patient is important, with further breakthrough analgesia being added to these medicines in the perioperative period. Wherever possible, chronic pain medications should be continued uninterrupted. Discontinuation can lead to extreme pain, anxiety and agitation. Chronic opiate therapy is a case in point – if unable to take oral medication, a continuous IV morphine background infusion (equivalent in rate to the 24-hour dose of opiate normally taken) can be prescribed, with a patient-controlled bolus for breakthrough pain postoperatively. Bolus doses of morphine for breakthrough pain may sometimes have to be increased dramatically in opioid-tolerant patients. Opioid patches (e.g. fentanyl and buprenorphine) may be continued as normal throughout the perioperative period, with breakthrough analgesia prescribed in addition to the patch. Absorption from patches may, however, be unpredictable if there are alterations in skin blood flow.

Opiate dependence, including prescribed methadone, can also lead to significant opiate tolerance, and vastly increased requirements for opiates should be anticipated. Methadone administration should be continued as usual, or replaced with parenteral opiate if the patient is unable to absorb orally. In patients who are recovering opiate addicts, it is advisable to clarify their feelings about the use of opiates in the perioperative periods, as they may wish to try and avoid them. It is often helpful to involve the hospital's acute or chronic pain team in the management of opiate-dependent patients.

Anti-emetic medication

Postoperative nausea and vomiting (PONV) is common and unpleasant, and may cause significant psychological distress, physical damage and prolong hospitalisation. Risk factors for PONV are listed in Table 12.6.

Low-risk patients do not require anti-emetic therapy unless they would suffer significant sequelae from vomiting as a result of the type of surgery they have undergone, for example, oesophageal surgery or jaw wiring. Monotherapy is indicated for patients with a moderate risk. A multi-modal approach (two or three agents) is of benefit in the prevention of PONV in high-risk patients.[22] Various classes of drugs acting on different receptor systems can be utilised (Table 12.7). Pre-emptive anti-emetic therapy may have a role in patients at high risk of PONV. In addition certain patients may find non-pharmacological interventions for PONV (e.g. acupressure bracelets) helpful.

Table 12.6 Risk factors for postoperative nausea and vomiting

Patient factors

Female

Non-smoker

History of PONV/motion sickness

Children age 2 to puberty (increasing with age)

Anaesthetic factors

Intra- and postoperative opiate use

Administration of volatile anaesthetic agents and nitrous oxide

Surgical factors

Prolonged surgery

Type of surgery (laparoscopy/laparotomy, abdominoplasty, ENT, ophthalmic, neurosurgery, breast, plastic, gynaecological)

Table 12.7 Anti-emetic medication

Class	Drug	Dose	Route
H1-antagonists	Cyclizine	50mg *tds*	IV / IM
5-HT3 antagonists	Ondansetron	4mg *qds*	IV / IM
	Granisetron	1mg *od*	IV
Butyrophenones (mostly D2-antagonists)	Haloperidol	1.25mg *once*	IV
Phenothiazines (anti-cholinergic, anti-histaminergic, anti-dopaminergic)	Prochlorperazine	12.5mg *tds*	IM
	(Buccastem®)	3–6mg *bd*	Buccal
Corticosteroids	Dexamethasone	8mg *once*	IV

Substance dependence

Nicotine replacement

Patients should be strongly discouraged from smoking tobacco in the perioperative period, as it increases airway sensitivity, respiratory secretions, blood carbon monoxide levels, and decreases oxygen-carrying capacity. However, withdrawal from nicotine can cause anxiety and agitation in certain patients and nicotine replacement therapy may be useful. Options available include patches, gum, lozenges and nasal spray. Up to 80mg of nicotine can be administered in a 24-hour period.

Non-prescription drug use and abuse

Consumption of non-prescription substances (e.g. alcohol or tobacco, cannabis, cocaine, ecstasy) can cause a number of problems in the perioperative period. Issues arise with both acute intake and intoxication with these substances, and with long-standing repeated use.

Acute intoxication with alcohol or psychoactive drugs is a contra-indication to surgery unless the condition is immediately life- or limb-threatening because of the risks of airway compromise, pulmonary aspiration, respiratory depression, cardiovascular instability, altered consciousness and aggression, and disrupted body temperature control.

Chronic drug misuse, in particular excessive alcohol consumption, is common world-wide. Specific problems that may influence the perioperative course include:

- chronic lung disease caused by exposure to tobacco, cannabis and other inhaled substances
- vascular disease, cardiomyopathy, hypertension
- malnutrition, muscle wasting
- liver dysfunction
- increased or decreased tolerance to sedative medications
- psychiatric illness (depression, anxiety, psychoses) and neurological disease (e.g. peripheral neuropathy, cerebellar ataxia)
- acute withdrawal syndromes (best characterised by delirium tremens with alcohol withdrawal), agitation and aggression
- increased pain experience with tolerance to analgesics.

In the case of chronic alcohol misuse, the administration of vitamin supplements (oral thiamine and B_{12} Co-strong, or the intravenous vitamin preparation Pabrinex) is recommended in the perioperative period, starting as long as is feasible prior to major surgery.

Delirium tremens (DT) is a potentially fatal condition of physical and psychological withdrawal in patients with alcohol dependence syndrome. Table 12.8 reproduces a well-validated assessment tool (CIWA-Ar, the Clinical Institute Withdrawal Assessment Regime) for assessing the risk of developing DT, as well as stratifying the severity of DT. Pre-emptive use of benzodiazepine drugs (e.g. chlordiazepoxide or diazepam) is recommended for patients at risk of developing DT perioperatively, and many hospitals have their own guidelines in place.[2]

Table 12.8 Alcohol withdrawal assessment scale

Nausea and vomiting

Ask 'Do you feel sick in the stomach? Have you vomited?'
Observation

0 No nausea and no vomiting

1 Mild nausea with no vomiting

2

3

4 Intermittent nausea, with dry retching

5

6

7 Constant nausea, frequent dry retching and vomiting

Tactile disturbances

Ask 'Have you any itching, pins and needles sensations, any burning. any numbness or do you feel bugs crawling on or under your skin?" *Observation*

0 None

1 Very mild itching, pins and needles, burning or numbness

2 Mild itching, pins and needles, burning or numbness

3 Moderate itching, pins and needles, burning or numbness

4 Moderately severe hallucinations

5 Severe hallucinations

6 Extremely severe hallucinations

7 Continuous hallucinations

Tremor

Arms extended, elbows slightly flexed and fingers spread. *Observation*

0 No tremor

1 Not visible, but can be felt fingertip to fingertip

2

3

4 Moderate

5

6

7 Severe, even with arms not extended

Auditory disturbances

Ask 'Are you more aware of sounds around you? Are they harsh? Do they frighten you? Are you hearing anything that is disturbing to you? Are you hearing things you know are not there?' *Observation*

0 Not present

1 Very mild sensitivity

2 Mild sensitivity

3 Moderate sensitivity

4 Moderately severe hallucinations

5 Severe hallucinations

6 Extremely severe hallucinations

7 Continuous hallucinations

Paroxysmal sweats

Observation

0 No sweat visible

1

2

3

4 Beads of sweat obvious on forehead

5

6

7 Drenching sweats

Visual disturbances

Ask 'Does the light appear to be too bright? Is its colour different? Does it hurt your eyes? Are you seeing things you know are not there?' *Observation*

0 Not present

1 Very mild sensitivity

2 Mild sensitivity

3 Moderate sensitivity

4 Moderately severe hallucinations

5 Severe hallucinations

6 Extremely severe hallucinations

7 Continuous hallucinations

Anxiety

Ask 'Do you feel nervous?' *Observation*
1 Mildly anxious
2
3
4 Moderately anxious or guarded so anxiety is inferred
5
6
7 Equivalent to acute panic states as seen In severe delirium or acute schizophrenic reactions

Headache, fullness in the head

Ask 'Does your head feel different? Does it feel as though there is a band around your head?' Do not rate for dizziness or light headedness. Otherwise rate severity. *Observation*
0 Not present
1 Very mild
2 Mild
3 Moderate
4 Moderately severe
5 Severe
6 Very severe
7 Extremely severe

Agitation

Observation

0 Normal activity
1 Somewhat more than normal activity
2
3
4 Moderately fidgety and restless
5
7 Paces back and forth during most of the Interview or constantly thrashes about

Orientation and clouding of sensorium

Ask 'What day is this? Where are you? Who am I?' *Observation*
0 Orientated and can do serial additions
Ask person to perform serial addition of 3s up to 30, e.g. 3.6.9...
1 Cannot do serial addition or is uncertain about date
2 Disorientated for date by no more than 2 calendar days
3 Disorientated for date by more than 2 calendar days
4 Disorientated for place and/or person

Herbal medicines, including traditional Chinese medicines

Complementary therapies (see Table 12.9 for a selection) are often overlooked by clinicians and patients alike. Often the doses, multiple constituent chemicals, contaminants and exact pharmacological effects of these preparations are unknown.

The adverse effects of these complementary therapies are usually related to excessive bleeding (mild) and delayed recovery from anaesthetics. The American Society of Anesthesiologists advises stopping herbal medicines two weeks before surgery,[24] although cancellation of surgery in a patient found to be taking these therapies is probably not warranted, given the relatively mild effects encountered.[25]

CONCLUSION

All those involved in perioperative care should take a detailed drug history to include both prescribed and other drugs, and recognise which drugs may interfere with the perioperative course. In general most medications can be continued with minimal interruption in the perioperative period, although some changes to the route of administration may be required. Occasionally specialist advice is needed for complex cases.

Table 12.9 Complementary therapies

Therapy	Uses	Potential problems
Garlic	Hypertension, hypercholesterolaemia	Increased bleeding
Gingko	Dementia, peripheral vascular disease	Increased bleeding
Valerian, Kava	Sedation	Excessive somnolence
Grapefruit	Various uses	Alter hepatic drug metabolism, QT interval prolongation
Ephedra	Stimulant, various	Cardiovascular disturbance
St John's Wort	Depression and anxiety	Sedation, confusion, withdrawal

REFERENCES

1. D. Redelmeier, D. Scales and A. Kopp (2005). Beta-blockers for elective surgery in elderly patients: population based, retrospective cohort study. *British Medical Journal* **331**: 932–8.

2. S. Bolsin and M. Colson (2005). Beta-blockers for patients at risk of cardiac events during non-cardiac surgery. *British Medical Journal* **331**: 919–20.

3. W. Burger, J-M. Chemnitius, G.D. Kneissl and G. Rucker (2005). Low-dose aspirin for secondary cardiovascular prevention – cardiovascular risks after its perioperative withdrawal versus bleeding risks with its continuation – review and meta-analysis. *Journal of Internal Medicine* **257**: 399–414.

4. T.T. Horlocker, H. Benzon, D.L. Brown, F.K. Enneking, J.A. Heit, M.F. Mulroy, R.W. Rosenquist, J. Rowlingson, M. Tryba and C.S. Yuan (2003). Regional anaesthesia in the anticoagulated patient: defining the risks (the Second ASRA Consensus Conference on Neuraxial Anesthesia and Anticoagulation). *Regional Anesthesia and Pain Management* **28**: 172–97.

5. D.E. Newby and A.F. Nimmo (2004). Editorial II: Prevention of cardiac complications of non-cardiac surgery: stenosis and thrombosis. *British Journal of Anaesthesia 92*: 628–32.

6. C. Marcucci, P.G. Chassot, J.P. Gardaz et al. (2004). Fatal myocardial infarction after lung resection in a patient with prophylactic preoperative coronary stenting. *British Journal of Anaesthesia* **92**: 743–7.

7. A.H. Gershlick and G. Richardson (2006). Drug eluting stents. *British Medical Journal* **333**: 1233–4.

8. D.R. Spahn, S.J. Howell, A. Delabays and P.G. Chassot (2006). Coronary stents and perioperative anti-platelet regimen: dilemma of bleeding and stent thrombosis. *British Journal of Anaesthesia* **96**: 675–7.

9. B. Williams, N.R. Poulter, M.J. Brown, M. Davis, G.T. McInnes, J.F. Potter, P.S. Sever and S.M. Thom. BHS guidelines working party, for the British Hypertension Society (2004). British Hypertension Society guidelines for hypertension management 2004 (BHS-IV): summary. *British Medical Journal* **328**: 634–40.

10. S.J. Howell, J.W. Sear and P. Foex (2004). Hypertension, hypertensive heart disease and perioperative cardiac risk. *British Journal of Anaesthesia* **92**: 570–83.

11. D.R. Spahn and H.J. Priebe (2004). Editorial II: Preoperative hypertension: remain wary? 'Yes' - cancel surgery? 'No'. *British Journal of Anaesthesia* **92**: 461–4.

12. L.A. Fleisher, J.A. Beckman, K.A. Brown, H. Calkins, E. Chaikof, K.E. Fleischmann KE. *et al.* (2006). ACC/AHA 2006 Guideline update on perioperative cardiovascular evaluation for non-cardiac surgery: focused update on perioperative beta-blocker therapy. A report of the American College of Cardiology/American Heart Association Task Force on practice guidelines (writing committee to update the 2002 guidelines on perioperative cardiovascular evaluation for non-cardiac surgery). *Circulation* **113**: 2662–74.

13. P.J. Devereaux, W.S. Beattie, P.T.L. Choi, N.H. Badner, G.H. Guyatt, J.C. Villar et al. (2005). How strong is the evidence for the use of perioperative beta-blockers in non-cardiac surgery? Systematic review and meta-analysis of randomised controlled trials. *British Medical Journal* **331**: 313–21.

14. B.M. Biccard, J.W. Sear and P. Foex (2005). Statin therapy: a potentially useful perioperative intervention in patients with cardiovascular disease. *Anaesthesia* **60**: 1106–14.

15. J.R. Kersten and L.A. Fleisher (2006). Statins. The next advance in cardiac protection. *Anesthesiology* **105**: 1079–80.

16. G. Van den Berghe, P. Wouters, F. Weekers, C. Verwaest, F. Bruyninckx, M. Scheetz *et al.* (2001). Intensive insulin therapy in critically ill patients. *New England Journal of Medicine* **345**: 1359–67.

17. H.J. Robertshaw and G.M. Hall (2006). Diabetes mellitus: anaesthetic management. *Anaesthesia* **61**: 1187–90.

18. G. Nicholson, J.M. Burrin and G.M. Hall (1998). Peri-operative steroid supplementation. *Anaesthesia* **53**: 1091–104.

19. D.R. Errington, A.M. Severn and J. Meara (2002). Parkinson's disease. BJA CEPD *Reviews* **2**: 69–73.

20. G. Nicholson, A.C. Pereira and G.M. Hall (2002). Parkinson's disease and anaesthesia. *British Journal of Anaesthesia* **89**: 904–16.

21. T. Asai (2004). Who is at increased risk of pulmonary aspiration? *British Journal of Anaesthesia* **93**: 497–500.

22. T.J. Gan, T. Meyer, C.C. Apfel, F. Chung, P.J. Davis, S. Eubanks et al. (2003). Consensus guidelines for managing postoperative nausea and vomiting. *Anesthesia and Analgesia* **97**: 62–71.

23. J.T. Sullivan, K. Sykora, J. Schneiderman, C.A. Naranjo and E.M. Sellers (1989). Assessment of alcohol withdrawal: the revised Clinical Institute Withdrawal Assessment for Alcohol scale (CIWA-Ar). *British Journal of Addiction* **84**: 1353–7.

24. P.J. Hodges and P.C.A. Kam (2002). The perioperative implications of herbal medicines. *Anaesthesia* **57**: 889–99.

25. J. Moss and C-S. Yuan (2006). Herbal medicines and perioperative care. *Anesthesiology* **105**: 441–2.

26. The British Thoracic Society and the Scottish Intercollegiate Guidelines Network (2003). British guideline on the management of asthma. *Thorax* **58**: i1-94.

13 Considerations in the preoperative assessment of paediatric patients

Simon Moore

SUMMARY

This chapter will cover the following:

- **introduction and definitions**
- **anatomical and physiological considerations**
- **psychological considerations**
- **practicalities of anaesthetising children**
- **postoperative care.**

INTRODUCTION

When assessing a paediatric patient preoperatively it is important to be aware of the considerable differences that exist in terms of anatomy, physiology, pharmacology and psychology, when compared to the adult patient. The younger the patient, the more pronounced these differences will be. It is also important to note that children vary enormously in weight, size, shape, intellectual ability and emotional response.

Special consideration will need to be given to neonates, ex-premature infants and those with congenital abnormalities. Ideally these patients will be dealt with in a tertiary paediatric centre, but may present to a district general hospital in an emergency situation. The approach to the elective and emergency situation follows the same broad pattern but time constraints will inevitably leave less time for thorough psychological preparation when inevitably the focus is on the adequacy of airway, breathing and circulation.

Definitions

- Neonates are babies less than 44 weeks post-conception.
- Infants are less than one year old.

- A child is between one and 12 years old.
- An adolescent is between 13 and 19 years old.
- A premature infant is an infant born before 37 weeks post-conception.
- Low birth weight is a birth weight of less than 2500g.

Anatomical and physiological considerations

A. Airway and respiratory system

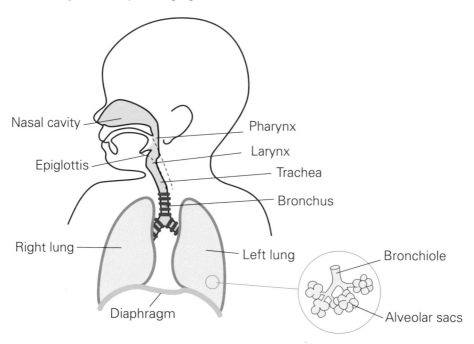

Figure 13.1 Paediatric airway and respiratory system

Anatomy

The anatomy of the airway and respiratory system has some of the most pronounced differences between adult and child. The head is relatively large and the neck is short. Coupled with this, the tongue is large and can obstruct the pharynx, leading to airway obstruction. An oral airway may be needed to aid ventilation.

Neonates are mainly nose breathers so any decrease in the already narrow nasal passages (50% of total airway resistance) from secretions or oedema can have a significant effect on gas flow and the work of breathing. Careful consideration should be given to any child with coryzal symptoms (see preoperative visit section below).

The larynx is anterior and cephalad (C3-C4). Positioning for intubation will therefore be different from that of an adult, as a 'sniffing the morning air' position in a neonate or infant will impair visualisation of the glottis. The use of a head ring to stabilise the head, or a roll under the shoulders, aids intubation. The epiglottis is long, stiff and U-shaped. A straight blade is often easier for intubation, as it lifts the epiglottis away from the cords. It must be remembered that the posterior part of the epiglottis is innervated by the vagus nerve; therefore intubation with a straight blade can lead to a bradycardia.

The paediatric airway is narrowest at the cricoid cartilage, just below the vocal cords. Here, the trachea is lined with pseudo-stratified ciliated epithelium, loosely bound to the underlying alveolar tissue. Any trauma which results in oedema will impede gas flow. The trachea is short (5cm in the neonate) so endotracheal tubes have to be placed and secured carefully to avoid an endo-bronchial intubation. The tracheal cartilages are soft and easily compressed and can collapse if breathing is attempted against an obstructed airway. The right main bronchus is larger than the left and less acutely angled at origin. This invariably leads to right-sided endo-bronchial intubation (see Figure 13.2).

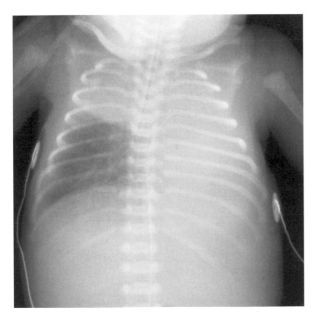

Figure 13.2 Malpositioned endotracheal tube – tube has passed along the right main bronchus distal to the origin of the right upper lobe bronchus with subsequent collapse of the left lung and right upper lobe.

Reproduced with kind permission from: Dr Richard Hopkins, Consultant Radiologist and Editor of Hopkins, R., Peden, C. & Ghandi, S.: *Radiology for anaesthesia and intensive care* (2nd edition), Cambridge Medical

The ribs are horizontal rather than bucket handle as in adults. Ventilation is therefore mainly diagphragmatic. Bulky viscera or gastrointestinal obstruction, leading to gas-filled bowel, can impede diaphragmatic excursion, leading to respiratory embarrassment.

The chest wall is very compliant and is pulled inward by the lungs, decreasing functional residual capacity (FRC). Closing capacity (CC) exceeds FRC during normal respiration in neonates, infants and children up to the age of six to eight years. Applying continuous positive airway pressure (CPAP) intraoperatively improves oxygenation and reduces the work of breathing.

At birth the tracheo-bronchial tree is developed to the terminal bronchioles. The alveoli are thick walled and number 20 million. By the age of six, the number of alveoli has increased to 300 million. Further growth is seen as an increase in the size of the alveoli and airways.

Physiology

Oxygen consumption is markedly raised in paediatric patients, and can exceed 6ml/kg/min in infants, i.e. double the adult value of 3–4ml/kg/min. To meet this increased demand, alveolar minute ventilation is increased via an increase in respiratory rate (tidal volume is the same as in adults at 7ml/kg). This leaves infants vulnerable to hypoxaemia in a very short space of time if there is any upper airway obstruction.

The maturation of neuronal respiratory control is related to post-conceptual age rather than postnatal age. Both hypoxic and hypercapnic drives are not well developed in neonates and infants. Importantly, hypoxia and hypercapnia cause respiratory depression in this age group. Postoperative apnoea occurs commonly in the preterm neonate.

Respiration is diaphragmatic, sinusoidal and continuous in nature rather than periodic, as seen in older children and adults.

B. Cardiovascular and haematology system

A basic understanding of the foetal circulation and the circulatory changes that occur at birth is important in understanding the response to conditions of severe hypoxia, hypercapnia, hypothermia and acidosis that can occur over the first few weeks of life. Essentially in these stressful conditions reversion to a foetal 'transitional' circulation can occur if conditions are not improved.

In the foetus little blood flow occurs to the pulmonary circulation, as the resistance to flow is high in the collapsed lungs. Blood flows from right to left atria via the patent foramen ovale and from the pulmonary artery to the aorta via the ductus arteriosus. This arrangement results in relatively oxygen-rich blood reaching the brain. At birth as the lungs become aerated, pulmonary vascular resistance falls, both directly and as a result of increasing oxygen tension, leading to an increase in pulmonary blood flow through the lungs to the left atrium. Pressure within the left atrium becomes higher than that in the right, and the foramen ovale begins to close. Systemic vascular resistance rises as blood flow to the placenta ceases. Aortic pressure rises above that in the pulmonary artery and blood flow in the ductus arteriosus reverses. The increased arterial oxygen tension leads to constriction of the ductus arteriosus over the first few days. In hypoxic conditions, these flow changes can reverse and potentially lead to a spiralling hypoxaemic decline.

At birth the right ventricle is more thick walled than the left, which is fibrous and noncompliant. This low compliance limits stroke volume (1.5ml/kg), and the high cardiac output (300ml/kg/min) is heart rate dependent. The practical importance of this is that the response to volume therapy is blunted because stroke volume cannot increase greatly to improve cardiac output. After birth the left ventricle enlarges disproportionately with the adult ratio of myocardial thickness established by about three to six months. By the age of two years, myocardial function and response to fluid are similar to those of an adult. Systemic vascular resistance rises after birth and continues to do so until adulthood, reflected in blood pressure changes (see Table 13.1). Pulmonary artery pressure, pulmonary vascular resistance and pulmonary blood flow approach adult values by four to six weeks. The autonomic innervation of the heart is incomplete in the newborn with relative lack of sympathetic elements, predisposing the neonatal heart to bradycardia.

Table 13.1 Cardiovascular and haematological physiological variables

Age	Neonate	Infant	1 year	5 year	Adult
Systolic BP (mmHg)	65	90	95	95	120
Heart rate (beats/min)	130	120	120	90	77
Blood volume (ml/kg)	90	85	80	75	70
Haemoglobin (g/dl)	17	11	12	13	14

Foetal haemoglobin HbF, which makes up 70–90% of haemoglobin at birth, is not able to deliver oxygen as efficiently to tissues as normal haemoglobin because it holds on to oxygen more avidly (less 2,3 Bisphosphoglycerate). The high haemoglobin level (13–19g/dl, depending on the degree of placental transfusion) and high cardiac output compensate for this. Within three months, the levels of HbF drop to around 15% and HbA predominates. Haemoglobin levels drop over three to six months to 9–12g/dl as the increase in circulating volume increases more rapidly than the bone marrow activity (physiological anaemia).

Vitamin K dependent clotting factors (II, VII, IX, X) and platelet function are deficient in the first few months. Vitamin K is given at birth to prevent haemorrhagic disease of the newborn.

C. Renal system and fluid management

Renal vascular resistance is high immediately after birth. It decreases rapidly and is low by two weeks. Glomerular filtration rate and renal blood flow are therefore low in the neonate and increase steadily throughout childhood, reaching adult levels around the age of two. Concentrating capacity of the infant kidney is less than that of an adult. Maximum urine osmolality is 600–700mOsm/kg, compared to 1200mOsm/kg in the adult. Despite the low glomerular filtration rate, infant kidneys can handle large water loads because of their low concentrating capacity.

After a free water load infants can excrete a markedly dilute urine of 50mOsm/kg compared to a maximally dilute urine of 70–100mOsm/kg in adults.

Table 13.2 Glomerular filtration rates by age

Age	ml/min/1.73 m2 *
1–2 days	20–25
1 week	35–40
3 months	55–60
Adult	120

* Glomerular filtration rate is indexed to body surface area; this is inexact because of the relatively high body surface area of neonates and infants.

The loop of Henle is short and this affects the kidneys' ability to retain sodium via the ascending limb of the loop. Even with a low glomerular filtration rate, a net loss of sodium can occur. Carbonic anhydrase is present in the proximal tubules at birth, but is scanty in the distal tubules. There are also lower concentrations of buffering ions and this, in combination with the decreased carbonic anhydrase, decreases the kidneys' ability to excrete acid.

Dehydration is poorly tolerated as children have large insensible losses due to the large surface area to weight ratio. There is a larger proportion of extra cellular fluid in children – 40% body weight compared to 20% in adults.

Fluid management in the paediatric surgical patient can be divided into three categories: deficit therapy, maintenance therapy and replacement therapy, all aimed at maintaining a urine output of 1–2ml/kg/hour. As with any prescribed treatment, fluid therapy should be monitored and adjusted according to response. Plasma electrolytes and glucose should be checked at least every 24 hours (more frequently in neonates).

Deficit therapy

Deficit therapy is the management of fluid and electrolyte losses prior to the patient's admission. This is a major consideration for patients presenting as emergencies following trauma or infective episodes of diarrhoea and vomiting.

Fluid deficit can be estimated from the history, examination and electrolyte evaluation. Examination includes an evaluation of the eyes and fontanelles (may be sunken), skin colour, turgor and temperature, character and rate of peripheral pulse, respiratory rate, mental state and capillary refill time. Initial fluid boluses of 20ml/kg crystalloid or 10ml/kg colloid followed by reassessment may be necessary. A fall in blood pressure is a sign of uncompensated hypovolaemic shock.

Maintenance therapy
Maintenance fluid requirements are calculated as shown below, on an hourly basis depending on body weight. They replace the fluid the child would normally have been drinking.

- 4ml/kg for the first 10kg body weight
- 2ml/kg for the next 10kg body weight
- 1ml/kg for each kg above 20kg body weight.

After most minor to moderate surgery, children will go back to drinking normally fairly quickly.

Replacement therapy
After major surgery or trauma, blood may need to be replaced. Also 'third space' losses will need replacing. This refers to fluid lost from the circulation, in the form of oedema, into the bowel and by evaporation. This is normally calculated as 7–10ml/kg/hour of surgery. Children, like adults, generally show a stress response to surgery, with a rise in blood glucose even if no glucose-containing fluid is given. There is an increase in antidiuretic hormone (ADH) secretion, leading to retention of water by the kidneys.

Most fluid is replaced as Hartmann's solution with colloid or blood used as necessary. Use of 0.9% sodium chloride and dextrose solutions depends on the requirements of the child. The routine prescription of hypotonic solutions such as 4% glucose/0.18% saline in the perioperative period is no longer acceptable practice with its attendant risk of hyponatraemia.

D. Gastrointestinal system

Hepatic enzyme systems are initially immature. Barbiturates and opioids, for example, have a longer duration of action and neonates are more prone to jaundice (glucuronyl transferase system is poorly developed). Carbohydrate reserves are low in neonates and they are more prone to hypoglycaemia. Regular blood glucose measurements should be performed and hypoglycaemia treated with 10% glucose. Hyperglycaemia is usually iatrogenic and can result in neurological damage

E. Temperature control

Neonates and infants have a large surface area to weight ratio, which increases heat loss. They also have minimal subcutaneous fat and poorly developed shivering, sweating and vasoconstriction mechanisms. Brown fat, which requires more oxygen for metabolism, is used for non-shivering thermogenesis in the neonate.

Heat loss during anaesthesia is mainly via radiation but can also be attributed to convection, conduction and evaporation. Low body temperature increases the duration of action of drugs, decreases platelet function and increases the risk of infection. It also causes respiratory depression, acidosis and decreased cardiac function. Children having prolonged intra-abdominal surgery, with a large surface area exposed to the operating theatre environment, are particularly vulnerable.

F. Central nervous system

The neonatal blood brain barrier is poorly formed. Drugs such as barbiturates, opioids, antibiotics and bilirubin cross the blood brain barrier easily, causing a prolonged and variable duration of action. The minimum aveolar concentration (MAC) of volatile agents is lower in neonates due to a relatively higher proportion of fat in the neonatal brain. MAC then peaks at one year (50% higher than adult values) decreasing thereafter, reaching adult levels by puberty.

Neonates can appreciate pain and this is associated with increased heart rate, blood pressure and a neuro-endocrine response. There is also evidence to suggest that infants who experience painful stimuli have an increased sensitivity to pain when older, possibly as a result of changes in the central nervous system.

Psychology

Children vary in their intellectual ability and emotional response. Some knowledge of child development will be helpful in understanding their fears and behaviour and will enable the perioperative team to take an appropriate approach to the child's surgery. Hospitalisation and medical procedures have profound emotional consequences for infants and children and behavioural disturbances can occur long after the event. The most important determinant of the impact of hospitalisation is age.

- Infants under six months are generally not upset by separation from parents.
- Children of six months to four years are much more upset by hospitalisations, primarily because of separation from family and familiar surroundings.
- School age children are more concerned with the procedure itself.

Factors other than age also influence the child's emotional response, such as length of stay, type of procedure and parental reaction. '[B]eing unable to choose parents for your patients, you must make do with those who come with the child'.[1]

Therefore for elective procedures adequate time must be set aside for psychological preparation for both children and parents. This may involve a visit to the hospital, play simulation, video presentations and age-specific literature for the child to read. Long-term behavioural benefits have been demonstrated in patients who participate in such preoperative preparation. A previous theatre experience may have gone badly and these children may benefit from a more thorough preoperative psychological preparation.

Even with a thorough approach it is still sometimes difficult to predict how children will cope once in theatre. Some who appear quite calm and understanding of the process on the ward preoperatively may react badly once in the anaesthetic room.

Practicalities for anaesthetising children

A. Preoperative visit

Use this important time to develop rapport and gain the confidence of both child and parents. Answer any questions in simple language and avoid wearing a white coat. Question the child directly, if possible, but include the parents in any discussion. Explain the approach to induction of anaesthesia and inform and obtain consent for the use of suppositories. Discuss postoperative pain management and any local anaesthetic procedures that will be performed. Take a thorough history and examine the child as necessary. Review the case notes, observation charts and any investigations performed. Prescribe premedication and local anaesthetic creams if necessary. Ensure adequate consent has been obtained. 'At age 16 a young person can be treated as an adult and can be presumed to have capacity'[1] to consent to any treatment. A child under 16 may also have capacity to decide on any treatment if they have an understanding of what is involved. For further details on consent, the General Medical Council (GMC) has produced guidance, available at: http://www.gmc-uk.org/guidance/current/library/consent.asp

Anaesthetic and medical history

The following items should be addressed when taking a history:

i. Problems with previous anaesthetics including postoperative nausea and vomiting (PONV), poor pain relief, difficult venous access.

ii. Family history to exclude malignant hyperthermia (MH) and Suxamethonium apnoea.

iii. Current or previous medical problems. If a significant history is obtained, communication with other healthcare professionals may be necessary to establish the current disease status. If a child presents with signs of an upper respiratory tract infection (URTI) try to establish whether this is the start or end of the cold. If at the start postpone surgery for two weeks. If the child is considered postviral, surgery is probably safe. Any child with a productive cough, pyrexia or constitutional illness should be postponed.

iv. Neonatal history.

v. Current medications.

vi. Allergies.

vii. Recent immunisations: surgery should be avoided for one week after DTP and Hib and two weeks after MMR.

viii. Check for the presence of loose teeth.

ix. Ensure the child adequately fasted:

- 6 hours for solids and milk if more than 12 months of age
- 4 hours for breast milk and formula feeds if less than 12 months of age
- 2 hours for unlimited clear fluids (as this decreases gastric acidity and volume).

There is an increased incidence of nausea and vomiting with long fasting periods.

Examination

Conduct a physical examination as appropriate, concentrating on the airway and cardio-respiratory systems. Children must be weighed, as the child's weight determines the dosage of drug to be administered. In the absence of actual weight, the following equations will give an approximate estimated weight to allow clinicians to calculate appropriate drug dosages especially in emergency situations:

- For children aged 3–12 months: weight (in kg) = [age (in months) + 9] / 2
- For children aged 1–6 yrs: weight (in kg) = [age (in years) + 4] x 2

Investigations

The following investigations should be considered for the following groups of patients:

- haemoglobin – large expected blood loss, premature infants, systemic disease, congenital heart disease
- electrolytes – renal or metabolic disease, intravenous fluids, dehydration
- chest X-ray – active respiratory disease, scoliosis, congenital heart disease.

Pre-medication and topical anaesthetics

- Analgesics – Drugs such as paracetamol, ibuprofen or codeine phosphate, given more than a half an hour preoperatively, are useful for shorter procedures, as they will have had time to reach an effective therapeutic level for the intra- and postoperative period.

- Sedation – Sedation should not be given as a matter of routine as it is unpleasant to take, difficult to time, can fail or cause agitation and may delay recovery and discharge. However, it may be necessary in an excessively anxious child or a child with a previous unpleasant anaesthetic or hospital experience. Oral midazolam (0.5mg/kg), given 30 minutes preoperatively, is widely prescribed. Adding Calpol or a sweetener, such as fruit juice, helps reduce the bitter taste. Alternative agents include oral ketamine (5–6mg/kg) (with or without midazolam), clonidine (4mg/kg), trimeprazine (2mg/kg), promethazine (1mg/kg), chloral hydrate (50mg/kg to a maximum of 1g) and temazepam (0.5–1mg/kg)(for older children).

- Anticholinergic drugs – Vagal blocking drugs (atropine, hyoscine, glycopyrrolate) are no longer given routinely but atropine should be immediately available to use if it becomes necessary. Atropine is the preferred anticholinergic in children, as it is most effective at blocking the cardiac vagus nerve (0.02mg/kg). The same dose can be given orally 90 minutes preop or intramuscular 30 minutes preop. It can also be given through the tracheal tube in the same dose diluted in saline to 2ml in an emergency.

- Topical anaesthetics – Local anaesthetic cream is applied to identifiable veins on those children for whom an intravenous induction is planned. EMLA cream is a eutectic mixture of 5% lignocaine and 5% prilocaine in a 1:1 ratio. It needs to be applied one hour prior to cannulation and lasts 30–60 mins. It also produces vasoconstriction and there is a risk of methaemoglobinaemia (prilocaine) in children less than one year old. Ametop is a 4% gel formulation of the ester local anaesthetic, amethocaine, and has a shorter onset time of 45 minutes. It is less readily absorbed across mucous membranes and does not cause methaemoglobinaemia. It also has the advantage of a prolonged duration of action (four hours) after the cream is removed. It causes local erythema and vasodilatation, making cannulation easier. It is more likely, however to cause allergic reactions and should be removed after 90 minutes.

B. Preparation for anaesthesia

As with any anaesthetic, the preparation starts prior to the preoperative visit when the anaesthetist finds out what patients are on the operating list. Occasionally at a district general hospital, there may be paediatric patients who are not on a dedicated paediatric list. If this is the case, the child must be operated on 'first on the list', so the starvation period is not extended.

The anaesthetic plan will have been formulated with the child and his or her parents during the preoperative visit. During this visit it is a good idea to decide which parent, if either, will accompany the child to the anaesthetic room. If one of the parents is present for induction, a member of staff must be available to escort the parent back to the ward from the anaesthetic room. This can be a very stressful experience for the parent.

Prior to the child arriving in the anaesthetic room, drug doses should be calculated according to the weight of the child. Emergency drugs, such as atropine and suxamethonium, should be drawn up in dilutions that are familiar.

All equipment should be ready and checked. Airways, facemasks, laryngeal masks, endotracheal tubes, laryngoscopes and blades and breathing circuits appropriate to the age and weight of the patient. Alternate sizes of all of the above should also be readily available.

Most anaesthetists use uncuffed tubes until the age of approximately eight years to reduce the risk of subglottic stenosis (the narrowest part of the paediatric airway is at the level of the cricoid cartilage). A small leak should be present; if the leak is too big, ventilation will be compromised. Cuffed tubes are available down to 5.5mm. Tube sizes and lengths can be estimated as follows:

- Tube size = age/4 + 4.5
- Tube length = age/2 + 12

These are guides to sizes and tubes should be checked for a leak, and length should be checked by auscultating the chest.

Laryngeal mask sizes relate to weight as follows:

- size 1 – up to 5kg
- size 1.5 – 5–10kg
- size 2 – 10–20kg
- size 2.5 – 20–30kg
- size 3 – over 30kg

Endotracheal tubes and laryngeal mask airways should be secured with tape fixed to the less mobile maxilla.

As discussed earlier, children lose heat rapidly. The theatre should be at an appropriate temperature. Optimal ambient temperature to prevent heat loss is 32°C for neonates and 28°C for adolescents and adults. Warming devices (mattress, forced air warmers and fluids) and padding should also be prepared. Use of a circle breathing system will also help to conserve heat.

The plan should be made known to the operating department practitioner or anaesthetic nurse.

C. Induction of anaesthesia

1) Intravenous

Placing an intravenous cannula has been made easier with the advent of local anaesthetic creams (see pages 262–3). Veins on the back of the hand or inner wrist are the easiest to find. Alternatives include the long saphenous vein, other veins on the dorsum of the foot and antecubital fossa in older children. The child can be placed on the parent's lap or on the trolley and the hand concealed from the child's view. The arm may be squeezed gently by an anaesthetic assistant or by the anaesthetist with the non-cannulating hand. The child should be distracted in some way or asked to cough during the cannulation attempt. Intravenous induction can be undertaken with propofol, thiopentone or ketamine.

2. Inhalational

Sevoflurane is the current volatile agent of choice due to its non-irritant nature, rapid onset and relative haemodynamic stability. It can be given either with a high initial concentration (8%) or increased gradually, usually with the addition of nitrous oxide. Halothane is an alternative volatile agent which may still be used in some centres. A variety of techniques can be used in performing an inhalational induction and it is important to develop a fluid approach depending on how the child and parents react. The child may be placed supine on the trolley or on the parent's lap. They may wish to hold the mask themselves or have the parent hold the mask. A clear, flavoured mask is less intimidating than a black mask. A cupped hand method may also be used. Warn parents that the child's head will become floppy and explain there is an excitatory phase accompanied by abnormal movements. Once anaesthesia is achieved, a skilled assistant will need to maintain the child's airway while intravenous access is obtained. A correctly sized (size from the corner of the mouth to the angle of the jaw) oropharyngeal airway may be used. Airways should not be inverted during insertion, as there is a risk of damage to the palate.

D. Maintenance

Techniques using nitrous oxide, oxygen and either sevoflurane, isoflurane or desflurane are accepted methods of maintaining anaesthesia in children. Sevoflurane and desflurane have a more rapid offset than isoflurane but do show more emergence agitation than the latter.

Total intravenous anaesthesia (TIVA) has advantages for patients at high risk of vomiting, such as, children undergoing strabismus surgery or surgery to the middle ear. Maintenance of anaesthesia with propofol has been shown to have significant anti-emetic effect.

The pharmacokinetics of propofol in children differs from adults. A three compartment model is applicable to children with a volume of distribution that is 50% larger than adults. Clearance is up to twice that of adults. Clinically this means that a higher initial bolus dose is needed to reach a given plasma concentration and increased infusion rates to maintain steady state plasma concentrations.

Neonates and infants are more sensitive than adults to non-depolarising muscle relaxants, though initial doses are similar, due to a larger volume of distribution. Duration of action may be prolonged in neonates due to decreased glomerular filtration rate and hepatic clearance. Larger doses of suxamethonium (2mg/kg for infants) are similarly required due to the larger volume of distribution.

Postoperative care

Children should be recovered in a designated paediatric recovery area (which can be within the adult recovery room), with easy access to appropriate equipment and correctly sized blood pressure cuffs and pulse oximeters. Staff should have received training in recovery of paediatric patients and provide one-to-one care. The area should be kept warm to prevent hypothermia and provision should be made for a parent or carer to rejoin their children as soon as they are awake. The usual standards of handover and discharge criteria apply.

Postoperative pain relief is provided by a standard multimodal approach with paracetamol and NSAIDs widely prescribed for minor cases. The rectal loading dose should be at least 30mg/kg, followed by 15mg/kg six hourly. Aspirin should not be used in children under the age of 12 years because of the association with Reye's syndrome. For moderate to severe pain, codeine or oromorph can be added. Morphine infusions, nurse-controlled analgesia or patient-controlled analgesia pumps can also be used if closely supervised by appropriately trained ward staff.

Local anaesthetic techniques including wound infiltration and specific regional blocks should always be considered as part of the multimodal approach to pain relief (see below).

Postoperative nausea and vomiting can be appropriately managed with the use of combinations of 5-HT3 antagonists with low dose dexamethasone. Children at particular risk, such as those undergoing tonsillectomy or squint surgery, should receive prophylactic ondansetron (0.1mg/kg IV) at induction of anaesthesia.

Regional anaesthesia

Most children would not tolerate surgery under a regional technique alone. However, such a technique is a very useful adjunct to general anaesthesia for postoperative pain relief. Tetracaine eye drops can be used after strabismus surgery and lidocaine ointment is useful after circumcision.

Wound infiltration with local anaesthetic is easy to perform and very effective. Some older children will tolerate procedures such as naevi removal with local infiltration alone.

Peripheral nerve blocks are also used as an adjunct to general anaesthesia. A penile nerve block is used after circumcision, minor hypospadias repair and other penile procedures. Ilioinguinal–iliohypogastric nerve blocks are effective analgesia for inguinal herniotomy and for the groin incision for orchidopexy.

Epidurals in children are beyond the remit of the district general hospital (DGH). There are not enough staff trained on the paediatric ward in a DGH to safely look after epidurals. Surgery requiring that level of postoperative pain relief should be done at a tertiary centre.

Caudal extradural anaesthesia (CEA) is a widely used, simple, safe and effective technique for intraoperative and postoperative analgesia. It is especially suited to the paediatric population due to the relative ease with which landmarks can be identified, the higher dermatomal block that can be achieved and the greater spread of local anaesthetic, due to less tightly packed epidural fat. The potential for lower limb weakness with caudal anaesthesia can be minimised with weaker local anaesthetic solutions. One of the drawbacks of the single shot caudal is that effective analgesia only lasts for a few hours. Addition of NMDA antagonists, such as ketamine 0.5mg/kg or alpha-2 agonists, such as clonidine 1-2μg/kg can double or even quadruple the duration of the analgesia.

REFERENCE

1. Mellish, R. (1969). Preparation of a child for hospitalization and surgery. *Paediatric Clinics of North America* **16** (3): 543–53.

FURTHER READING

A.R. Aitkenhead and R.M. Jones (1996). *Clinical Anaesthesia*. Oxford: Churchill Livingstone.

K.G. Allman and I.H. Wilson (2006). *Oxford Handbook of Anaesthesia* (2nd edn). Oxford: Oxford University Press. 758–87.

L.J. Brennan (1999). Modern day-case anaesthesia for children. *British Journal of Anaesthesia* **83**: 91–103.

Chidanande-Swamy, M. and Mallikarjum, D. (2004). Applied aspects of anatomy and physiology of relevance to paediatric anaesthesia. *Indian Journal of Anaesthesia* **48**(5): 333–9.

General Medical Council (2008). *Consent: Patients and Doctors Making Decisions Together*. London: GMC.

R. Hopkins, C. Peden and S. Gandhi (2003). *Radiology for Anaesthesia and Intensive Care*. London: Greenwich Medical Media.

L. Rusy and E. Usaleva (1998). 'Paediatric Anaesthesia Review Update'. *Anaesthesia* issue 8. Available at: http://www.nda.ox.ac.uk/wfsa/html/u08/u08_003.html

C.L. Snyder, T.L. Spilde and H. Rice (2008). Fluid Management for the Paediatric Surgical Patient. Available at: http://emedicine.medscape.com/article/936511-overview (updated 24 January 2008).

D.J. Steward and J. Lerman (1975). *Manual of Pediatric Anesthesia* (5th edn). London: Churchill Livingston.

S.M. Yentis, N.P. Hirsch and G.B. Smith (2009). *Anaesthesia and Intensive Care A to Z: An Encyclopedia of Principles and Practice*. (4th edn) Oxford: Churchill Livingstone.

INTERNET RESOURCES

www.childrenscentralcal.org

www.gmc-uk.org/guidance/ethical_guidance/children_guidance_appendix_1.asp

14 Preoperative assessment and day case surgery

Ian Smith
Clare Hammond

SUMMARY

This chapter will describe:
- **the current trends in day case surgery**
- **patient selection and clinical approaches to care**
- **future developments in day case practice.**

INTRODUCTION

Preassessment before day surgery should aim to identify all those patients for whom, because of medical conditions or social circumstances, successful discharge on the day of operation would be unlikely or unsafe, or where complications thereafter would be highly probable. As with other forms of preassessment, every attempt should be made to ensure that the patient is optimally treated before elective surgery. Patients who, once optimally treated, are still likely to experience complications or will be difficult to manage during the operative period or in the early stages of recovery may still be suitable candidates for day surgery, provided these problems will have resolved by the time of intended discharge.

Day surgery can trace its origins back to the early 1900s,[1] but it did not become particularly common until the late 1980s and has recently undergone a further expansion. Day surgery was once seen as a highly selective and specialised form of care, which was unsafe and undesirable in all but the fittest patients. As the practice has expanded, especially in North America and northern Europe, increasing experience and evidence show that this is not the case. Day surgery offers patients numerous clinical benefits[2] and should be seen as the treatment of choice[3,4] or default option, for a wide range of surgical procedures.[5]

It is beyond the scope of this chapter to consider all of the surgical procedures suitable for day surgery (for a comprehensive selection, see the British Association of Day Surgery's *Directory of Procedures*[5]), but the advent of minimally invasive surgery means that much is now possible. Surgical prejudices must be challenged, paying particular attention to the likely timing of postoperative complications. Complications which occur early, and which would be detected by careful postoperative observation and a thorough review prior to discharge, or else which only occur after several days, when even inpatients would be at home, should not prevent day surgery.

Mechanism of day surgery preassessment

Once the decision to operate has been made, and if the intended surgical procedure is possible to perform as a day case, it should be the preassessment team who decide the individual patient's final management.[2,4,6,7] Day surgery should be considered as the default option,[3,6] with inpatient care selected only if there are unsuitable social circumstances or legitimate medical concerns (see Figure 14.1). Current medical and social criteria for day surgery[7-9] will be discussed later in this chapter.

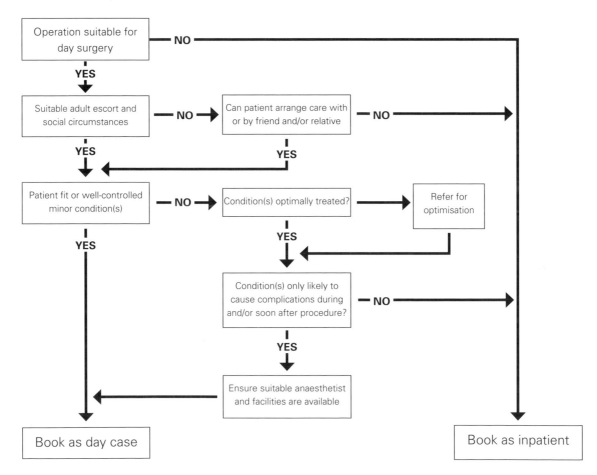

Figure 14.1
Basic principles for the preassessment and selection of day case patients

Day surgery preassessment may be broken down into three components. First, there is the information gathering and health assessment necessary to determine the patient's level of fitness and whether or not they are optimally treated. This process is essentially similar to other forms of preassessment before elective surgery. The second component is the decision as to whether the optimised patient is a suitable candidate for day surgery, or if they would be better managed as an inpatient. This requires specialist knowledge of the postoperative course of numerous procedures, as well as some of the specialised anaesthetic techniques which can be used to good effect in certain higher risk patients. The third component is information giving, since much of the success of day surgery comes from developing a positive mental attitude and preparing the patient to be able to cope outside the hospital environment. Patients need to be given a realistic idea of how much postoperative pain they will have and how this will be managed, as well as what support they will require and when they can safely resume various activities.

There is currently a preference for centralising all preassessment services, as this concentrates the valuable resource of nurses trained in health assessment. Centralised preassessment is also consistent with the default to day surgery philosophy, with every patient at least being considered for this form of care. However, the other two components of day surgery preassessment, as outlined above, are highly specialised and there are considerable advantages if preassessment is performed within the facility where day surgery will take place.[8] Here will be found many nurses with the necessary specialist skills and ready access to specialist anaesthetists (and surgeons) who can usually give an instant opinion on the more difficult cases. Suitable preoperative information will also be available and there is an opportunity for the patient (and perhaps their carer) to familiarise themselves with the surgical facility. Despite the logistical advantages of centralised preassessment, there are definite advantages to segregating preassessment for services where day care is unlikely, such as cardiac, colorectal and major orthopaedic surgery, from those where it is a probable form of care. Alternatively, day surgery preassessment may function well as a 'team within a team'.

Assessing fitness for day surgery

The health assessment of adults (preassessment of children for day surgery follows essentially the same principles as for any paediatric preassessment and is not considered in this chapter) presenting for day surgery is a clinical process which relies most heavily on the patient history. Although much attention is focused on acquiring clinical skills, such as chest auscultation, in the authors' opinion this is rarely helpful. For example, a previously unknown cardiac murmur is unlikely to represent significant cardiac risk (or indicate the need for endocarditis prophylaxis) in the absence of any symptoms or physical limitation. Similarly, screening investigations rarely detect pathology which will significantly alter the intended management or eventual outcome. For example, ECGs are rarely abnormal (to a degree to cause concern or alter management) in the absence of symptoms or other cardiovascular risk factors, even in the elderly.[10] Even screening for sickle cells is probably unnecessary in adults; the disease (which may very well dictate modification in anaesthetic or surgical management) should be clinically evident by adult life, whereas the presence of the trait (which is clinically undetectable) requires no change in management.

Obtaining the patient history can be achieved in a variety of ways, but most conveniently involves some sort of questionnaire (for an example, see AAGBI (2005)[8]). These can be completed at a face-to-face interview, over the telephone or internet, or can be sent home with the patient and returned by post. The format usually involves basic screening questions, with supplementary questions asked, if appropriate. Computerised versions can exploit the concept of selective questioning to a far greater degree and can also calculate perioperative risk and advise on appropriate management automatically.

Preassessment should ideally allow enough time to investigate and optimise patients, but not be so far in advance as to permit the patient's condition to deteriorate further.[6] It is most convenient for the patient if preassessment, or at least an initial health screen, is performed at the time of the surgical outpatients clinic and, with the move towards the 18-week wait, such a 'one-stop shop' will have to become the norm. Not all patients will require a formal face-to-face consultation as part of their health assessment, however, and screening questionnaires are often used to identify these healthier patients. Nevertheless, most patients will still benefit from the type of information which can be provided by a preassessment service.

Social selection criteria

The residual effects of general anaesthesia or sedation, combined with the sedative effects of some analgesic medications and the discomfort and dysfunction produced by the surgical procedure, mean that the patient's fine judgement may be impaired for some time after surgery and they can be at risk from everyday activities. Patients must therefore be discharged into the care of a responsible adult who can ensure they remain safe and also summon help in the unlikely event of a serious problem. A somewhat arbitrary period of 24 hours is commonly recommended,[11] although considerably longer may be required after some operations or in more frail individuals. Conversely, an escort is usually unnecessary after operations conducted under local anaesthesia, unless the surgery itself is significantly disabling. Patients also need easy access to a telephone, to summon assistance, and should have reasonable access to emergency care.

With an ageing population and increasing break-up of the family unit, many more patients now live alone, making them potentially unsuitable for day surgery. However, in many cases, adequate preparation time can allow them to make suitable arrangements to be accompanied by, or to stay with, a friend or family member. Such arrangements mean that these patients are not denied the benefits of day surgery, not least being the significant reduction in postoperative confusion in the elderly compared with inpatient care.[12]

In the United Kingdom, most patients will live within a few miles of their nearest hospital. However, if they have to stay with a relative postoperatively or need access to specialised surgical services which are not available locally, they may be contemplating a much longer journey after day surgery. It is common to limit the recommended travelling time to an hour or less, but longer journeys are more common in countries with widely scattered populations. In Norway, for example, patients may often travel up to 300 miles by air or four to six hours by road.[13] The available evidence suggests that travelling long distances is safe, provided that emergency care is available at the final destination. The patient must also be aware that the journey may be somewhat unpleasant, due to residual discomfort from the surgery and the possibility of postoperative nausea and vomiting (PONV).

Medical selection criteria

It is tempting to apply various criteria and cut-offs to day surgery selection, and such an approach has certainly been practised in the past.[14] However, most limits of this type are somewhat arbitrary and rarely supported by sound evidence. In addition, there will always be patients who fall outside the exclusion criteria in whom day surgery would be both desirable and safe, while others might be unsuitable only through an interaction of several variables, none of which alone would be a contra-indication.

The modern approach[7,8] is to consider the patient as a whole and assess their suitability according to their physiological status and overall fitness, rather than relying on arbitrary limits, such as age, ASA status or BMI. The interaction between the patient and the proposed surgery, as well as the intended anaesthetic and analgesic techniques, are also important in reaching a final decision.

ASA status

The American Society of Anesthesiologists (ASA) classification is a useful 'shorthand' for describing chronic health and is a good example of an arbitrary limit. It has previously been common to exclude patients graded ASA 3 and above from day surgery. Certainly, patients of ASA 3 do experience more complications during the intraoperative period than those of ASA grades 1 and 2[15] but, crucially, once these have been effectively managed, problems are no more likely in the medium-to-late recovery period. Furthermore, complications and the need to seek assistance from primary care are no more common in ASA 3 patients after discharge from day surgery.[16] ASA 4 patients have a condition which represents a constant threat to life, yet a small number may still be suitable for some surgery on a day case basis under very specific circumstances, especially if the procedure can be performed under local or regional anaesthesia. In all cases, the specific condition(s) should always be assessed on an individual basis and specialist anaesthetic advice is advisable.

Obesity

Obese patients present numerous problems with manual handling, venous access, airway management, pulmonary ventilation, surgical access and so on, but none of these difficulties should preclude day surgery, since they would be equally problematic with inpatient management. Problems which would be directly relevant to day surgery include delayed respiratory depression or airway obstruction, poor pain management and delayed wound healing, but none of these problems begin to occur until the body mass index (BMI) is well in excess of 40kg/m². Yet many far less obese patients have previously been denied day surgery, a good example of not considering the nature and timing of complications, only their overall incidence.

Patients with a BMI of up to 35kg/m² should always be acceptable for day surgery (in the absence of other problems), while patients with a BMI of 35–40kg/m² should be acceptable for most procedures.[7] Even greater degrees of obesity are acceptable in some countries[17] and many feel that obesity should not be an absolute contra-indication, provided the right level of expertise and facilities are available.[8] Increasing numbers of obese patients are now safely undergoing day surgery and even gastric banding procedures for the morbidly obese have been performed as day cases.[18]

Day surgery – associated with short-acting medications, excellent pain relief achieved with non-opioid analgesia and early ambulation – offers clear benefits for obese patients who may be at particular risk in the hospital environment. However, obesity is also commonly associated with sleep apnoea, cardiac dysfunction and overall poor fitness, conditions which may independently make day surgery unsafe.

Diabetes mellitus

Diabetes is associated with end-organ disease in the cardiovascular, renal and autonomic systems and preassessment should carefully screen for evidence of these by way of a careful history, blood tests and ECG. Any abnormalities should be investigated and managed in their own right.

Preassessment should also consider the stability of diabetic control as poor glycaemic control increases the chances of wound infection and the likelihood of perioperative hyper- or hypoglycaemia, all of which are undesirable in day surgery. While random blood sugars are unhelpful, records of recent blood and urinalysis results are more informative and glycosylated haemoglobin provides evidence of stability over the past few months.

Perioperative glycaemic control is remarkably simple in stable diabetic day case patients, who are best managed in a way that interferes as little as possible with their usual regimen (see Figure 14.2). Normal medications (including metformin) should be continued up to, and including, the night before surgery,[19] which should be scheduled first on the morning operating list. Patients should omit their morning oral hypoglycaemic agent or insulin and aim to resume normal diet and medication as soon as possible after surgery.[20] The success of this strategy is most likely after relatively short procedures. Local or regional anaesthesia are preferable, but general anaesthesia is possible, provided a technique associated with minimal postoperative sedation, nausea and vomiting is used; multimodal anti-emetics may also be required. This approach can be adapted for afternoon surgery by allowing a light breakfast and morning short-acting hypoglycaemic therapy, but there is less time available to ensure a full return to normal and to manage unexpected difficulties. Therefore, diabetic patients should be managed during morning sessions whenever possible. Sliding scales and other complex regimens are unnecessary, and have no advantages, for stable patients undergoing relatively minor surgery, but may be required for more complex cases or when a simple regimen has failed, for example due to prolonged nausea.

Figure 14.2 Key principles for the management of diabetic day case patients
reproduced from BADS (2005),[33] with permission

Minor surgery in the morning

(In this context, a minor surgical procedure is defined as one where the patient is expected to resume oral intake within an hour or so of surgery)

Consider reducing long-acting insulin (insulatard, monotard, humulin I, ultratard or hypurin lente) taken before bed by $1/3$ on night before surgery.

Omit morning insulin and/or oral hypoglycaemics.

☐

On arrival in day surgery unit

Blood glucose <5mmol/l: Notify anaesthetist.

Patients on insulin or sulphonylurea: Consider infusion of 5% glucose at 100ml/hr and monitor blood glucose hourly.

Blood glucose 5–13mmol/l: Monitor only.

Blood glucose >13mmol/l: Check for intercurrent infection. Consider postponing surgery.

☐

After surgery

Give delayed breakfast with usual morning insulin/oral hypoglycaemics.

Blood glucose should be in range 5–13 mmol/l prior to discharge.

Minor surgery in the afternoon

(In this context, a minor surgical procedure is defined as one where the patient is expected to resume oral intake within an hour or so of surgery)

Normal diet and insulin and/or oral hypoglycaemics on day before surgery

☐

Morning of surgery

Half normal dose of morning insulin with light breakfast.

Oral hypoglycaemic drugs to be taken as normal with light breakfast.

Usual fasting rules (e.g., light breakfast before 8am, clear fluids until 11am).

☐

On arrival in day surgery unit

Blood glucose <5mmol/l: Notify anaesthetist.

Patients on insulin or sulphonylurea: Consider infusion of 5% glucose at 100ml/hr and monitor blood glucose hourly.

Blood glucose 5–13mmol/l: Monitor only.

Blood glucose >13mmol/l: Check for intercurrent infection.

Consider postponing surgery.

☐

After surgery

Give delayed lunch with any diabetic tablets or insulin normally taken at that time of day.

If patient injects insulin at least twice daily and does not normally take insulin with lunch, give ¹/₄ total daily dose (must be rapid acting, e.g. human soluble, human velosulin, novorapid, actrapid or humalog).

Blood glucose should be in range 5–13 mmol/l prior to discharge.

Cardiovascular diseases

Hypertension is a common condition with long-term health implications, but it appears to increase perioperative risk only slightly,[21] despite being associated with an increase in immediate cardiovascular complications. When hypertension is suspected at preassessment, the diagnosis should be confirmed and treatment instigated for the long-term benefit of the patient. Issuing patients with home blood pressure monitors is a rapid way for the preassessment team to distinguish true hypertension from the white-coat syndrome, thereby reducing the burden on the patient's GP.[22] Surgery need not be delayed, however, unless the blood pressure is excessively high (for example the systolic pressure exceeds 180mmHg and/or the diastolic pressure is 110mmHg or more) and even here there is little evidence to suggest greatly increased risk if urgent surgery is still performed.[21]

Known hypertensives should have their control optimised and antihypertensive medications should be continued throughout the perioperative period. There is currently some controversy concerning angiotensin converting enzyme (ACE) inhibitors (e.g. ramipril, enalapril), with many anaesthetists advocating that these should not be given on the day of surgery because they are associated with perioperative hypotension. A similar view was once held concerning beta-blockers, but it is now known that the benefits of continued treatment outweigh the apparent disadvantages. Similarly with ACE inhibitors, the degree of hypotension is generally mild and easily correctable with simple measures,[23] while ACE inhibitors also convey benefits, including a degree of cardioprotection, attenuated sympathetic responses and improved renal function.[24] The authors prefer to continue ACE inhibitors, which also simplifies patient instructions and reduces confusion.

Ischaemic heart disease

Cardiovascular risk is significantly increased by severe angina, heart failure and previous myocardial infarction. Diabetes and peripheral vascular disease also increase risk, but to a lesser extent, while the intensity of the surgical procedure must also be considered. The assessment of cardiac risk is mainly clinical, primarily through the patient history. Good exercise tolerance, especially the ability to climb a flight of stairs without any symptoms, usually indicates that day surgery will be an acceptable option.

Angina at rest or on minimal effort is a contra-indication to day surgery, but patients with stable (and optimally controlled) angina are acceptable, provided there are no other major risk factors. It is imperative that established beta-blockade is continued through the perioperative period.[25]

Patients who have suffered a myocardial infarction or who have undergone revascularisation procedures, such as bypass grafts or stenting, are at increased risk for a period of six weeks[26] to three months[27] afterwards and elective surgery should be delayed until this interval has elapsed. It is common to defer day surgery for six months after previous myocardial infarction,[7] adding a margin of safety which may be overcautious. Once again, cardiac medications should be continued during the perioperative period. Patients with drug-eluting stents present particular problems, since these require anti-platelet medication (usually with clopidogrel and aspirin) to be continued for at least a year. These medications *should not be stopped* simply to facilitate surgery, since interruption of therapy is associated with an exceptionally high likelihood of stent stenosis and death.[28] Unless surgery can be deferred for a long time, an increased risk of bleeding may have to be accepted. Careful liaison between cardiologist, surgeon and anaesthetist is therefore essential in these cases.

Careful assessment by a cardiologist is also required in the comparatively uncommon case of heart transplant recipients. While these patients may be able to undergo day surgery if they are stable,[25] not surprisingly there is little evidence available to support this practice. Acute rejection is a constant risk which is difficult to detect and the patient will not feel the pain of angina, since the transplanted heart no longer has a nerve supply.

Respiratory diseases

Asthma

Well-controlled asthmatics with good exercise tolerance should have no problem with day surgery. Recent exacerbations, especially those requiring hospital admission or systemic steroids, generally warrant a delay in elective surgery. The assessment of asthmatic patients is still essentially clinical; peak expiratory flow may be helpful, but other lung function tests are not usually necessary. Postoperative adverse respiratory events are up to five times more common in asthmatic patients,[29] but these generally occur early and should have resolved well before the time of discharge.

A history of safe use of non-steroidal anti-inflammatory drugs (NSAIDs) should be sought, as these drugs trigger bronchospasm in less than 5% of asthmatics and it is foolish to withhold these useful drugs in patients who have taken them in the past without problems. The risks and benefits of NSAIDs must be balanced for the individual patient in the absence of such a history.

Chronic obstructive pulmonary disease (COPD)

Like asthma, COPD increases the risk of postoperative pulmonary complications, but the majority are relatively short-lived or minor and do not increase the length of stay in recovery after day surgery.[30] Postoperative complications are more likely if patients continue to smoke or have experienced respiratory symptoms within the last month, and especially if they are symptomatic at the time of admission.[31] Under these circumstances, elective surgery should probably be delayed, unless a local or regional anaesthetic technique is an option.

The most useful assessment tool for respiratory disease is exercise tolerance; spirometry is not predictive of adverse events in the absence of symptoms.[25] Patients with dyspnoea at rest or on minimal exertion (such as household activities) are generally unsuitable for day surgery, although they may still be acceptable if the procedure can be completed using regional or local anaesthesia.

Smoking cessation should be encouraged at preassessment. Ideally this should be for at least six to eight weeks, to reduce respiratory and wound complications, although shorter periods of even a few hours are enough to reduce carbon monoxide levels and improve oxygen carriage.

Acute upper respiratory tract infections (URTIs)

URTIs are common, especially in the winter months, and they are not effectively prevented by preassessment. However, day surgery should be relatively safe if the URTI is mild and patients are afebrile without signs of lower respiratory tract involvement. Other sources of respiratory irritation, such as smoking, asthma, COPD and the likely need for tracheal intubation should all be considered and may influence the decision to postpone surgery. Patients should be rescheduled if they are febrile or unwell, or if their surgery will involve the airway. Patients with chronic respiratory conditions should be advised, at preassessment, to contact their GP and the day surgery unit for advice if they develop signs of a URTI within a few days of planned day surgery.

Obstructive sleep apnoea

Obstructive sleep apnoea (OSA) is associated with gross obesity and is increasing in prevalence. Not surprisingly, OSA is associated with difficulty in tracheal intubation and airway management in general, but there is also an increase in hypertension, dysrhythmias and the risk of sudden death.[25] The risk of perioperative complications increases in proportion to the severity of the OSA, as well as with the invasiveness of the surgery and the requirement for perioperative opioids and sedatives.[32]

The diagnosis of OSA is confirmed by formal sleep studies, but should be suspected in anyone who is grossly obese with a large collar size (>17 inches in men, >16 inches in women), loud or frequent snoring and daytime hypersomnolence.[32] Patients who have had surgery aimed at correcting OSA should not be assumed to be cured unless they have subsequently had a negative sleep study and/or all symptoms have resolved. The main non-surgical treatment is the use of some form of continuous positive airway pressure (CPAP) device, which is worn during all sleep periods.

There is insufficient evidence on which (if any) patients with OSA may be suitable for day surgery, but expert opinion[32] suggests that this should be safe for superficial surgery performed under local or regional anaesthesia. There is less certainty when general anaesthesia is required, but general agreement that airway surgery (including uvulopalatopharyngoplasty) and laparoscopic surgery to the upper abdomen should be managed as inpatient procedures.

It is advisable that an experienced anaesthetist be consulted over any patient with OSA, since even the most straightforward may present perioperative difficulties and skilled individuals and full back-up facilities must always be available; these patients are probably not suitable to be managed in freestanding day units. Local and regional anaesthetics are clearly preferable; if general anaesthesia is contemplated, it should be with short-acting drugs and the avoidance of opioids. Patients should be instructed to bring their CPAP device with them and this should be worn during all sleep before surgery and reintroduced as soon as possible after the operation. Patients should also be warned that their stay on the day unit is likely to be longer than average, since these patients should not be discharged until they have returned to baseline levels of oxygen saturation on room air and have been shown not to become obstructed when left alone.

Miscellaneous conditions

Severe liver disease and end stage renal failure on dialysis both generally contra-indicate day surgery,[7] although simple procedures may be possible under local anaesthesia. A good example is the formation of a fistula for haemodialysis, which is frequently performed as a day case under a regional limb block.

Epilepsy does not contra-indicate day surgery, provided it is stable and well controlled.[7] Less stable patients may also be acceptable under some circumstances; while it is more likely that they will experience a fit in the early postoperative period, this is an event which they and their carers will already be very experienced at coping with in the home environment.

Preassessment nurses should always seek the advice of an anaesthetist in patients with a history of previous or family problems with anaesthesia (e.g. succinylcholine apnoea, difficult tracheal intubation, neuromuscular disorders, malignant hyperpyrexia). These conditions can all be safely managed in the day case setting providing appropriate techniques are used and the right individuals and equipment are available.

Patients with learning difficulties are well-suited to day surgery, since they benefit from minimal separation from their normal environment. These patients may be difficult to manage on the day, however, and ideally should be accompanied by their family or usual carers.

Chronic medications

Preassessment is an excellent opportunity to offer advice on chronic medications, most of which confer significant benefits and should not be withheld on the day of surgery. The principles are broadly similar to inpatient surgery, but earlier ambulation may alter the balance of risks and benefits. For example, oral contraceptives should not routinely be stopped before day surgery since the thromboembolic risk from unwanted pregnancy is greater than that of remaining on therapy, at least for the majority of patients and procedures. Local guidelines should be agreed for which (if any) patients need to stop oral contraceptives.

There may also be less need to stop anticoagulants, since many day surgery procedures are associated with a low risk of bleeding. However, this is obviously changing as more ambitious procedures are undertaken and individual risk assessments will be needed. In some cases, it may be prudent to delay surgery until anticoagulation is no longer required.

Day surgery may be difficult in alcoholic patients, where preoperative abstinence may be difficult to enforce. In contrast, it may be advantageous for opioid addicts, as non-opioid analgesia (a common principle of day surgery care) is especially desirable in this group. Other recreational drug use does not present major problems for day surgery with the exception of recent use of MDMA ('ecstasy') and cocaine, which contra-indicate any elective surgery.

CONCLUSION

Preassessment of potential day case patients should follow the same basic principles of information gathering as for any elective surgery. However, specialist skills are necessary to understand how the various co-morbidities will interact with the proposed surgery and likely anaesthetic technique. Where these interactions will produce only early perioperative complications, the patient's management may be complex, but day surgery will ultimately be safe and successful. However, complications occurring late in the recovery process will suggest that an inpatient stay may be more beneficial. In addition to these very specialised judgements, preassessment of day case patients presents an invaluable opportunity for information giving and to begin to prepare the patient to care for themselves in a familiar home environment after surgery. Day surgery preassessment requires a highly skilled and specialist team.

REFERENCES

1. J.H. Nicoll (1909). The surgery of infancy. *British Medical Journal* **2**: 753–4.

2. I. Smith, T. Cooke, I. Jackson and R. Fitzpatrick (2006). Rising to the challenges of achieving day surgery targets. *Anaesthesia* **61**: 1191–9.

3. Department of Health NHS Modernisation Agency (2004). *Ten high impact changes for service improvement and delivery*. London: HMSO.

4. Department of Health NHS Modernisation Agency (2004). *Day surgery – making it mainstream*. London: HMSO.

5. British Association of Day Surgery (2006). *BADS Directory of Procedures*. London: BADS.

6. Department of Health NHS Modernisation Agency (2004). D*ay Surgery – A Good Practice Guide*. London: HMSO.

7. NHS Modernisation Agency (2002). *National Good Practice Guidelines on Pre-operative Assessment for Day Surgery*. London: HMSO.

8. Association of Anaesthetists of Great Britain and Ireland (2005). *Day Surgery*. Revised edition. London: AAGBI.

9. V. Gudimetla and I. Smith (2006). Pre-operative screening and selection of adult day surgery patients. In P. Lemos, P. Jarrett and B. Philip (eds) *Day Surgery Development and Practice*. Porto: International Association for Ambulatory Surgery, pp. 125–37.

10. L.C. Callaghan, N.D. Edwards and C.S. Reilly (1995). Utilisation of the pre-operative ECG. *Anaesthesia* **50**: 488–90.

11. I. Smith I. (2001). Postoperative instructions: good compliance, but is the advice sound? (Editorial). *Anaesthesia* **56**: 405–7.

12. J. Canet, J. Raeder, L.S. Rasmussen, M. Enlund, H.M. Kuipers, C.D. Hanning, J. Jolles, K. Kortilla, V.D. Siersma, C. Dodds, H. Abildstrom, J.R. Sneyd, P. Vila, T. Johnson, L. Muñoz Corsini, J.H. Silverstein, I.K. Nielsen and J.T. Moller, The ISPOCD2 investigators. (2003). Cognitive dysfunction after minor surgery in the elderly. *Acta Anaesthesiologica Scandinavica* **47**: 1204–10.

13. J. Raeder (2007). Extended recovery and hospital hotels in sparsely populated areas. Paper presented at the 7th International Congress on Ambulatory Surgery, International Association for Ambulatory Surgery, Amsterdam.

14. Royal College of Surgeons of England (1992). *Commission on the Provision of Surgical Services. Guidelines for Day Case Surgery*. London: HMSO.

15. F. Chung, G. Mezei and D. Tong (1999). Pre-existing medical conditions as predictors of adverse events in day-case surgery. *British Journal of Anaesthesia* **83**: 262–70.

16. G.L. Ansell and J.E. Montgomery (2004). Outcome of ASA III patients undergoing day case surgery. *British Journal of Anaesthesia* **92**: 71–4.

17. Z. Friedman, D.T. Wong and F. Chung (2003). What are the ambulatory surgical patient selection criteria in Canada? (abstract). *Canadian Journal of Anaesthesia* **50**(Supplement): A16.

18. F.S. Servin (2006). Ambulatory anesthesia for the obese patient. *Current Opinion in Anaesthesiology* **19**(6): 597–9.

19. G.L. Bryson, F. Chung, R.G. Cox, M-J. Crowe, J. Fuller, C. Henderson, B.A. Finegan, Z. Friedman, D.R. Miller and J. van Vlymen, for the Canadian Ambulatory Anesthesia Research and Education (CAARE) Group (2004). Patient selection in ambulatory anesthesia – an evidence-based review: Part II. *Canadian Journal of Anaesthesia* **51**: 782–94.

20. British Association of Day Surgery (2004). *Day Surgery and the Diabetic Patient* (revised edition). London: British Association of Day Surgery (available from www.bads.co.uk).

21. S.J. Howell, J.W. Sear and P. Foëx (2004). Hypertension, hypertensive heart disease and perioperative cardiac risk. *British Journal of Anaesthesia* **92**: 570–83.

22. K. Venkatesan, D. Mercer and K. Hickmott (2006). Reduction of unnecessary cancellation of patients in day surgery due to high blood pressure. *Journal of One-day Surgery* **16**(4): 86–9.

23. T. Comfere, J. Sprung, M.M. Kumar, M. Draper, D.P. Wilson, B.A. Williams, D.R. Danielson, L. Liedl and D.O. Warner (2005). Angiotensin system inhibitors in a general surgical population. *Anesthesia and Analgesia* **100**: 636–44.

24. D.W. Pigott, C. Nagle, K. Allman, S. Westaby and R.D. Evans (2000). Effect of omitting regular ACE inhibitor medication before cardiac surgery on haemodynamic variables and vasoactive drug requirements. *British Journal of Anaesthesia* **83**: 715–20.

25. G.L. Bryson, F. Chung, B.A. Finegan, Z. Friedman, D.R. Miller, J. van Vlymen, R.G. Cox, M-J. Crowe, J. Fuller and C. Henderson, for the Canadian Ambulatory Anesthesia Research and Education (CAARE) Group (2004). Patient selection in ambulatory anesthesia – an evidence-based review: Part I. *Canadian Journal of Anaesthesia* **51**: 768–81.

26. K.A. Eagle, P.B. Berger, H. Calkins, B.R. Chaitman, G.A. Ewy, K.E. Fleischmann, L.A. Fleisher, J.B. Froehlich, R.J. Gusberg, J.A. Leppo, T. Ryan, R.C. Schlant and W.L. Winters, Jr, American College of Cardiology, American Heart Association Task Force (2002). ACC/AHA Guideline update for perioperative cardiovascular evaluation for noncardiac surgery – executive summary: a report of the American College of Cardiology/American Heart Association Task Force on Practice Guidelines. *Circulation* **105**: 1257–67.

27. P.G. Chassot, A. Delabays and D.R. Spahn (2002). Preoperative evaluation of patients with, or at risk of, coronary artery disease undergoing non-cardiac surgery (review). *British Journal of Anaesthesia* **89**: 747–59.

28. G.M. Howard-Alpe, J. deBono, L. Hudsmith, W.P. Orr, P. Foëx and J.W. Sear (2007). Coronary artery stents and non-cardiac surgery. *British Journal of Anaesthesia* **98**: 560–74.

29. F. Chung and G. Mezei (1999). Adverse outcomes in ambulatory anesthesia. *Canadian Journal of Anaesthesia* **46**(5 part 2): R18–34.

30. F. Chung and G. Mezei (1999). Factors contributing to a prolonged stay after ambulatory surgery. *Anesthesia and Analgesia* **89**(6): 1352–9.

31. D.O. Warner, M.A. Warner, R.D. Barnes, K.P. Offord, D.R. Schroeder, D.T. Gray and J.W. Yunginger (1996). Perioperative respiratory complications in patients with asthma. *Anesthesiology* **85**(3): 460–7.

32. American Society of Anesthesiologists (2006). Practice guidelines for the perioperative management of patients with obstructive sleep apnea. *Anesthesiology* **104**: 1081–93.

33. British Association of Day Surgery (2005). Key principles for the management of diabetic day case patients. *Journal of One-day Surgery* **15**(2): 42–3.

15 Preparation for discharge

Liz Lees

SUMMARY

This chapter will describe:

- **the importance of discharge planning and impact of perioperative scheduling**
- **key policy drivers for early discharge**
- **the challenges in active discharge planning process**
- **developing effective discharge bundles**
- **managing complex discharges**
- **coordinating discharge with multi-agencies.**

INTRODUCTION

This chapter will explore the optimal discharge process for patients undergoing surgical procedures and provide an in-depth analysis of discharge planning, including the contemporary perspectives of the nurse's role in facilitating patient discharge from hospital. It is also acknowledged that nurses facilitate the process of discharge from many other healthcare settings, and the principles of practice discussed are transferable across many areas.

The chapter begins by discussing the potential challenges when discharging surgical patients. It offers a detailed overview of the governmental policies creating the impetus to modernise discharge processes. Perspectives such as change management, bed management and team working, which influence the process of discharging patients from hospital, are discussed. Moreover, leadership, responsibility and accountability will be explored in relation to expanding the nurse's discharge planning role. A distinction will be drawn between nurse-led and nurse-facilitated discharge from hospital. This distinction will be supported by principles of good practice, including protocols that should enable the discharge process to operate in a timely manner. Furthermore, competency and educational development and supplementary approaches will also be explored. Throughout the chapter, examples will be used to identify some of the systems and processes that need to be in place, if we are to assist nurses in their role as a focal point for discharge planning.

Core elements supporting best practice in discharging patients include:

- hospital policy guidance
- change management processes
- proactive discharge planning
- excellent multi-disciplinary team working
- information technology: transparency and information sharing
- excellent pharmacy support
- nursing leadership skills
- ward coordination: role and functions
- good skills in patient assessment
- discharge training: sustained
- competency development
- timely patient information.

The challenges for discharging surgical patients

Surgery is often referred to as planned activity constituting the 'bread and butter' of a hospital's core business. Consequently it must be supported by processes and practices at a strategic level which control the flow and overall patient capacity.[1] Conversely, the business of medicine is generally unplanned activity and the patient demand/flow is relatively unpredictable, making it impossible to include a preadmission phase. Notwithstanding, surgical patients do present as emergencies and these patients can be more challenging, with the added complexity of recovery from invasive procedures, and emergency presentation precludes any preparation for discharge. To ensure such emergency patients are expedited efficiently from hospital, systems must be in place to act quickly and ensure consistency with 'normal' preadmission processes, postadmission.

While the complexity of the discharge process may be regarded as simpler for young and relatively independent patients requiring surgical interventions, one miscommunication or error can be just as catastrophic for the patient and organisation, such as forgetting to prescribe or administer bowel preparation preoperatively. A miscommunication with letters (especially if the patient has moved address or GP) may result in cancelled surgical procedures and operations. From experience it is often a misplaced laissez faire attitude to the 'simple discharge' which may result in a failed discharge, poor patient experience or readmission.

The discharge process must be actively managed to reduce and control the number of variables, which will in turn increase the likely positive outcome for the patient. Moreover, greater collaboration is required to share best practice in caring for patients with complex discharge needs. Furthermore, care of patients should involve appropriate practitioners at the outset of care regardless of professional base; for example, a patient having had surgery may need specialist mental health and elderly care support. To address discharge planning challenges in detail requires a thorough understanding of each stage in the discharge process, namely:

● point of referral (emergency or elective)

● preoperative management

● admission (likely investigations and recovery time)

● rehabilitation and enablement (early involvement of the multi-disciplinary team)

● predischarge preparations (bespoke details to individualise plans)

● day of discharge

● follow-up care.

There are many policy documents driving different perspectives of care; those that specifically address the surgical component are briefly outlined below.

Spotlight on surgery

The *NHS Plan* (2000) stated that 75% of all surgical interventions will be carried out as day cases[1]. The drive towards shorter lengths of stay widely advocates access, booking and choice at the centre of care planning for surgical patients.[2] Following this, a specific guide detailing patient condition groups and operational guidance for their management was published.[3] In the move towards redesigning surgical services, four main considerations were suggested, which could easily be applied to discharge planning, namely, increasing the volume of patients whose care is managed in primary care, use of care protocols, commissioning of services and carrying out minor procedures in primary settings. It also states that moving towards more day surgery 'should not impact upon the work of GPs and primary care'.[3] While it offers brief guidance on discharge planning it somewhat oversimplifies the whole process. A key aspect that must be addressed when embracing such policy is to ensure sufficient supply of primary care and social services to support aftercare, following discharge. For example, we have an ageing population, whose needs may be overlooked without the involvement of experienced practitioners who understand the 'simply risky' elements to discharge planning that cannot always be anticipated and thereby managed in advance of surgical procedures. The multifaceted elements associated with ageing may mean such patients are not managed consistently, for example, with different processes for inpatients and day surgery.

Discharge policy: key changes

The principles underpinning discharge planning remain largely unchanged despite large-scale organisational NHS changes since its inception. Perhaps the core challenges affecting the discharge process arise from: rising numbers of emergency admissions, changing patterns for patient referrals, shorter lengths of patient stay and the acuity of patients admitted to hospital. In addition, the gradual and sustained advances in new roles have played a large part in adapting the nursing response to changing clinical practices, including discharge planning. For example, discharge planners and coordinators are now commonplace. However, the changing NHS has altered patient/carer needs and expectations, and thus the commissioning of services, stimulating further changes in discharge planning practice.[4,5,6] Therefore policy documents are placing more emphasis on changes required in specific areas of discharge practice and, in particular, the nurse's contribution to those.[7] Some of the key areas are discussed below.

Chief Nursing Officer's ten key roles for nurses

From a nursing perspective, the Chief Nursing Officer of England responded to the NHS Plan with the ten key roles.[1] This creates new opportunities for some and increased responsibilities for others, depending on the extent to which nurses are proactively involved in discharge planning and implementation of discharge. This change process will stimulate development of new organisational policies, protocols and training, which will serve to protect both the employing organisation and individual practitioner in expanding their role and taking on new practices.[8] It will also promote the development of new teams and instigate innovative ways of working to benefit the patient. Finally, the scale of change will elicit integrated working practices outside the hospital in different organisations that deliver health and social care.

In most cases policy stimulates new ways of working; in others it may provide additional support to a change already being practised by nurses. Yet the case of discharge planning policy appeared to revive interest in the focus of the nurse's role, most notably after the announcement of the Chief Nursing Officer's ten key roles for nursing.[1] The inclusion of the key role 'admitting and discharging patients' has elevated discharge practices from arguably an everyday matter to a high–profile part of patient care. The journey to achieving this key role in practice is dependent upon many different organisational facets impacting upon many professional groups, and adjusting responsibility for discharge planning.

Single Assessment Process

The concept of the Single Assessment Process (SAP) was introduced after the *National Service Framework for Older People* was published in 2001.[9,10] It is aimed at all clinical areas where the care of older patients is taking place. While the process of implementation was initially arduous, its intention to simplify and integrate assessments formed the precursor for new ways of working between health and social care. Best Practice documents raised the profile of health and social care working together, requiring a step outside the nurse's traditional role in hospital, to integrate not only professional practices but organisational systems, to guide the patient's discharge.[11] Concurrently, changes in the funding aspects of patients delayed in hospital, while waiting for social care arrangements to be put in place, brought about another process known as recharging.[12] While this requires nursing responsibility to instigate, through its inextricable links with the discharge process, arguably it has been seen as a separate or parallel process. Enquiries in the surgical setting have revealed that the SAP is seen to sit outside 'usual discharge practice'. The advantages of completing the SAP are therefore outweighed by its lack of integration within hospital information technology systems and a lack of understanding of the overall benefits it could bring to patients. One key area of consideration should be to ensure that information technology systems interface and information can be exchanged between systems without the need for duplication of data entry. The biggest impact of the SAP is slowly but surely being realised through the action of estimating dates of medical fitness to discharge and perhaps estimating the length of stay or discharge date itself.

Key named discharge planners

A noteworthy, inspiring guidance document, namely *Freedom to Practise*, combined emergency care policy with case examples of patient care from the point of referral to the point of discharge; it included mechanisms to facilitate nurse leadership in the discharge processes.[13] Its radical approach placed tangible support behind traditionally bureaucratic processes, which often seem distanced from the reality of everyday clinical practice. A second area of policy focus, reiterated in several policy documents, recommends the practice of developing key named persons to act as discharge coordinators at ward level. This suggestion was meant to provide members of the multi-disciplinary team and other agencies with a named person to liaise with, who would coordinate the discharge plan.[14]

Discharge checklists

Discharge policy was further refined by its specific focus on 'discharge checklists' as part of the process. Once more the policy guidance was virtually 'directive', reinforced at hospital board level through its inclusion as a measurable facet of Trust performance in the Clinical Negligence Scheme for Trusts.[15] The CNST stipulates a named person in the discharge plan and the use of a checklist providing a quantifiable audit trail, to determine the components of discharge that have taken place.

Reasserting the nurse's role – nurse-facilitated discharge

Finally, another toolkit was introduced, which would reassert and embrace the nurse's role in facilitating timely discharge from hospital.[16] This aspect is addressed in detail later in the chapter; timely discharge combines the concept of estimating dates for discharge, nurse led or facilitated discharge, and improving all processes (by removing blocks) relating to a simple discharge. Almost all hospitals have adopted some parts of the redesign suggested, yet standardisation and lean approaches continue to rely on innovative practitioners rather than strategically resourced approaches. Inevitably, national evidence of published projects reveals disparate practice is rife, ranging from well-developed highly innovative local policy and protocols to small-scale projects with little strategic support to sustain good practice. Organisational readiness is imperative in order to support nurses, who alone cannot achieve the scale of change required to embrace the concept of nurse-facilitated discharges. It is the inextricable links with other practitioners that are vital in balancing policy, understanding and embracing this concept.

The sustainable introduction of new or innovative ways of delivering discharge practice rests firmly with systematic introduction of new processes. This impacts directly on the nursing profession, though nurses may perceive this to be dominated by new paperwork and systems of collecting data.

A few words about change

Despite this positive perspective, 'change' is quite a frightening prospect for some professionals and not necessarily readily adopted in the area of discharge practice. In health care, professions may attempt to maintain control by keeping the status quo as well as through professional protectionism. This is often reinforced by oppressive strategies deliberately used to slow down the pace of change, especially if the change is seen to adversely impact upon role development.[17] If a method of facilitating this change is not used, often it is easy to misinterpret the implications, giving rise to tension. To counterbalance possible misapprehension and fragmented practices (reactive to proactive discharge planning) organisations should try to develop a culture of sustaining new practices, rather than adopting a 'must do by the end of' mentality, which may only serve to constrain development or shorten the shelf life of the change. Therefore, change must be managed effectively and preparation, planning and discussion are crucial to ensure success. This is particularly important when change is occurring because of wider agendas and priorities which may not seem apparent at practice level.

Processes which directly impact upon discharge planning

Bed management

Bed management is not a new concept; indeed it is a fundamental aspect of every hospital's working day.[18] So why is it perhaps seen as a separate role from that of clinical professionals? Posts of this nature were originally appointed to relieve pressure on the nurse's role, yet they most certainly require nursing input. The root of managing beds started in nursing, but perhaps the migration of this role into a separate management post mitigates against promoting clinical perspectives of care which proactively manage the process of patient admission and discharge. There are many texts written which explore capacity management and large organisational systems, yet perhaps because of their remoteness from clinical practice they tend to be seen as of little relevance. It could be argued that lack of bed capacity and intensive turnover of patients with a higher acuity creates untoward clinical pressure and is potentially at odds with 'caring for patients', creating a culture of counting patient throughput (in time) rather than measuring quality of care. A constructive way forward may be determined by asking what it is we want these roles to achieve. What approach should be used? Is a universal role the answer? This said, a variety of bed management models can be seen throughout the country, such as: non-clinical bed coordinators, strategic bed managers, computerised data entry systems (only as reliable as the person entering the data). I firmly believe that decision making based on clinical expertise is at the centre of managing beds.

An ideal model embraces the nurse's unique knowledge of the patient, with knowledge of systems and process, as part of a problem-solving approach. One model developed at the Heart of England NHS Foundation Trust in the UK involves a clinical coordinator. This serves to focus responsibility for the discharge and effect clinical coordination of patient's needs and to free the hospital bed earlier in the day. However, this approach is not without its problems. For example, all areas need to adopt a uniform approach to such roles to achieve a uniform degree of momentum across the organisation, placing as much pressure on the internal transfer of patients as on discharge. Cost-effectiveness needs to be explored, aligned with freed bed capacity while considering patient satisfaction and patient-centred care; without all this, discharge coordinators may be regarded as an expensive luxury, once again 'here today and gone tomorrow'.

Team working

Team work may be in a state of demise with a huge aspect of the nurse's role centred around coordinating a 'group' of staff rather than a 'team' of staff working together on a shift.[19] Understanding the difference between 'group' and 'team' is important if nurses are to begin to appreciate the root of some discharge planning problems. For example, a ward team can be defined as being made up of consistent staff members with clearly defined roles[20] belonging to that ward. In addition, a team will have a shared or common purpose,[19] such as achieving the discharge plan within a defined timescale. This is hugely important from the patient's perspective along what may be quite a complex route to discharge from hospital.[21] Perhaps the systems that are established to manage services lie at the roots of the demise of team work. Invariably, staff are moved to ensure safe staffing levels; agency and bank nurses, while crucially needed, are often used to 'top up levels of staff' to established levels per shift. Moreover, temporary wards with flexible capacity are often opened to serve times of additional pressure, with skeleton staffing and agency or bank nurses, who do not know each other's strengths or specialist knowledge base. Furthermore, such wards are often closed at relatively short notice, having a catastrophic effect on the essential communication and handover of the process of patient discharge plans. Effectively pulling together a discharge plan is a multi-professional and coordinated activity, but is more often than not facilitated by nurses. Organisational practices of this nature will constrain the development of nurses' knowledge, extend patient lengths of stay through fragmented communication and perhaps promote a lack of ownership of discharge planning.[22] The notion of a team involves accepting responsibility and growth in knowledge and skills.[19] It must be remembered that the team also includes allied health professionals and doctors. Hence, it could be argued that reducing junior doctors working hours and the shift away from ward-based teams of doctors has also fragmented our concept of a team. The final element of this disjointed picture is completed when patients are also selected as suitable for moving to 'flexible capacity wards' (often at short notice) where the continuum of care may also become fragmented, resulting in processes being missed altogether or duplicated. Nonetheless, it has moved responsibility to nurses who have the greatest patient contact spread over 24 hours a day, seven days a week. Perhaps nurses are in a position to assert some control by stating what it is they need (tools, resources) and how they need to work.[23] Without doubt, to achieve nurse-facilitated discharges effectively will require strong leadership from nursing.

Developing the culture: perspectives on leadership

'Passion, drive and commitment' are three essential aspects of developing a culture of nurse leadership irrespective of the particular subject being explored.[19] Passion about discharge planning may arise from an intimate knowledge of the subject and the desire to carry out the role. The drive may be helped by understanding the organisational goals; this will help nurses have a sense of ownership of the fundamental principles of proactively being involved in patient discharge. Drive and commitment go hand in hand, particularly regarding discharge planning, where ownership of the problem or issue, by tracking its progress until it is resolved, is crucial. For example, rather than leaving an issue to chance, handing it over to others or disowning the issue altogether, it will require follow-through, regardless of shift pattern or which professional it was handed to. Conversely, the patient acuity and complexity of care makes it notoriously difficult to keep track of 'who did what', 'what the result was', and 'its implications for patient care', ultimately impacting on the discharge plan and length of stay (see Box 15.1).

Box 15.1 Case example: what plan?

Junior doctors on an acute medical ward made a physiotherapy request for an oxygen saturation assessment and mobility assessment, only to discover that the physiotherapist had in fact already discharged the patient from her care earlier in the week. In this case the central facets of the discharge plan were not stated at the outset of care; while individual therapy referrals had been made, the notion of waiting in a queue for a series of single unconnected events to take place was evident, leaving the outcome, or desired outcome, uncertain/open-ended.

Hence, it requires a significant commitment from the nurse to take and accept responsibility, focusing upon creating discharge plans as a priority, amongst the many other aspects of nursing care that have to be delivered. Leading the plan requires sustained commitment to regularly review the patient's progress and to assert control. The change to leadership mentality demands that nurses question the way they organise themselves to deliver care.

Nurses assert that they feel overwhelmed with activities and tasks, but organisation and leadership help to create valuable time. For example, in the case of discharge planning and the busy acute hospital environment, perhaps we are too tied up in the individual task, rather than understanding where we are in the process and thereby which tasks will achieve the biggest impact in the time we have. There is an overwhelming need to be able to clarify with all professionals involved the patient's individual needs, over approximately what indicated time scale, in a discharge plan.[24,25,23] This must be supported by principles regarding the process and outcome desired (see Box 15.2). All of these contribute to the estimated date of discharge. Evidence from the case notes from patients who have had reasonably short lengths of stay

---

Box 15.2 The fundamental principles of discharge planning

1. Knowledge of disease process or condition
2. **Estimating how long recovery might take, or if recovery is a realistic outcome**
3. **Involving the patient and family and carers in the plan**
4. Proactively dealing with issues and difficulties that may arise
5. Communicating and documenting the plan to the team or group of staff
6. Making appropriate referrals and following through outcomes
7. Coordinating and owning the discharge information
8. Being decisive and carrying out activities
9. **Reviewing and updating the progress of the plan**
10. Disseminating accurate information to all involved

(perhaps less than three days) indicates three stages of the process (2, 3, 9) are quite commonly overlooked. If these three aspects were addressed routinely it is thought that nurses would assert a greater degree of control and ownership of the discharge process to benefit patient care. Nevertheless, leadership provided by nurse executives/directors must be actively engaged by experienced nurses to develop the appropriate infrastructure and to guide the processes required. Collectively such actions will promote the principles of partnership, working with the patient, family and multi-disciplinary team towards effective nurse-facilitated discharge practice.[16]

Contemporary practices: nurse-led?

There is debate regarding the terms 'nurse-led' and 'nurse-facilitated'. Nursing literature has focused a great deal of attention upon creating a definition for the subject of nurses leading the discharge process.[26,27] For some consultants and other healthcare practitioners, anecdotal evidence suggests that the name which is adopted is incredibly important. For example, 'nurse-led' implies a uni-disciplinary activity, which can serve to generate bad feeling and fear that patients will be discharged without appropriate management from medical and allied health professional colleagues. In nursing alone, it can cause ramifications, such as being seen as an exclusive role and the domain of only a privileged, adequately prepared/trained minority. Hence, while defining a concept can prove a time-consuming exercise, opening the debate does serve useful functions, such as unifying understanding and making explicit the intended goal(s). Moreover, in determining organisational discharge policy it paves the way to implement new and innovative practices.

Nurse-facilitated

This term refers to a set of behaviours or principles (see Box 15.2) required to complete the process. For example, a nurse-facilitated process could be defined as 'a process where nurses take responsibility for the proactive management of discharge of patients in their care from hospital'. The nurse will actively facilitate processes which help the discharge. Their acts or omissions will not serve to inhibit or delay the process of discharge from hospital.

Nurse-led

This term has been further defined as 'nurses leading the whole process of discharge following decisions made by nurses, using criteria, protocols or given set of principles' (adapted from Lees 2006[28]). Nurses are given the tools or bespoke instructions which allow them to make decisions within the parameters determined by the protocol. In this, protocols guide rather than make the decision for the nurse. It should always be remembered that there are exceptions to protocols, which need to be stated as decisions to act or not to act – known as exceptions.

Regardless of which name is adopted, this role should not be seen as unique to nursing roles (nurse specialists or nurse consultants), nor should it be thought that it can be conducted in isolation without the support of all appropriate members of the interdisciplinary team.

Perhaps some of the fear felt by a range of other healthcare practitioners can be managed appropriately if the concept is explored in terms of explicit factors, such as what *is not* desirable and what *is* the desired outcome, as stated below.

Nurses facilitating discharge should NOT:

- Carry out a series of instructions as indicated by the medical team. This is arguably what the nurse or MDT would do ordinarily.
- Decide a patient is fit for discharge without consultation with relevant professionals involved with the patient's care.
- Defer discharge decisions to wait for the doctor to make a decision, for which the nurse has had the relevant training/knowledge.

- Discharge a patient according to different rules, depending on who is in charge of the ward and on duty.
- Discharge patients without adequate preparation to accommodate bed capacity issues.

Nurses facilitating discharge SHOULD:

- Initiate and lead the discharge process with involvement of all relevant professionals to expedite discharges, assist bed and capacity management across the whole hospital.
- Carry out regular and ongoing patient assessments/evaluation to assist timely and appropriate discharges.
- Be progress chasers for results of investigations, which require his/her decision to expedite discharge.
- Proactively engage the MDT at appropriate points in the patient's care.
- Proactively promote and discuss discharge decisions, in collaboration with family and MDT to promote discharges.
- Follow up the patient (in and out of hospital) and review progress, according to the plan.
- Act as the patient's advocate. (Adapted from Lees, 2004[27])

Box 15.3 A continuum of practice

1. Increasing knowledge
2. Increasing breadth of role
3. Increasing responsibility

Senior Practitioner:
receives referrals.

Experienced Nurse:
- writes discharge letter
- follows up the plan
- instigates the overall plan.

Competent Nurse:
- determines the outcomes (with everyone)
- rectifies issues to make plan work
- knows the process
- assesses and liaises.

It is suggested that nurses learn new ways of behaving and reframe their professional image, role and values. In reality nurses facilitating patient discharge from hospital are trying to achieve clearly defined roles and responsibilities along the multiple stages of the discharge process. This clarity will benefit patients firstly, and the organisation, a very close second. Inevitably a minority of NHS organisations developing the principles of nurse-facilitated discharge practice have changed their processes to the definitive extreme, transferring the vast majority of responsibility for patients' discharge, previously undertaken by doctors and therapists, on to nurses. Some nurses regard the expansion and gradual adjustment of their roles as the natural evolution of the caring process, while others argue that it is carrying out doctors' duties for a nurse's pay. Nonetheless, nurse-facilitated discharge provides a positive step forward for discharge practice development which places nurse-facilitated and nurse-led on a continuum of development (see Box 15.3, page 291). With this in mind, nurses need to have a good understanding regarding their parameters of practice and be aware of their individual responsibility and accountability.[29]

Box 15.3 attempts to visualise the nurse's progress through a trajectory of learning in practice, and perhaps begins to distinguish nurse-facilitated from nurse-led behaviours. Nevertheless, it is not necessarily easy to quantify through a series of increasing responsibilities, at which point the nurse may move along the trajectory towards that of a senior practitioner. In this case clinical exposure is crucial to experience the different facets required. To encourage nurses to take on greater responsibility requires a governed framework that promotes safe practice.

Responsibility and accountability

There is a reluctance to embrace nurse-facilitated discharge and this becomes apparent with practice and differing attitudes from ward to ward, within one organisation alone. Part of the reason, until recently, was the absence of organisational policies and protocols to support nursing actions in practice. There are no legal or professional reasons to prevent nurses from taking increasing responsibility for the discharge process, including the decision to discharge a patient.[16] Specifically, local policy is essential to confirm a place for nurse-facilitated discharge in practice settings, ensuring it is recognised at all levels of the organisation.[15]

Responsibility

Perhaps it is individual interpretation of the meaning of nurse-facilitated discharge that adds the extra dimension of caution that is self-limiting our practice. Evidence suggests that nurses fear the 'responsibility' of being left alone to contemplate a discharge decision, where perhaps not all issues are resolved or further clarity is required. Moreover, guarded behaviour is evident when nurses believe the responsibility is not 'theirs' to take. This issue is compounded when junior and senior members of the medical teams fear their patients will be discharged without their prior knowledge or consent. Conversely, in some areas it is considered an insult to nursing to suggest that they have ever practised any other way, and they do indeed lead and coordinate all discharges from hospital in their area of practice, with absolute support of medical colleagues. The responsibility to make decisions will vary tremendously depending on the expertise of the nurse facilitating the discharge. Equally, the same can be said of the junior medical team, who conversely may 'admit' patients as a safeguard, and delay a discharge decision, until their senior colleagues are present. Furthermore, the converse of nurse-facilitated discharge may occur with the inception of new protocols and policy; for example, they may serve to elicit safer discharges which are well informed and appropriate. In some cases this may mean patients are not discharged and the plan will be revisited. The most important aspects to be understood are outlined below:

- Knowledge of the patient is prerequisite.
- Training is required.
- Experience is essential.
- It is not a uni-disciplinary activity.
- The patient must be reviewed regularly in line with their changes and/or condition.
- The patient must be medically fit for discharge.

Accountability

The Nursing and Midwifery Council (NMC)[29] states the professional standards which underpin the foundation of practice. Central to these are nurses' decisions to act or not to act, and to act always in the best interest of the patient. These are guiding principles which can be applied to nurse-facilitated discharge from hospital. Understanding what nurse facilitation involves is vital in order to understand whether sufficient preparation has been undertaken. Equally, interpretation of the accountability framework – rather than fearing any consequences and possible removal from the register or litigation – is a good place to start work. Rudd and Smith[26] believe that nurses should proactively take the lead in coordinating discharge planning. Nurse-facilitated discharge involves assessing the patient, liaising with the multi-disciplinary team, and planning timely discharge based on the agreed plan of care.[13,16] Writing discharge letters, making follow-up calls and advising patients, carers and other professionals are also within the scope of the nurse's role in discharge planning.[29,16,13] Nevertheless, making decisions within agreed parameters requires experience in using professional judgement; and experience and judgement are not necessarily indicated by a nurse's pay banding or job title. Experience in the role through proven activities is desirable, although some discharge issues are multifaceted and require confidence to deal with effectively.

Competency development and successful implementation

The level of activity and momentum surrounding competency achievement within nursing (although this profession is by no means unique) is noteworthy and competency requires in-depth application to be achieved successfully in practice. The rounded development of NHS roles, through prerequisite knowledge and skills is now supported by the *NHS Knowledge and Skills Framework* (KSF).[30] Competencies underpin the framework and should provide the necessary detail in order to encourage individual practitioners to develop through different levels of the trajectory.[31] This in turn will support 'expanded' practice to support new services. However, competency 'development' is often misinterpreted as task-orientated, implying that training is required to enable a series of individual tasks to be performed. These 'extended' practices are then hurriedly introduced, thus producing a sometimes superficial and constrained approach to developing the practice needs of the workforce.[32] Perhaps consequently the NHS has a history of short-term change projects.

Moreover, the short-term projects do not necessarily interlink with established services and as a result can be stand-alone, frequently marginalising the person, role and service.

It has been suggested that the first stage towards creation of appropriate competencies is through a thorough understanding of discharge planning in context, for example, the team, the service the patient is being 'discharged from and to', together with other interfacing roles/services.[33] Conversely, it is perfectly possible that all the individuals comprising a whole ward team will never be fully competent. This is where competence at the three levels suggested by the Royal College of Nursing (RCN), competent, experienced and senior practitioner, is most relevant. Furthermore the concept of team competence (previously probably best known as 'skill mix') safeguards individual practitioners while they advance, adjust or expand their practice through the skills/career trajectory. In this sense the notion of team competence accepts the responsibility of the team members to support each other to develop practice; nurse-facilitated discharge should not remain the domain of a select few.

Box 15.4 Example of nurse-facilitated discharge skills set for an older person

- Mechanisms which share the discharge process with patients and their carers
- Understanding services available for older people
- Demonstrable knowledge ofi ntermediate care and social care services
- Understanding of chronic disease management
- Understanding the tools available, which will assist discharge planning
- Good communication, liaison and documentation skills
- Completing the Single Assessment Process (SAP)
- Conducting a range of relevant assessments: social, falls, frailty, abbreviated mental test scoring
- Making simple referrals (e.g. to district nursing, transport requests, etc)
- Engaging voluntary services and patient representatives
- Making appropriate referrals to intermediate care services
- Referral to social care services for instigation or restart of services
- Referral to Elderly Care Assessment Unit
- Submitting a section(2) and (5) form
- Follow up of patients

Implementing a competency framework for discharge practice should be achieved through a systematic replicable process, and to this end a skills analysis may prove to be the best place to start.[8] The process involves four key principles, namely:

1. plan the education required

2. develop discharge skills in practice (applied behaviour)

3. develop nurse-facilitated discharge (use skills and knowledge actively)

4. audit and research developments (engaging staff for future).

The majority of competencies already established are specific regarding the description of what has to be achieved, yet they are relatively high-level, generally lacking in detail and guidance on how they are to be best achieved and over what timescale. To implement competencies successfully requires a wide range of flexible learning opportunities and techniques (see Box 15.4) to aid individual learning styles.[34] For example, busy practitioners need support in practice from expert facilitation if they are to develop new knowledge, skills and competencies, which underpin new and developing multi-professional roles.[33,35] Box 15.5 (see page 296) offers an overview of how competency underpinning blood result interpretation might be achieved; this is cited as one of the six competencies that contribute towards nurse-facilitated discharge.

When the experiential learning is completed, assessing competencies should not be approached as a subjective self-assessment or 'tick box' exercise, adding to a wealth of meaningless papers in a dusty portfolio. On the contrary, competencies should be transparent, interactive, live and constantly evolving. Consequently, implementation of competencies can potentially open up a can of worms, highlighting the huge responsibility that needs to be embraced, shared and sustained by employees and employers alike. For example, following the development of competencies, staff will need support (time out) for the updating/maintenance and adjustment of competence; accepting, that is, that practice does not remain static. Moreover, foundation work, such as undertaking a training needs analysis, which supports competence, may not have been systematically developed in the first place. Hence remedial action will be required before competency development can be fully undertaken. Furthermore, education and subsequent competencies can only offer a small semblance of assurance, interfacing with clinical supervision and governance plans, towards reduction of clinical risks and improvement in quality of patient care. Competencies are needed to support and protect practitioners if they are to develop holistic new areas of practice with confidence.

Supplementary approaches to identify and develop skills

The greater the range of approaches employed, the more likely any programme is to be sustainable in the longer term. For example, traditional approaches to didactic learning are becoming outmoded and are being replaced with a sharp focus on delivering results in the workplace and encouraging staff from different professional backgrounds to acquire skills and competencies in a flexible manner.

Five approaches, stemming from the personal development plan, are suggested:

1. staff rotations (experiential learning)

2. undertaking non-clinical existing learning opportunities (agreed as part of *KSF*)

3. undertaking formal education at universities (didactic/academic)

Box 15.5 Achieving competency in blood results interpretation

Stages involved (6)

1. Attendance at one lead lecture set at post-registration level for 'experienced nurses' [31]. Read and understand underpinning information sources related to blood results.

(Learning objective: to gain prerequisite base line knowledge regarding commonly requested blood investigations).

2. Participation in the process of reporting blood results received in your practice area by separating blood results into: A. Results within universally accepted normal ranges.

B. Results outside universally accepted normal ranges

(Learning objective: to participate in the process and familiarise self with results received, which may be outside normal range)

3. Participate in a ward round where the patient's results are discussed in the context of the overall condition/diagnosis/working diagnosis. Alternatively, if a ward round is not taking place, conduct a discussion with a member of the consultant's medical team.

(Learning objective: to begin to apply knowledge and results together; to further personal understanding of appropriate connections between diagnosis, treatment and nursing care required)

4. Complete continual professional development document (CPD) with case studies, participating in reflective practice.

(Learning objective: to document evidence of 'on the job learning' that has taken place and identify areas for further development required)

5. Proactively network with other colleagues while also undertaking programme of learning related to blood results reporting, by feeding back learning at a ward teaching session with peers.

(Learning objective: to build confidence in own decision making and reporting skills and provide a feedback loop for discussion of pertinent issues arising)

6. Participation in oral discussion with senior level doctor in area of blood results reporting pertinent to role and subsequent declaration of competence through completed competency document. Key phrases that are important to identify with participant to gauge understanding.

1) Effective and timely discharge of individuals with complex care needs is important if their quality of life is to be promoted and if effective use of resources is to be maximised.

2) Discharge planning for those with complex care needs usually occurs within a more global context, involving multiple on-going and underlying health and social care needs, whereby arrangements, which form a key component in the continuity of community care, must be put in place before successful transfer or discharge to another service or home can occur.

3) Effective discharge of those with complex discharge requirements requires a whole systems approach.

4) Effective discharge places the individual at the centre of the discharge process, promoting continuity of care through adequate information and communication flow between patients, carers and services so as to ensure optimal outcomes for individuals.

5) The effective discharge of those with complex care needs is a challenging and skilled process, requiring staff to have grasped the key principles and to have developed sophisticated skills.

(Learning objective: to accept responsibility for level of competency achieved and acknowledge 'life long learning for other areas of practice').

4. secondments to gain specific skills or experience as a stepping stone into new roles

5. completion of new clinical skills as part of sets (to be accredited as CATs in the future).

Two areas requiring further exploration are staff rotations and developing broad clinical skills.

Experiential learning

Regardless of how much is said in the literature about nurses employing good assessment skills, a suitable model of assessment is also required to support the practitioner, in practice.[36] It is suggested that commonly used nursing models may require adaptation to take into full account social perspectives, which will allow for proactive planning regardless of whether the patient is being treated in day surgery or on the ward. In some cases, surgery will have developed protocols, pathways and documentation which prompt the pertinent discharge planning factors to be explored. This approach alone may not be sufficient to deliver actual skills in practice and is often treated as a form-filling exercise, without the depth of knowledge or implications from lack of knowledge, being realised. Staff rotations to other areas of practice, to learn about the complexities of discharge planning, are rarely employed. Elderly care assessment units, rehabilitation units and areas where multi-disciplinary team meetings are held, provide ideal places to learn acute skills in assessment and planning, especially links with intermediate care services, all of which should be considered for the surgical patient requiring post-discharge rehabilitation and support.

So what is a skill set?

To enable a cohesive nurse facilitation of the many services used in discharging patients from hospital, 'skill sets' could be established, by grouping together the particular competencies, skills required (if competencies are not yet developed) and training opportunities into a set, which holistically addresses the needs and interests of the patient. While individual skills can be learned through supplementary approaches, these are best applied holistically to patient care. For example, there is a danger of creating a silo mentality regarding skills, especially those related to specialist areas of practice. Hence, a discharge planning skill set may require the inclusion of supplementary competencies not traditionally associated with discharge planning. As services become more cosmopolitan, spanning boundaries, discharge may equate to 'transfer of care', (where patients are transferred into other services) and knowledge of other interfacing services will be required.

An example could be: a discharge skill set for an older person (see Box 15.4, page 294), which may comprise; knowledge, comprehension, application and evaluation throughout services, pertinent assessments leading to referrals/good liaison abilities (which should not be taken for granted).

Despite the best of ideas to bring about new skills, development is often constrained through lack of a consistent organisationally supported approach. Hence access points into skill sets would need to be instigated from the point of recruitment into an organisation, moving away from an ad hoc approach towards fairly apportioning study time required for each person. Furthermore, it is essential to determine what knowledge, skills and experience in discharge planning staff possess on arrival to promote professional growth. If not, stagnation or regression may occur if their skills and abilities are not effectively utilised from the outset of employment.

Implementation and surgery

In summary, while any of the methods outlined below can be engaged, clarity regarding which approach is used is essential to drive practice forward.

Several methods can advance nurse-led discharge, namely:

- bespoke discharge management plans (useful in emergency admissions)
- discharge checklists with variance measured against the norm (all areas)
- protocol- or criteria-driven discharges (useful for specific condition groups and day surgery)
- care pathways with integrated discharge points (for specific operations or procedures spanning different organisations delivering the care).

It can be argued that one approach across a whole organisation will not realise the implementation of nurse-facilitated discharges. To some extent the approach selected will depend upon the organisational readiness and area of practice. For example, Trauma and Orthopaedics, General Surgery and Gynaecology were the first disciplines to express an interest in developing systems to support nurses to facilitate discharge. In each case, while the discharge process was clearly stated as part of a care pathway, the detail underpinning the 'how' still required work. In some instances this required the addition of a protocol with discharge parameters aligned to the greater majority of patients with a particular condition or following a particular procedure/operation.

Principles of good practice for surgery (protocols)

While there are huge interfaces between discharge practice across different hospital settings, some useful principles for surgical patients were stated when developing protocols, in the *Waiting, Booking and Choice* document (p. 5, 2.5, iii)[3]:

The discharge protocol should include:

- Assess the patient's fitness for discharge
- Ensure the patients and carers understand the constraints on fitness following an anaesthetic
- Include the provision of written information about the side effects or complications, and of medication to be taken
- Include a supply of postoperative analgesia and written information on how to take it
- Make arrangements for outpatient follow-up if appropriate
- Check that an emergency contact number has been given and that the patient knows how to use it should a problem arise.

In addition, the Royal College of Nursing (RCN) produced discharge information for nurses working in day surgery settings; this outlines detailed information regarding physiological, psychological and social needs of patients (Fact sheet 4)[37].

Conversely, acutely ill patients presenting as emergencies may have many potential variables, which are less suited to a protocol-managed approach. In this case a criteria-led approach, with the post-take ward round providing a management plan and estimated date of discharge, has provided the central structure. However, the management plan alone provides a reductionist approach, where nurses may be tempted to rely only on the plan (in a fast-moving acute environment) and not use the tools available to them, such as the SAP or other assessments that have been carried out since admission. Regardless of approach or speciality it is worth remembering that the patient enters into a discharge process once they are admitted to hospital and this approach should not be undermined by the discharge viewed as one task or a simple checklist of activities.

Follow-up of patients

The use of telephone follow-up is advocated for the care of surgical patients to provide postoperative support. The patient should be contacted by telephone 24 hours after surgery and nurses should provide an on-call commitment to do this.[38,3] Once again the exact method to be employed will depend upon the type of surgery that has been performed. General principles will include medication management, particularly in the case of analgesia and the risk of bleeding and infection post surgery.[39] Although evidence suggests follow-up of surgical patients from day surgery is relatively commonplace, an area of untapped opportunity exists in emergency care settings.[40] Increasingly patients are transferred directly from emergency care on to lists for day surgery. Follow-up from such settings may ensure patients are adequately informed in the comfort of their own home, when they are perhaps better able to address specific queries they may have and this in turn may increase the compliance with the care activities anticipated.[41]

Patient involvement in the process

Without doubt, central to the success of nurse-facilitated discharge is nurses' relationship with the patients they care for. Increasingly nurses are being asked to employ practices which provide evidence of the patient's involvement in their care. Many supporting systems are evolving, and some have always been better than others. Noticeboards, patient information leaflets, patient focus groups and satisfaction surveys are common. In the case of complex discharges the patient's involvement has always been a pivotal part of the discharge liaison nurse's role. Yet, conversely, for simple discharges it could be argued there are varying degrees of patient involvement from superficial to highly involved and that we have a long way to go to develop relationships which truly achieve patient empowerment.[42] Evidence of patient involvement in the discharge plan is required,[43,15,7] and this can be achieved in its simplest form through meaningful conversations that are documented in the patient's records. Chronic disease management and admission prevention through case management and new roles in the community are also allied in the role of discharge planning; in relation to this the promotion of 'self-care' strategies features as a distinct and evolving part of the nurse's role.[43] While these are not new concepts, as with nurse-facilitated discharge, the best chance of implementation may rest with the way the concept is packaged and the profile it is afforded alongside other key developments. If these aspects are effectively brought together they will form a powerful mixture to firmly involve the patient in discharge planning. Some further practical tips are offered below as examples.

Tips

- Identifying how you can help your patients learn from each other
- Involving the patient in their plan
- The provision of regular information
- Having a nurse on the ward round to reinforce good professional communication.
- Meeting the family and carers; taking time to meet during visiting periods
- Patient-led discharge checklists
- Giving clear ideas regarding date of discharge as soon after admission as practical
- Guiding doctors and other professionals on ways of getting involved
- The greatest of plans can be made by professionals but if they have not been discussed or shared with the patient they are not likely to be executed with any success.

CONCLUSION

At present discharge planning is very high profile across the NHS, with systems and practices playing constant catch-up to integrate policy into practice settings. Nurse-facilitated discharge from hospital is multifaceted. I feel we are at the beginning of something very important in the history of nursing. The timing is apt to bring about the change along with new systems of working to support far-reaching NHS changes. If not, at the very least we should be able to look back (over time) and realise, irrespective of the exact terminology used or policy that frames nurse-facilitated discharge, our actions will improve care for our patients. To this end it relies upon knowledge way beyond discharge planning, across expert knowledge bases and different organisational agendas. Healthcare professionals working in a hospital setting must draw on their experience and share this openly to provide the best care during the patient's acute phase, through an integrated approach, both professionally and organisationally. Nurse-facilitated discharge practice involves effectively preventing uncoordinated care delivery, regardless of organisational base, in the best interests of the patient.

REFERENCES

1. Department of Health (2000). *The NHS Plan: A Plan for Improvement, a Plan for Reform.* London: Department of Health.

2. Department of Health(2001). *Tackling Cancelled Operations.* London: NHS Modernisation Agency, Department of Health.

3. Department of Health (2002). *Day Surgery: An Operational Guide: Waiting, Booking and Choice.* London: Department of Health.

4. Department of Health (2002). *Discharge Planning: Model Discharge Documentation.* London: Department of Health.

5. Department of Health (2005). *Creating a Patient Led NHS: Delivering the Improvement Plan.* London: Department of Health.

6. Department of Health (2005). *Commissioning a Patient Led NHS.* London: Department of Health.

7. Department of Health (2003). *Effectiveness of Inpatient Discharge Procedure.* London: Department of Health.

8. L. Lees and K. Emmerson (2006). Identifying discharge practice training needs. *Nursing Standard* **20**(29): 47–51. Available at: www.nursing-standard.co.uk

9. Department of Health (2001). *The National Service Framework for Older People.* London: Department of Health.

10. Department of Health (2001). *The Single Assessment Process Consultation Papers and Process: An Introduction to Single Assessment.* London: Department of Health.

11. Department of Health (2002). *Health and Social Care Joint Unit and Change Agent Team, Discharge from Hospital: A Good Practice Checklist.* London: Department of Health. Available at: http://www.dh.gov.uk/assetRoot/04/12/62/50/04126250.pdf

12. Department of Health (2003). *The Community Care (Delayed Discharges) Act LAC/2003 Guidance for Implementation.* London: Department of Health.

13. Department of Health and Royal College of Nursing (2003). *Freedom to Practise: Dispelling the Myths.* London: Department of Health.

14. Department of Health (2003). *Discharge from Hospital: Pathway, Process and Practice.* London: Department of Health.

15. Department of Health (2003). *Making Amends: Proposals for Clinical Negligence Reforms.* London: Department of Health.

16. Department of Health (2004). *Achieving Timely 'Simple' Discharge from Hospital.* London: Department of Health.

17. K. Leason (2003). Delay tactics. *Nursing Standard* **17**(24): 16–17.

18. National Audit Office (2003). *Ensuring the Effective Discharge of Older Patients from NHS Acute Hospitals.* London: The Stationery Office.

20. R. Belbin (1993). *Team Roles at Work.* Oxford: Butterworth Heinemann.

21. Tierney, A. J. (2006). Commentary on Dunnion ME & Kelly HW (2005) From the emergency department to home: Discharge planning and communication of information between an emergency department and primary care sector following discharge of older people from an emergency department of a rural general hospital. *Journal of Clinical Nursing* **14**, 776-785 and *Journal of Clinical Nursing* **15**(6) 789–79.

22. J. Pethybridge (2004). How team working influences discharge planning from hospital: a study of four multi-disciplinary teams in an acute hospital in England. *Journal of Interprofessional Care* **18**(1): 29–41.

23. L. Kuockkanen and H. Leino-Kilpi (2000). Power and empowerment in nursing: three theoretical approaches. *Journal of Advanced Nursing* **31**(1): 235–41.

24. L. Lees, G. Allen and D. O'Brien (2006). Using post-take ward rounds to facilitate simple discharge. *Nursing Times* **102**(18): 28–30. Available at: www.nursingtimes.net

25. L. Lees and C. Holmes (2005). Estimating date of discharge at ward level: a pilot study. *Nursing Standard* **19**(17): 40–3.

26. C. Rudd and J. Smith (2002). Discharge planning. *Nursing Standard* **17**(5): 33–7.

27. L. Lees (2004). Making nurse led discharge work to improve patient care. *Nursing Times* **100**(37): 30–2. Available at: www.nursingtimes.net

28. L. Lees (2006). Emergency Care Briefing Paper: Modernising Discharge from Hospital, updated version January. National Electronic Library for Health, available at: http://libraries.nelh.nhs.uk/emergency/viewResource.asp?uri=http%3A//libraries.nelh.nhs.uk/common/resources/%3Fid%3D63696andcategoryID=1414

29. Nursing and Midwifery Council (2008). *The NMC Code of Professional Conduct: Standards for Conduct, Performance and Ethics.* London: Nursing and Midwifery Council.

30. Department of Health (2004b). *The NHS Knowledge and Skills Framework (NHS KSF) and the Development Review Process.* London: Department of Health.

31. Royal College of Nursing (2006). Core Career and Competency Framework. www.rcn.org.uk/resources/corecompetencies. Last accessed 15 May 2006.

32. T. Bargargliotti, M. Luttrell and C. Lenburg (1999). Reducing threats to the implementation of a competency based performance assessment system. *Journal of Issues in Nursing* **4**(2) www.nursingworld.org (last accessed February 2010).

33. H. Barr (1998). Competent to collaborate: towards a competency based model for inter-professional education. *Journal of Inter-Professional Care* **12**(2): 181.

34. M. Williams (2003). Assessment of portfolios in professional education. *Nursing Standard* **18**(8): 33–7.

35. A. Jones (1999). The place of judgement in competency-based assessment. *Journal of Vocational Education and Training* **51**(1): 145–60.

36. L. Lees (2005). A framework to promote the holistic assessment of older people in emergency care. *Journal of Older People's Nursing* **16**(10): 16–21. Available at: www.nursingolderpeople.co.uk

37. Royal College of Nursing (2004). Sheet 4. Discharge Planning. Day Surgery. Royal College of Nursing, Cavendish Square, London. www.rcn.org.uk

38. M. Brennan (1992). Nursing process in telephone advice. *Nursing Management* **23**(5): 62–4.

39. S.J. Closs (1997). Discharge communications between hospital and the community healthcare staff; a selective review. *Herald Social Care Community* **5**: 181–7.

40. J.R. Nelson (2001). The importance of post discharge telephone follow up for hospitalists: A view from the trenches. *American Journal of Medicine* **111**(9b): 43s–44s.

41. L. Lees (2004). Improving the quality of patient discharge from emergency settings. *British Journal of Nursing* **13**(7): 412–21.

42. D. Brown, C. McWilliam and C. Ward-Griffin (2006). Client-centred empowering partnership in nursing. *Journal of Advanced Nursing* **53**(2): 160–8.

43. Department of Health (2005). *Supporting People with Long Term Conditions: Liberating the Talents of Nursing Caring for People with Long Term Conditions.* London: Stationery Office.

44. H. Rushforth and E.A. Glasper (1999). Implications of nursing role expansion for professional practice. *British Journal of Nursing* **8**: 22.

45. M. Williams (2003). Assessment of portfolios in professional education. *Nursing Standard* **18**(8): 33–7.

16 Consent and the perioperative patient

Christine Hughes

SUMMARY

This chapter will cover:
- **an overview of the legal framework for consent**
- **a good practice approach to consent in the surgical patient**
- **implications for consenting adults and children**
- **the role that advanced practitioners can play in the consent process.**

INTRODUCTION

This chapter discusses the legalities of obtaining informed consent to invasive procedures in the adult, child, unconscious and mentally incapacitated patient. Refusal and withdrawal of consent from a legal stance is also addressed. The process of gaining consent is discussed and the use of procedure-specific consent forms, which inform the patient of common yet significant risks associated with the planned procedure. The provision of information is acknowledged as being a vital aspect of the consent process and one in which professionals can have input with the patient and family.

The chapter concludes with a discussion of the developing role of advanced practitioners who may be involved in the consent process as part of their role in the management of the perioperative patient and aspects of training required for non-medical consent takers.

To give one's consent can be defined as to 'agree', 'allow', or 'give permission'.[1] In relation to consent to intervention within the healthcare setting, consent to treatment or procedure involves a process of ensuring that the patient is equipped to make an informed decision regarding treatment and is provided with the relevant information to do so. The aim of the consent process is that the patient develops an understanding of the benefits, risks and any alternative treatments to the proposed procedure in order that valid consent can be deemed to have been obtained.

We discuss below some of the complicated issues surrounding the process of obtaining consent for health professionals across the multi-disciplinary team including doctors, nurses and allied professionals during their daily interaction with patients,. Consent can be implied, given verbally or written – all of equal importance within the process. The legal aspects of gaining consent from the adult, child, unconscious and mentally incapacitated patient will be discussed with regard to the capacity of the individual to understand and consequently ensure that consent is valid.

Refusal and withdrawal of consent to intervention can pose difficult dilemmas for healthcare professionals in ensuring a satisfactory outcome for the patient. Healthcare professionals face challenges as to how to act in patients' best interest while ensuring that their rights to refuse or withdraw consent are met. Legal decisions can appear complicated and confusing.

Consent can also be seen as a process of providing information and gaining patient understanding of that information – a well-informed patient is able to make important decisions regarding their treatment. Patients today are often more informed about their illness than traditionally has been the case because of an increase in media attention as well as the availability of information, especially on the Internet, which is accessible to a wide range of individuals.

The use of procedure-specific consent forms may help to reduce subjectivity and variance in discussion of risks with the patient. In conjunction with these issues. The changing roles of the extended practitioner within the nursing sphere will be debated in relation to the consent process and provision of patient information, as will training requirements for non-medical consent takers.

Legal aspects

The mentally competent adult (aged 18 or over) has a right to give consent prior to any touch of his person within present common or civil law of the land.[2] This is a set of principles applied across the country which recognise an individual's right to protect their body against invasion by another person.

It is vital that consent is valid; in order to be valid the patient must be empowered to make an autonomous decision about their health and lifestyle.[3]

Consent to intervention may be implied non-verbally or given verbally, which is what happens in everyday practice. It is not always necessary or indeed realistic to gain written consent to every physical intervention carried out by the healthcare professional. However, any form of consent should be recorded within patient documentation.

The patient must be mentally able and correctly informed by a suitably competent and knowledgeable person regarding the procedure. The consent must be given voluntarily, not being subject to coercion or influence of others. Therefore, the professional must first ascertain when seeking consent that the patient has the capacity to understand and retain the information. At this point, consideration must be given to the fact that patients' decisions can be affected by stress, illness and medication[2,4] and the patient may understandably be nervous and fearful.

If a person is touched without implicit consent, or without any lawful means of ascertaining consent, he has the right of civil or criminal action as trespass to himself may have occurred. This may amount to battery or trespass in the law courts – when the person is actually touched. A case of assault may be brought if he believes he will be touched without consent.[2]

Although the patient may imply or give verbal consent to a variety of daily interventions there may be significant risks associated with a more invasive procedure such as surgical intervention, for which written consent should be sought.[5] The Department of Health states that consent can be implied[6] for example, when a patient holds their arm out for a blood sample to be taken. However, it remains pertinent that health professionals provide information to the patient and seek permission prior to proceeding with any invasive procedure. The patient and the professional may have conflicting perceptions as to the nature of the planned intervention.

It is important not to dismiss the need to gain consent for what often appears to the health professional as a routine procedure, such as inserting a urinary catheter. Assumptions should not be made that the patient gives permission for any intervention to take place on their person. The patient has a right to information and to question why any intervention is to be carried out and to information and explanation regarding any of the associated risks.

The General Medical Council[7] warns that care should be taken by the practitioner in relying on implied consent. For example, a patient may be lying on an examination couch in a clinic, but this does not mean that the patient understands what the healthcare professional proposes to do or why, nor does it mean that they give consent to the professional's planned intervention. Therefore the professional must be aware that implied consent is not given solely by the patient arriving at the hospital.[2]

The unconscious patient

The unconscious patient may be treated by necessity. In this situation common law recognises that the professional must act in the best interest of the patient in relation to the standard and duty of care accepted within the profession. This is not implied consent, it is a necessity,[2] as the unconscious patient is not able to imply anything. The professional must, therefore, be able to defend their actions. It is wise to discuss the management and risks of a procedure with a relative or close friend if possible, in order to ascertain any details which may affect clinical judgement, even though these persons are unable to give consent for another.[8]

Written consent

Although it is accepted that implied or verbal consent is acceptable for many everyday interventions, written consent is, without doubt, superior to a verbal agreement which can later be refuted, as there is often no documented evidence of a conversation taking place. Word of mouth can be much more difficult to prove in a court of law and is therefore unreliable and open to dispute.[2]

Consider the example in Box 16.1.

Box 16.1 Example 1

Janet is a 43-year-old woman who is admitted to theatre for repair of epigastric hernia and removal of lesion on right cheek under general anaesthetic. After anaesthesia was administered the patient was taken into the Theatre area where it was noted by the Theatre Sister that the consent form stated epigastric hernia repair but omitted to indicate removal of lesion on cheek – although this additional procedure was written on the operating theatre list. The Senior Registrar insisted that he had discussed removal of the lesion with the patient on the ward preoperatively but had inadvertently omitted to write this on the consent form. What could be the outcome of this situation if removal of the lesion had been carried out?

Janet may have denied that the discussion with the Registrar took place. If she subsequently suffered a complication such as scarring or infection, she might deny any prior discussion or understanding of the associated risks. Although this type of situation is uncomfortable for the professional who is then often at the mercy of a disappointed or angry patient, any invasive procedure such as surgery should not be carried out without appropriate attention to the consent process unless in a life or death situation where action in the patient's best interests could be justified.

Although it is rarely a requirement of law that written consent is obtained, it is recognised as best practice to obtain patients' signatures when planning to carry out invasive procedures,[5] including the following interventions:

- general anaesthetic, regional anaesthesia or sedation
- a complex procedure in which significant risks apply, such as surgical procedures
- intervention which may have consequences for future lifestyle, social life, employment or quality of life.

A signature on a consent form is evidence that the patient has given consent, but it is not proof of valid consent.[6] Therefore, validity may be questioned if the patient did not give consent voluntarily or was not provided with adequate information to make an informed decision.

Should there be dispute regarding consent, a court of law may ask whether the 'reasonable' patient would have given consent had they been aware of the risks. The law may view absence of documented proof of information provided and discussion of associated risks as a failure in the practitioner's duty of care.[8]

Refusal and withdrawal of consent

If a patient refuses to consent to treatment, they have every right to do so.[2] However, the health professional should seek to ascertain the patient's reasoning for this decision and discuss the implications of refusal or withdrawal of intervention, providing support and information to ensure that the patient has based their decision on correct information and understands the possible implications of their actions.

Refusal of any treatment or intervention should be clearly documented in the patient's notes. The patient's autonomy must be respected – it is an individual's right to decide, even if the outcome may cause harm to themselves.[7] There are no statutory powers which force an individual who is mentally competent to receive intervention against their will, which can be a dilemma for medical staff when issues of this nature arise, for example, pertaining to the pregnant woman. A woman who is mentally competent but refuses intervention for reasons such as religious grounds or even irrational reasons may not be overruled by the courts – even if her actions result in death or disability of infant.[2] Being of sound mind and maturity still remains the general principle.[8] However, if the patient is deemed mentally incapacitated in some way, intervention may then be declared by the law court under the Mental Health Act 1983.[2]

Box 16.2 Example 2

A pregnant woman who refused treatment for pre-eclampsia was detained under Section 2 of the Mental Health Act 1983. The High Court declared that a caesarean section should be carried out. This procedure subsequently went ahead. The woman then claimed at the Court of Appeal that she was wrongly detained under the Mental Health Act and therefore the caesarean section should not have been carried out against her will. She won her case.

Guidelines were subsequently produced to check the validity of patients' refusal of intervention and steps to check mental capacity and ability to make informed decisions, free from coercion and influence.[2]

It is accepted that when a patient gives valid consent, this is valid indefinitely unless withdrawn by the patient; therefore, no specific time limit is designated from signature to procedure.[6] However, it is good practice to confirm the patient's wishes if significant time has lapsed since the initial process. The patient is entitled to withdraw consent at any time both before and during a procedure. If withdrawal of consent during a procedure would pose a significant risk to the life of the patient, then the practitioner may be justified in continuing until the immediate risk is no longer applicable.[6]

Children and young persons

Children under the age of 16 are now able to give consent if they have sufficient comprehension of what is proposed; this is known as Gillick competent – if the professional concludes during discussion that the child has the capacity to make decisions and has sufficient understanding of the proposed treatment. It is good practice to involve family members in these discussions if possible so as to aid understanding and informed decision-making. If the individual lacks capacity to consent, the parent or person with parental responsibility may give consent on the child's behalf.[6]

However, if the Gillick competent child objects to treatment, the parent or person with parental responsibility or indeed the Court may be a sufficient authority to act against the child's wishes.[9] The refusal to give consent by a minor can be very complex. Although refusal may be overruled by those with parental responsibility or by the Court of Law, consideration of the psychological and physical welfare of the child must be deliberated over as a basis for this decision[6] and should be given careful consideration, especially if the child is older, more mature, capable of fully understanding the implications[9] and therefore making decisions.

A person aged 16 or 17 is entitled to give their consent as an adult would, and as indicated in Section 8[1] Family Law Act 1969.[10] Refusal by a 16- or 17-year-old can be overridden by a Court of Law; in this instance it may be appropriate to use the Mental Health Act 1983.[9]

Box 16.3 Example 3

A 16-year-old girl who suffered from anorexia nervosa refused all treatment despite a severe deterioration in her condition. The Court of Appeal ruled that she be treated in a specialist unit against her will under the Mental Health Act 1983. They deemed that the disease process destroys the ability to make an informed decision.[8]

While it is deemed correct that a child can understand and agree to intervention, refusal of intervention is difficult for us to accept, as we then question the ability of the minor to appreciate risks. The fear of having the procedure may be overwhelming for the child for them to appreciate the risks, and therefore agreeing to it being undertaken. However, this may be problematic as the condition could worsen to the point that treatment options are limited and incompatible with a good prognosis or surgical outcome.

Mentally incompetent patients

It must be considered that a patient with mental health problems may be perfectly able to comprehend and make decisions to give, refuse or retract consent to intervention. In the case of an individual who does not have the capacity to understand information and subsequently give consent, two doctors may take this responsibility on behalf of the patient, acting in the patient's best interest. Family or close friends may be helpful in advising health professionals of the patient's wishes,[6] and should be involved in discussion when possible in the interest of their relative. However, consent cannot be given on behalf of another adult.

Box 16.4 Example 4

Sandra is a 45-year-old woman with learning difficulties, who was an elective admission to the surgical ward for right hemicolectomy for an adenocarcinoma of the colon. Sandra was accompanied by her brother Jonathon, who was her advocate and carer. Jonathon explained that Sandra was a very independent woman despite her learning difficulties and verified that she was fully able to comprehend and make informed decisions about treatment.

Therefore, the postoperative management plan, benefits and risks of surgery were discussed with Sandra in a manner that she could comprehend; all her questions were answered fully and her brother, who was present throughout the discussion, was aware of plans and could give Sandra the support she required.

The consent process

Obtaining a patient's consent for a surgical procedure should be viewed by health professionals as a 'process'.[6] This process should take place over a period of time, especially when major surgery is to be embarked upon, to allow the patient to digest information and options and develop an understanding to allow an informed decision to be made. However, it is accepted that this may not be possible, for example, in the emergency situation.

It may be appropriate to initiate the consent process on first meeting, for example, at an outpatients' clinic where elective surgery is often primarily discussed. At this stage, benefits, risks, alternative treatments and the consequences of no surgical intervention can be discussed. Written information can also be offered to support the discussion. The consent form can be signed at this stage and a copy given to the patient, including the name and contact number of the health professional involved in the process. However, the patient must then be given the opportunity to ask further questions and clarify information as required on admission to hospital.

The early implementation of the consent process may not only be of benefit to the patient but to the surgical team. Within the expanding climate of day case surgery and reduced length of hospital stays, time management can be an issue. If the patient has been fully informed and has consented to the procedure prior to hospital admission, the chance of a rushed and unsatisfactory consent process due to time constraints may be reduced. Discussing associated surgical risks immediately prior to surgery is not ideal when the patient is anxious and possibly aware of time constraints placed upon health professionals. Obtaining consent solely on the day of surgery is not a practice recommended in the literature.[6]

It may be inappropriate for a patient who is to undergo more complex surgery or those who are given bad news in the clinic area, to discuss risks in detail at this point in time. The patient would be unlikely to retain this important information due to emotional stress and would therefore be unable to digest the information and make an informed decision. Therefore further discussion should be arranged at a later time. However the process of information giving and support can commence at this stage.

In order for the patient to retain their autonomy they must be involved in a two-way conversation and should be able to understand what is being discussed.[11] Obtaining consent does not just mean the written record but the quality of the verbal interaction between the professional and the patient. Solely being offered a consent form to sign without discussion and opportunity to ask questions is not adequate according to the law. Historically the focus was often in gaining the patient's signature on the consent form rather than ensuring patient comprehension of associated risk.[12,13] Patients were even asked to sign consent forms in the operating theatre area on occasions – a practice which is considered unacceptable today.

It is essential that informed consent be based on 'knowledge of the nature, risks, consequences and alternatives associated with the proposed therapy' (p. 396).[8] It is often useful to discuss levels of risk in terms of accepted percentages to reduce misconceptions between patient and professional. For example, informing the patient of a 3% risk of recurrence following mesh repair of inguinal hernia is clear and concise and not subject to misinterpretation. This can be indicated on the consent form and documented in the patient's notes or clinic letter for clarification.

Procedure-specific consent forms

Many hospitals have moved towards using procedure-specific consent forms, which reduce the risk of illegibility and ensure that all significant risks related to the procedure are documented.[3] Generic consent forms are subject to variance in the risks discussed and documented. However, procedure-specific consent forms do not necessarily equate to patient understanding of the identified risks or indeed the doctor discussing them at all. It could be argued that the patient should read and understand all risks before signing the consent form. In reality, the patient believes and trusts the doctor and will often sign the consent form with little understanding of what risks are involved.[3] This is clearly inappropriate and morally unacceptable, though time restraints, patients' mental and physical condition, suitability of environment and patient understanding all play a part in the dilemmas faced by those involved in consent process.

One of the most common consent issues between a patient and surgeon is viewed as being 'failure to warn'.[14] A standardised consent form can warn the patient of rare but potentially serious or life-threatening complications, of which, if they are to make an informed decision, they need to be aware.[14]

There is a moral and ethical obligation on the part of the health professional to provide information, as the individual has the right to make health choices and retain their autonomy.

Box 16.5 Example 5

A dentist carried out invasive treatment on eight patients, none of whom it was alleged had received sufficient information to make an informed decision. It was later found that the treatments were unnecessary as the dentist had carried out these procedures on healthy teeth.

The dentist was subsequently charged with assault, being deemed by the judge to have acted in ill-faith and to have deliberately withheld information from the patients.[15]

Patients' understanding of the consent process

Within today's healthcare environment, the power of knowledge should no longer be held solely in the hands of the doctor. Information should not be withheld because the doctor or nurse thinks the patient does not need to know, or would be unable to comprehend.[3] It is the responsibility of the health professional to provide information in the most pertinent manner suited to the individual's level of understanding.

This requires honesty; trying to hide facts in an attempt to protect the patient from upset is no longer acceptable. If there is a risk of death or severe disability, then this must be addressed in order to fully inform the patient. The author would suggest, however, that there is a fine line between providing all this information and causing immense fear and stress to the patient.

One could argue that patients today are more aware of health matters than in the past and are better informed about disease and surgical procedures. This may be due to increased media coverage and access to the Internet. Therefore patients may actively seek consent or joint decision-making, which involves discussion and agreement between patient and healthcare professionals based on patients' wishes.[5]

A prospective study[16] was carried out to examine patients' understanding of the consent process. Understanding was found to be limited – these patients viewed the consent form as ritualistic and bureaucratic, its place to protect the hospital and doctors from litigation. Patients had little concept that the intention of the consent process was actually to inform and protect them. This raises questions as to the disparity between models of consent and patients' perceptions, and how far the process can address patients' autonomy and rights. Informed consent is, therefore, a vital element in making the consent process valid.[4]

Although the patient may actively seek information and understanding, this does not necessarily mean that the patient fully understands. Comprehension arises from explanation, use of diagrams, written information, repetition of information, verification of patient understanding and the opportunity for the patient to ask further questions at a later date.

A study, in which questionnaires were sent to doctors, nurses and patients to compare perceptions of patient information offered, concluded that medical and nursing teams greatly underestimated the amount and type of information patients required concerning their condition.[17] The study also highlighted that the more educated the patient, the more information they required. It could be argued that the more educated patient has the capacity to formulate appropriate and direct questions. It must not be assumed, however, that a patient who chooses not to question, refrains because they fully understand. Lack of information can cause anxiety and a feeling of helplessness.[18]

In contrast, the practitioner may be faced with the patient for whom too much information is anxiety provoking. The ability to judge this often depends on professional judgement, experience, and assessment of the individual's receptiveness to information given during two-way discussion. The professional must heed patients' verbal and non-verbal signs, body language and tone of voice, which can convey level of understanding, and ensure that the discussion is directed at the appropriate level. A record should be made within patients' notes of the type of information given; refusal of information or to discuss related risk must also be clearly documented.

Who can take consent?

Any healthcare professional having direct contact with a patient must gain consent whether it be implied, verbal or written and indeed must do so on a daily basis while caring for their patient. It is the responsibility of the clinician providing the treatment to ensure that valid consent to more invasive procedures such as surgery is carried out within the guidelines, as the consultant is ultimately responsible for the patient's welfare by law. However, the clinician may delegate the process of obtaining consent to a healthcare professional, only if that delegated individual is deemed to be a willing, competent and knowledgeable practitioner.[6,19]

The anaesthetist or a suitably competent member of the anaesthetic team should also discuss risks related to chosen method of anaesthesia and obtain consent from the patient. Associated risks related to an intervention, for example, epidural for postoperative pain relief, should be discussed with the patient, as should any alternatives such as patient-controlled analgesia. Written information can be used to support this decision.

A study published in 2006[20] used questionnaires to ascertain the changing practice of anaesthetists with regard to the use of thoracic epidurals. Data collected via questionnaire in 1997, which was then repeated in 2004, was analysed, and it was concluded that there was a considerable change in practice relating to the consent process over this period of time. This was demonstrated by a shift from the majority believing that they had gained patient consent by discussing matters of anaesthesia to the recognition that specific associated risks must be directly discussed with the patient and documented in the notes. This shift was thought to have been influenced by the Kennedy Report which followed the inquiry into paediatric heart surgery at Bristol Royal Infirmary.[2]

The role of the advanced practitioner

There has been much debate regarding the scope of advanced or extended roles in nursing over the past two decades – those which cross boundaries between nursing and medicine. New roles have evolved due to a focus on improving the quality of care for patients, developing careers of senior nurses (supported by professional nursing bodies and changing political agendas), such as the reduction of junior doctors' hours. Patient satisfaction has been noted to improve with nurse specialist intervention[21] though further audit of the roles would be useful if related to patient outcomes and satisfaction.

Box 16.6 Changing roles

Within the surgical speciality, roles such as the surgical care practitioner (SCP) and more recently the perioperative specialist practitioner (PSP) have been developed in response to the political agendas and to meet the demands of present day healthcare.

The PSP programme at St Mary's Hospital, London, in conjunction with Imperial College, London, is now in its fifth year. Throughout the United Kingdom the PSP has a varied and adaptable role, which Trusts have embraced and developed to improve patient satisfaction.

The Nursing and Midwifery Council[22] supports the notion of advanced nursing practice, where the practitioner is, within their sphere of practice, clinically competent to make complex clinical decisions using expert clinical judgements independently, though more often as part of the team. The advanced practitioner is an essential team member who can be not only viewed as a source of continual contact for the patient and development of services,[21] but is also equipped with the knowledge and skills to discuss the individual management plan with the patient and relatives.

Surgical practitioners today can help provide more holistic management of the patient during the perioperative period than initial roles allowed and will have many advantages for the patient, medical and nursing colleagues alike in education, training, information and the provision of quality care.[23] The advanced practitioner role and clinical experience can often be utilised as a resource for teaching and training various designations of healthcare professionals such as nurses and junior doctors and can involve teaching of Foundation 1 and 2 surgical house officers regarding surgical management of patients, therefore contradicting the argument that such roles detract from doctors' training.[24]

The consent process may not be given high priority at times, due to time constraints, and can therefore be left to junior doctors who may have little experience or knowledge of the risks associated with a particular surgical procedure or the choices open to patients. The author would argue that this is clearly unacceptable and can be detrimental to the patient if they are misinformed and misled. Doctors are under greater pressure in today's climate in relation to litigation, meeting government targets, increased specialisation and changes within working hours and some see new nursing roles as an added stressor.[25] However, it can be suggested that practitioners in new roles can be beneficial in certain surgical settings, allowing doctors to focus on more complicated clinical issues.[26] Opposition to these developing roles by doctors, nurses and indeed managers may be due to lack of understanding of the role and professional jealousy.[27] This hostility often comes from those who misunderstand the ethos and intention of these extended roles.

The debate regarding changing roles would be better focused on who is best placed to deliver patient care within various settings, with the focus on improvement of the patient's perioperative experience.[28] It can be argued that nurse-led consent may be the way forward in increased efficiency within the clinic environment, resulting in a more streamlined service for patients.[29] The author would argue however that nurse-led consent to surgical intervention must only be delegated to those with specific knowledge, skills and competencies to undertake this important process and with the support of a Consultant Surgeon.

Box 16.7 The PSP role

The author is a perioperative specialist practitioner (PSP) in the general/colorectal specialty within East Cheshire Trust and is a permanent member of the surgical team. This role involves the management of patients throughout the perioperative journey, from initial clinic appointment to discharge and includes extended skills such as physical examination, history taking, ordering and interpreting diagnostic tests, patient education and family support to name but a few. The PSP has a varied role within the Trust between theatre, ward, clinic and endoscopy areas. At present six PSPs and one surgical care practitioner (SCP) are employed within the Trust across General Surgical and Orthopaedic specialties, though their individual roles may differ. One element of training within the PSP model[30] incorporates communication and consent issues, including attendance at legal workshops and study days as part of the training programme. Competence to take consent to surgical intervention within the clinical area is then assessed by a consultant surgeon in accordance with the local hospital policy.

Training for non-medical consent takers

The practitioner involved in the consent process must possess the knowledge and skills to assess the individual patient for any additional risks posed due to their pre-existing co-morbidity[4] and may need to liaise with members of the multi-disciplinary team if potential problems are highlighted. Nurses carrying out an extended role would be judged on their competence to perform at the level of the doctor if they have been adequately trained and possess the appropriate knowledge to do so. Therefore the advanced practitioner practising at a senior house officer level may be judged as such in a court of law. In cases of negligence the 'Bolam test' would apply, where the practitioner would be judged on the standard of 'the ordinary skilled man exercising and professing to have that special skill'.[2] As a professional, there must be recognition of role boundaries and the knowledge and ability to recognise when support is required.

Educational programmes and retaining competence regarding consent issues are also recognised as important by local authorities and various authors and must be subject to audit.[4,5,31] It is vital that the Trust ensures that all aspects of consent are reflected within the individual's role profile and that the practitioner completes training and retains competencies according to Trust policy and remains updated on issues relating to consent. The Trust should carry out a regular audit of the consent process to ensure that the it is carried out in a safe and satisfactory manner, in accordance with policy and the patient's best interests, making any change to policy where necessary. Any issues relating to consent will be discussed during the consent steering group meetings within the Trust.

CONCLUSION

Consent has many facets relating to the legal aspects of gaining consent to intervention, be it implied, given verbally or by written consent form. It is essential that consent is gained from an individual who has been offered adequate and appropriate information to allow them to make an informed decision which is not subject to coercion from others and therefore given voluntarily. In order to be valid, the patient must have the capacity to understand the proposed course of action and any risks associated with it, so they should be aware of any treatment options or possible consequences of no intervention at all.

The mentally capacitated adult has the right to give consent to any touch of their body; violating this right in any way can be deemed as trespass, battery or assault in a court of law. The right to refuse or withdraw consent is the prerogative of the adult. This may be overruled by a court under the Mental Health Act 1983 if the patient is deemed incapacitated in some way. The unconscious patient cannot give consent nor can they imply it. Therefore it is the responsibility of the professional to act in the patient's best interests and to do no more, and no less, than would be expected of a professional in their role.

The child under 16 years of age can be involved in the consent process if they are deemed to be Gillick competent – the parent or those with parental responsibility can give consent to treatment of the minor. Refusal to consent by a minor may be overruled by a parent or by a court of law acting in the child's interest or by application of the Mental Health Act 1983 if required, though the reasons for refusal must be carefully considered.

Those who are mentally incapacitated may be able to give consent to intervention; this will depend on the individual's capacity to understand and retain information. If the individual cannot consent then two doctors can do so on the patient's behalf.

Implied consent should not be assumed. Any intervention should be discussed with the patient and their understanding and agreement sought. Written consent is viewed as superior when carrying out more invasive procedures such as surgery, which has significant associated risks. However, gaining a signature on a consent form is not considered valid consent alone – patient awareness and understanding of associated risk and treatment options is also necessary.

Consent can be viewed as a process where discussion, questioning and exchange of information can take place. This can begin early in the professional relationship to ensure that the patient is fully equipped to make an informed decision regarding treatment.

Patients are now better informed than historically regarding surgery and disease process, due to increased media attention, and may actively seek information and specific treatments. Directing information at the appropriate level for patient comprehension is vital in order to ensure that the individual is fully equipped to make informed decisions regarding the benefits, risks and any alternative treatments when faced with surgical intervention. Procedure-specific, as opposed to generic, consent forms can reduce discrepancies in signifying associated risks and illegibility of handwriting, which can cause misconceptions and misunderstanding.

The healthcare profession is constantly involved in the consent process, usually in the form of implied and verbal consent, in their daily interaction with patients. Gaining written consent to more invasive procedures, such as surgical intervention, is the responsibility of the surgeon. However, this can be delegated to a responsible and adequately knowledgeable professional who is deemed competent to deal with it.

Extended roles within nursing and allied professions have crossed boundaries into more traditional medical roles, in order to meet the demands of the modern-day health service. Positions such as the SCP and PSP within Trusts are examples of these developing roles within the surgical speciality. These roles have been seen to improve service to patients and can be a teaching resource for nursing, medical and allied professionals. New roles continue to be the topic of discussion, debate and question within the nursing and medical professions and within the media and will continue to be so as the demands on healthcare providers change. New roles often cross boundaries in nursing and medicine and can be subject to lack of understanding within the professional group as well as by patients.

However, the many expanding roles within the surgical speciality that have developed in recent years in the nursing and allied professions are arguably improving patient outcomes in terms of provision of information and support to the patient and family throughout the perioperative period. The process of providing information and patient understanding is vital, as a wel-informed patient is paramount in the consent process.

REFERENCES

1. *Oxford Dictionary Thesaurus and Wordpower Guide* (2003). Oxford: Oxford University Press.

2. B. Dimond (2002). *Legal Aspects of Nursing* (4th edn). London: Pearson Education Limited.

3. R. Worthington (2002). Clinical issues on consent: Some philosophical concerns. *Journal of Medical Ethics* **28**(6): 377–80.

4. H.A. Schofield, C. Viney and J. Evans (1997). Expanding practice and obtaining consent. *Professional Nurse* **13**(1): 12–16.

5. East Cheshire NHS Trust (2005). *Policy for consent to examination of treatment* (un-published).

6. Department of Health (2001). *Reference Guide to Consent for Examination or Treatment.* London: Department of Health.

7. General Medical Council (1998). *Seeking Patients' Consent: The Ethical Consideration.* London: GMC. Available at: http://www.gmc-uk.org/guidance/current/library.consent.asp (last accessed 20/03/07).

8. J.K. Mason and R.A. McCall-Smith (2005). *Law and Medical Ethics* (7th edn). London: Butterworths.

9. Department of Health and Welsh Office (1999). *Mental Health Act 1983 Code of Practice.* London: The Stationery Office.

10. Family Law Act 1969. Section 8. Available at: http://www.statutelaw.gov.uk/content.aspx?LegType=All+Primary&PageNumber=61&NavFrom=2&parentActiveTextDocId=1277000&ActiveTextDocId=1277000&filesize=143394

11. S. Humphreys (2005). Patient autonomy. Legal and ethical issues in the post anaesthetic care unit. *British Journal of Perioperative Nursing* **15**(1): 35–43.

12. British Medical Association (2001). *Report of the Consent Working Party.* Available at: http://bmahouse.co.uk/ap/nsf/consent (last accessed 23/03/07).

13. D.J. Mazur (2003). Influence of the law on risk and informed consent. *British Medical Journal* **327**: 731–4.

14. J. Adshead (2006). Procedure specific consent forms. *Medical Protection Society Casebook* **14**(3): 24.

15. P. Marquand (2000). *Introduction to Medical Law.* London: Butterworth-Heinemann.

16. A. Akkad, C. Jackson, S. Kenyon, M. Dixon-Woods, N. Taub and M. Habiba (2006). Patients' perceptions of written consent: questionnaire study. *British Medical Journal.* **333**: 528–9.

17. R. Sullivan, L.W. Menpace and R.M. White (2001). Truth-telling and patient diagnosis. *Journal of Medical Ethics* **27**: 192–7

18. S. Hughes (2002). The effects of giving patient pre-operative information. *Nursing Standard* **16**(28): 33–7.

19. S. Dowling, R. Martin, P. Skidmore, L. Doyal, A. Cameron and S. Lloyd (1994). Nurses taking on junior doctors' work: a confusion of accountability. *British Medical Journal* **312**: 1211–14.

20. S.H. Pennyfeather, S. Gilby, A. Danecki and G.N. Russell (2006). The changing practice of thoracic epidural anaesthesia in the United Kingdom: 1997–2004. *Journal of the Association of Anaesthetists of Great Britain and Ireland* **61**(4): 3.

21. J. Wilson and T. Bunnell (2007). A review of the merits of the nurse practitioner role. *Nursing Standard* **21**(18): 35–40

22. Nursing and Midwifery Council (2005). The proposed framework for the standard for post registration nursing. Available at: http://www.nmc-uk.org (last accessed 30/5/07).

23. M. Radford (2000). A framework for perioperative advanced practice. *British Journal of Perioperative Nursing* **10**(1): 50–4.

24. C. Shannon (2005). Doctors object to a wider role for surgical care practitioners. *British Medical Journal* **330**: 1103.

25. W.J.D. Murray (1999). Nurses in surgery – opportunity or threat? A personal view. *British Journal of Theatre Nursing* **9**(8): 365–8.

26. R. Kneebone and A. Darzi (2005). New professional roles in surgery. *British Medical Journal* **330**: 803–4.

27. L.P. Woods (1998). Implementing advanced nurse practice: identifying factors that facilitate and inhibit the process. *Journal of Clinical Nursing* **7**(3): 265–73.

28. S. Hopkins (1996). Junior doctors' hours and the expanding role of the nurse. *Nursing Times* **92**(14): 35–6.

29. M. Davies (2005). Nurse practitioner-led consent in day case cataract surgery. *Nursing Times* **101**(13): 30–2.

30. R.L. Kneebone, D.Nestel, J. Chrzanowska, A.E. Barnet and A. Darzi (2006). Innovative training for new surgical roles – the place of evaluation. *Medical Education* **40**(10): 987–94.

31. M. Davies (1998). *Textbook on Medical Law* (2nd edn). Hants: Ashford Colour Press.

17 Changing the preoperative process – a review of the evidence

Ross Kerridge

SUMMARY

This chapter will describe:

- **developing a model of perioperative care**
- **the implications of change for clinicians and managers**
- **managing expectation and risk in the change process.**

INTRODUCTION

The importance of appropriate preoperative and pre-anaesthetic patient assessment and preparation in order to assure patient safety has long been recognised, and has been confirmed by morbidity and mortality audits. In recent years, there has been an increased appreciation of the adverse effects of poor patient preparation on dimensions of quality other than safety, such as avoidable cancellations, process delays, inefficiency in the operating theatres, staff frustration, and patient dissatisfaction. Some of these effects may not be immediately apparent, but collectively produce a large negative impact on the quality of the health system. This is the inevitable result of a poorly designed and organised patient preparation system. Conceptually, it can be described as the 'iceberg of poor patient preparation' (Figure 17.1).

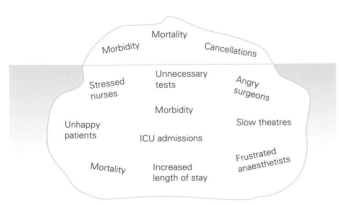

**Figure 17.1
The iceberg of poor patient preparation**

The traditional preoperative process

The traditional model of patient care for patients having surgery is based on the organisational structures developed in the hospitals of the late nineteenth century. In this model, it is presumed that the surgeon is in authoritative command of a small 'firm' that acts as a hierarchical team. This 'firm' was relatively autonomous with regard to the rest of the hospital – so that each surgeon or firm could have clinical practices that were unique to that firm. It was presumed unnecessary to involve other medical specialists in medical decision-making. The surgeon was regarded as omniscient, omni-competent, and omni-present – the traditional model assumes that the surgeon is always in control, and thus can and must be contacted (either directly or through a lower member of the hierarchy), whenever management decisions are to be made.

The traditional model required the members of the surgical team to have a broad understanding of all matters to do with perioperative patient care, as the surgeon (or delegate) was empowered and expected to make decisions regarding any patient care matter. It also required the members of the surgical team to have a comprehensive knowledge of everything regarding the patient's clinical care. These aspects of the traditional care model were major strengths, but were built on assumptions regarding the hospital workforce. It assumed that the patient was treated in one ward with a small stable number of nurses providing all the care on the ward. With regard to 'junior' members of the medical hierarchy, the traditional model implied a working style based on living in the hospital, and an expectation of being available and contactable at all times.

This traditional model had both strengths and weaknesses. The major strengths of the traditional model included a clear line of command and control – it was clear to everyone in the system that one person was in charge of all decision-making. There was also clarity of process – the steps involved in an episode of surgical care could be described linearly, and there were very few points of 'greyness' where there were obviously conflicting requirements in planning patient care.

The traditional model also existed in an environment that was different from that of today. Clinical information was less complex, as patients had fewer co-morbidities, inter-current therapies, and fewer results of investigations. The average length of stay was longer, and patients stayed on one ward for their entire hospital stay. Organisational process control (management of information) was substantially less. Information management was simpler due to the smaller number of clinicians and others involved in the care process. Finally, financial constraints and expectations of efficient process management were fewer. The results of poor patient preparation could be accommodated, by practices such as early admission, which are no longer accepted.

Conceptually, the traditional surgical process was hospital-based; most steps in the process occurred in hospital (see Figure 17.2). After the initial decision that the patient needed an operation, the patient was admitted to hospital, and the care process commenced with nursing and medical admission, investigations, preparation, and the procedure itself. Postoperative care tended to be reactive, so that discharge planning started when the decision was made that the patient could be discharged. Reflecting this system, the portrayal of hospitalisation in popular

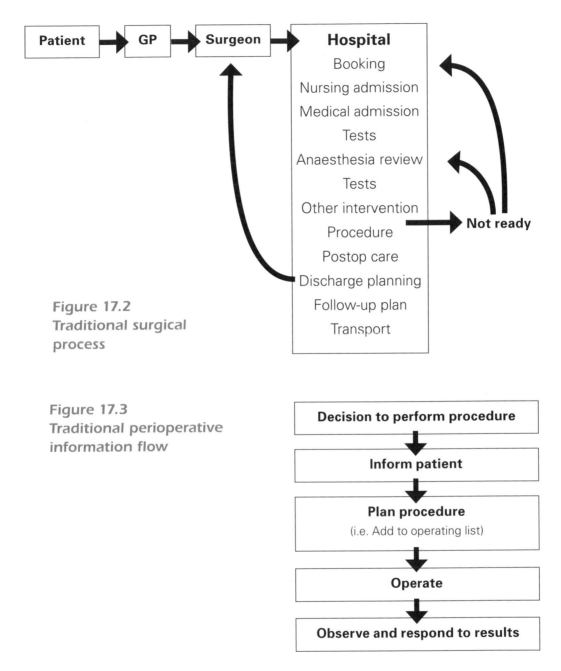

**Figure 17.2
Traditional surgical
process**

**Figure 17.3
Traditional perioperative
information flow**

culture has commonly featured the senior doctor announcing to the patient (and staff) 'you can go home today' as unexpected and welcome news.

The traditional process can also be viewed from an information management perspective (see Figure 17.3). The surgeon made the decision to operate at a particular time and informed the patient and the hospital. It was presumed that the patient's health issues, personal preferences, the equipment and other requirements, and the organisational constraints of the hospital could all be managed as secondary to the original decision to operate. It can be seen that the traditional process was conceptually simple and linear, with few points of interactive or conflicting requirements. Information flowed in one direction, as planning was reactive.

One possible exception arose with regard to anaesthetic management. In some countries (particularly in the British tradition), the anaesthetist was seen as professionally autonomous and independent of the surgeon, so that differing requirements or interpretations of information could result in a possible point of disagreement about clinical management. However, assessment for anaesthesia was the role of the procedural anaesthetist, who tended to become involved in care only shortly before surgery, and acted as a 'journeyman' or individualist practitioner. Decision-making options were thus often reduced to postponement or even cancellation – a tool of last resort used only when major patient safety issues were identified at the time of preoperative assessment by the anaesthetist.

The traditional process is failing

The traditional system is increasingly unable to deal with the complexities of modern patient care and the demands of the modern hospital workforce. These problems are becoming increasingly obvious, and despite its strengths, the traditional model is no longer sustainable. It is no longer possible for any single person to be omniscient and omni-competent with regard to all aspects of patient care. Multiple medical and non-medical specialists are involved in decision-making regarding patient care. Specialised knowledge is held by multiple semi-autonomous professions. The power hierarchy implied in the traditional model is neither appropriate nor acceptable in today's multi-disciplinary healthcare teams.

The individuals in the healthcare workforce are also changing. Nursing staff are better paid, have higher education levels, and have markedly different career and social expectations. The full-time (168 hours/week) commitment by medical staff that the traditional care model required is not compatible with current work- and life-style preferences. Allied health and ancillary staff are more commonly involved in patient care. The workforce is more specialised and fragmented, and more commonly working part-time. As a result, patient care is now delivered by multi-disciplinary teams including a much larger number of staff, many of whom will have only transient contact with the patient.

Apart from the changing health workforce, the organisational environment has also changed. Requirements for clinical information management are more critical as patients have more co-morbidities, and operations and surgical procedures are becoming more complex. This complexity is multiplied by patient care being geographically fragmented into specialised ward areas, particularly as length of stay is reduced.

The rise of hospital management has made clinical process control more detailed, increasing organisation information requirements. There is less tolerance of process inefficiencies and other indicators of poor quality. Finally, the patient is no longer a passive 'recipient' of the outcomes of surgical or other healthcare processes, but is an active 'partner in care' whose preferences and choices must be included in planning and preparation for procedures.

In order to deliver high-quality patient care for modern surgical and other procedures, with the modern health workforce, and in a changing hospital environment, there must be a fundamental redesign of the perioperative care process, and development of new roles for all health professionals in this process. Redesign of perioperative processes is occurring internationally with a wide variety of different changes, although common themes can be identified, which are discussed elsewhere (Chapter 18). Simultaneously, evidence is accumulating from disparate sources that can be used to guide decision-making as to how preoperative processes and systems should be designed. The remainder of this chapter will review the available evidence that can be used.

Using evidence for managerial decision-making

Evidence is variously required for the purposes of clinical science (i.e. classical clinical research), to monitor and improve patient outcomes on a day-to-day basis (i.e. audit and quality improvement activities) and to provide a 'hard' basis to support a business case to be put to health service management to guide investment of resources in the preoperative service. Obviously, these different applications of 'evidence' have differing requirements, both in the importance given to the various outcomes measured, and the expectations of 'scientific rigour' in the data collection and analysis.

Given that the change in perioperative care is an international phenomenon, what evidence is available? By the usual standards of evidence-based medicine, there is disappointingly little evidence that is generally (internationally) applicable to help make 'hard' decisions about the organisation and management of perioperative systems. This is a telling comment on the disparity between expectations of evidence in the 'scientific' world of clinical medicine and the standards expected in management. The most rigorous evidence deals with changing behaviours (and costs) in the area of preoperative testing. These various studies show clearly that an organised approach produces more appropriate care and saves costs (which is hardly surprising!), but doesn't clarify which organisational model is best. There is limited evidence concerning other issues, such as reductions in cancellations on day of surgery, but most of the published work in this area is limited by being strongly affected by local conditions affecting organisation of services. Nevertheless, 'evidence' from disparate sources is available, and this provides some 'hard' data on which to base future action.

It is useful to consider alternative strategies for analysing and presenting the data that is available. As noted above, management executives may be less concerned with 'scientific' data, and the subtleties of statistical analysis, than clinician/scientists. Furthermore, they may prefer to work from generalities to specifics by inductive reasoning, rather than the deductive processes of traditional scientific method. Conventional scientific analysis will start with 'an open mind', and gather data. Each piece of research evidence will be considered independently, and by deduction a general conclusion will be reached. Clinicians may tend to continue using this pattern when presenting data. Managers may prefer to use inductive methods, starting with a general theory or knowledge framework, and examining available data to draw conclusions using an inductive process. Selection of an appropriate framework is a key step in effectively presenting, analysing and using data inductively. This may be unfamiliar to traditional scientists, but is an effective strategy for using data in 'grey' areas such as clinical system redesign.

Presenting the available evidence in a quality framework

A useful framework for assessing changes in clinical care systems is the patient-centred model of quality in healthcare, including seven elements of safety, access, effectiveness, efficiency, timeliness, acceptability and appropriateness.[1]

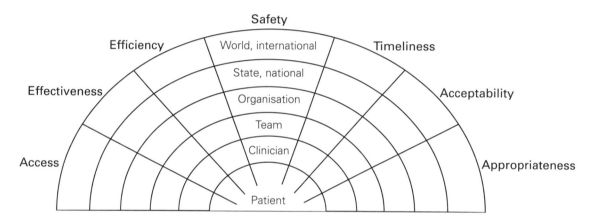

Figure 17.4 Seven elements of quality in healthcare

Using the framework shown in Figure 17.4, evidence gathered to guide change in perioperative systems can be categorised, assessed and presented against these various elements of quality. The following brief review of existing evidence is not intended to be comprehensive, but rather to provide examples of the use of disparate sources of evidence presented within the suggested quality framework.

Safety – Does it do no harm, and/or reduce harm being done?

'Inadequate preoperative assessment' has been consistently identified as a contributing factor in adverse patient outcomes in multiple studies such as NCEPOD in the UK, the Australian Incident Monitorin Study (AIMS)[2], and in in ongoing mortality reports in various jurisdictions[3] and continues to be identified in hospital investigations. At the Cleveland Clinic, a shift to preoperative patient assessment and preparation by a centralised anaesthesiology-led service, rather than assessment by different surgical teams, led to a reduction in intraoperative cardiac events.[4]

Improved preoperative assessment may enable safer antibiotic choices. At the Mayo Clinic, patients at the preoperative evaluation clinic with a self-reported penicillin allergy were investigated preoperatively by consultation and skin testing.[5] This enabled better identification of those who could be safely given beta-lactam antibiotics, reducing the use of vancomycin to only 16% of patients.

The results of implementation of a re-engineered elective surgery service in an Australian tertiary referral hospital setting were studied.[6] The hospital introduced pre-admission clinics and same day admission through a separate preoperative area. Previously, patients were admitted on the day before surgery through a surgical ward. There was no increase in adverse outcomes and an increase in patient satisfaction. Most interestingly, there was a major (almost 60%) reduction in indicators of surgical wound infection. This may be predominantly due to avoiding one night on a surgical ward preoperatively, although other factors may contribute.

For the purposes of guiding change initiatives at an institutional or organisational level, these general findings can be supplemented by locally produced reports of adverse patient outcomes due to poor patient preparation identified within the organisation.

Access – Is the patient able to access the clinical service provided?

A reduction in avoidable late cancellations and 'no-shows' of booked surgical patients is one of the most demonstrable benefits of improved preoperative preparation systems. This is probably best considered as addressing the 'access' element of the quality framework. Length of stay is also an 'access' issue, since it demonstrates that improved preparation systems can increase service provision within existing resources, and without adverse effects on other quality elements. This is one of the most powerful arguments for improved preoperative preparation.

Early reports of changed preoperative systems showed reduced cancellations and length of stay.[7,8] Some reports were equivocal.[9] More recent reports from other jurisdictions have confirmed this effect. In the Netherlands, outpatient preoperative evaluation reduced cancellations from 2.0% to 0.9% and increased same day admissions.[10] Reduction of avoidable cancellations by clinic-based preparation also improves theatre efficiency.[11,12] Reduction of cancellations can be linked to cost savings.[13] A recent survey of US Anaesthetists reported that cancellations and delays were substantially reduced in hospitals with preanaesthesia evaluation clinics, although problems persisted. Clinical information management deficiencies are a common cause of delays or cancellations.[14]

Apart from cancellations, hospital and operating theatre resources may be wasted by 'no-show' patients. A study in a US veterans' administration hospital showed that patient non-appearance could be strongly predicted from non-compliance with clinic visits and other hospital procedures.[15] By predicting such patients in advance, locally appropriate strategies can be implemented to avoid waste of resources and increase operating theatre utilisation.

The characterisation of various causes of cancellations or 'no-shows' will vary widely depending on the jurisdiction and local factors, in particular the funding characteristics of the patient service provision. That said, cancellations due to whatever cause are a common cause of waste of resources or increased costs. The complexities of economic and business process modelling to demonstrate this comprehensively make interpretation difficult.[16] As a result, the total impact of cancellations on theatre efficiency is commonly underestimated. Nevertheless, even 'simple' analysis, based on local audit, may produce powerful evidence of potential for improvement, and be used to emphasise the importance of improved patient preparation.

Even in optimised systems, some late cancellations will be unavoidable, such as those due to patients developing unexpected acute illnesses. A 'high-functioning' perioperative service will include a 'stand-by' list of patients who have been identified in advance as appropriate, available and willing to be called at short notice to substitute for these late cancellations.

Effectiveness – Does the treatment provided achieve the intended result?

With regard to preoperative assessment and preparation, what evidence is available that relates to the effectiveness of actions taken preoperatively? Some of the data refers to intermediate or surrogate outcomes, but there is increasing evidence that improved or redesigned systems for preoperative preparation result in increased effectiveness of actions at this stage in patient care.

Improved preparation systems also increase the effectiveness of preoperative testing by increasing the likelihood that results are interpreted correctly and acted upon more rigorously.[17] Importantly, medico-legal risk may be greater if a test is ordered and not acted upon than if it is not ordered at all.

Outpatient preoperative assessment clinics are an effective means to reduce preoperative anxiety.[18] Recent British experience supports the general effectiveness of consultant-led clinics for vascular surgery patients.[19]

A patient preparation system based on a multi-disciplinary clinic improved compliance with agreed guidelines giving beta-blockers perioperatively.[20] Similarly, a system approach to clinical process redesign improved appropriate antibiotic selection and administration, resulting in reduced surgical site infections.[21]

Many enthusiastic health professionals have encouraged patients to quit smoking, but the effectiveness of such actions in the absence of a systematic approach is unclear. In the author's hospital, the effectiveness of a multimodal preoperative smoking cessation programme including an interactive computer-based smoking assessment, brief advice, telephone follow-up, nicotine replacement therapy, and referral to follow-up telephone counselling has been evaluated. In a prospective randomised controlled trial, the programme resulted in 78% of smokers achieving preoperative cessation, with a three-month quit rate of 19%.[22] The programme was acceptable to patients and staff and cost-effective. Apart from interest with regard to smoking cessation, this is a demonstration of the potential for improved patient care by utilisation of new technology, system redesign, and an organised approach to preoperative preparation.

It is obvious that any treatment cannot be effective unless it is provided. The Institute for Healthcare Improvement has identified ten common patient care interventions for which there is evidence, but that are not routinely practised. An organised preoperative process may facilitate optimisation of patient healthcare with regard to these interventions.

Efficiency – Are unnecessary or ineffective actions avoided?

The efficiency of preoperative assessment and preparation systems has been most commonly evaluated by examining preoperative tests. This is a reflection of both a perception of widespread unnecessary preoperative testing, and the relative ease of studying the problem and effect of interventions.[23] Commonly this is studied by audit of patient testing against defined 'standards' such as preoperative testing guidelines.

Early reports of anaesthetist-led preoperative clinics showed reductions in unnecessary preoperative tests, with overall cost reductions.[24] These results have been replicated by many others.[25,26] The challenge of ensuring appropriate preoperative testing has been a major focus of discussion and a driver for system redesign, particularly in the USA.

Preoperative testing is only a minor part of preoperative preparation and perioperative patient care, and the emphasis on this visible and easily measurable aspect may be to the detriment of overall system improvement. (In 1974 in my first year as a medical student, it was said that 'Diagnosis is 90% history, 9% examination, and 1% tests'. This may have changed slightly but the message remains important.) Preoperative assessment requires clinicians to evaluate the patient by history and examination, not primarily by laboratory tests.[27]

In a widely noted British study that focused on the debate over different health disciplines in preoperative preparation clinics rather than process efficiency, nurses were shown to comply with testing guidelines more closely than 'junior' medical staff.[28] In this study the nurses had been specifically trained to work in the preoperative clinic setting, whereas the surgical housemen were working in the traditional model of care, with minimal setting-specific training. The study was criticised as an examination of the effect of workforce substitution to increase process efficiency, without considering whether the process was perpetuating unnecessary rituals.[29] The accuracy of trained nurses performing preoperative health assessment has also been studied.[30]

More recently, the use of a decision support system to assist trained nurses in making decisions with regard to preoperative investigations has been evaluated.[31] Performance was compared to a reference standard based on the recommendations of multiple consultant anaesthetists after blinded assessment of case histories. The combination of the decision support system and nurses' predictions achieved performance equivalent to consultant anaesthetists. Regardless of which health professionals are involved, these studies demonstrate that efficient and appropriate care is most readily achieved using a systemic approach with appropriately trained staff working in supervised teams.

In a US tertiary hospital setting, implementation of a multi-disciplinary preoperative assessment and testing clinic resulted in fewer preoperative cardiology consults. The ordering of consults was not audited against a 'gold standard' but the results were interpreted as showing that unnecessary consults were avoided without adverse outcomes.[32]

Apart from preoperative testing, the efficiency of preoperative preparation may be evaluated by reduction in unnecessary clinic visits, process rework, and duplication of documentation. These indicators are more difficult to study, and there are few such reports in the formal scientific publications, although they are commonly mentioned in the 'grey literature'.

The use of quality management techniques to improve the efficiency of the preoperative assessment clinic itself has been advocated, particularly at the Cleveland Clinic.[33] A recent report from the Netherlands discusses process management in preoperative clinic scheduling.[34] The generalisability of the particular conclusions is limited by local factors, but these reports provide useful direction as to improvement of quality and efficiency in preoperative services.

Timeliness – Is the service provided at the 'right' time?

'Traditional' surgical scheduling is based on clinical urgency. Existing scheduling systems can usually address clinical urgency appropriately. While clinical timeliness would generally be presumed to be of the highest priority, there may also be non-clinical factors that may determine optimal timing of surgery. Therefore 'timeliness' as an element of health service quality may also be determined by both organisational and patient factors. Optimising the scheduling of booked surgery may improve hospital processes by enabling proactive consideration of issues such as bed availability, planned utilisation of intensive care or high-dependency beds, improved operating theatre performance by aggregating or ordering cases appropriately, and assisting planning for equipment availability. From the patient's point of view, timeliness may include scheduling of surgery to consider employment, social, transport or 'simple' personal preferences. This may include the planned day of operation, and timing on the day.

A high-functioning perioperative service should identify both organisational and patients' non-clinical preferences regarding scheduling of surgery. Some centres have described experience with this in the 'grey literature'.[35,36]

Acceptable – Is the service acceptable to patients?

There have been few high-quality studies of patient satisfaction with clinic-based preoperative assessment and preparation services.[37,38] These few studies, and more general reports, have consistently reported high acceptability.[39,40] Recent work from the Netherlands has provided detailed evaluation of patient preferences in the preoperative assessment clinic using a purpose-designed questionnaire.[41]

The variation in types of clinics, especially internationally, makes comparison difficult. Patients' and health professionals' perspectives on the important indicators of acceptability differ. Delays and waiting in clinics is the strongest source of dissatisfaction; patients value communication and choice about the clinic and hospital processes, being given information, and education about their planned procedure. Education aids such as printed booklets or videos can be used to increase patient satisfaction and the acceptability of the service.[42]

A recurrent finding in patient surveys and qualitative interviews is that patients do not like being asked the same question multiple times, and that inconsistent communication is a major source of concern and complaint. These patient preferences are facilitated by a well-organised preoperative assessment and preparation process.

Most preadmission processes require some form of patient-completed health questionnaire. The development of electronic systems to improve the efficiency of this process has been reported by a number of groups. Patient acceptance of new technology has been seen as a constraint. A recent Canadian trial comparing paper and electronic questionnaires (PDA or touchscreen computer) found patients accepted electronic systems, and expressed a preference for computerised systems for future questionnaires.[43]

Anecdotal reports suggest that patients strongly prefer spending less time in hospital preoperatively. In the author's hospital, discharge surveys of patient satisfaction after inpatient surgery have consistently found that over 90% of patients would prefer to arrive in hospital three hours or less before a planned operation, if it was medically acceptable.

Appropriate – Is the choice of treatment appropriate for the patient?

As discussed earlier, recent changes in preoperative processes represent a shift from passive and reactive hospital processes to more proactive systems. Centralisation of preoperative preparation provides a platform for oversight of planned surgery well before admission to hospital. This may enable the development of better processes to ensure that planned care is appropriate.

Preoperative risk assessment can predict patients who are likely to have costly, prolonged or complex hospital treatment.[44] Further, improved preoperative assessment can identify patients at high risk who may benefit from higher-intensity perioperative care, and may also identify patients who should not have surgery at all.[45] Anecdotally, this is more likely to occur when performed early (as an outpatient) than immediately prior to proposed surgery, and established 'high-functioning' preoperative clinics report this latter function as a significant component of their work.

Patients identified at high or even moderate risk may be appropriately encouraged to address end-of-life issues. Some experiences with programmes to facilitate advance care planning in the preoperative clinic setting have been reported.[46]

Improved preoperative assessment and preparation also provides an opportunity to explore appropriate new patient treatments. It is already known that there are a number of potential preoperative interventions to improve patient outcomes that are currently under-utilised. These interventions may have been viewed as not feasible or logistically difficult, or they may simply not be known about by the relevant clinicians. The development of improved, centralised systems for early preoperative assessment by specialists in this field makes it feasible to apply this knowledge. A number of 'simple' examples of utilisation of the preoperative period to improve or to provide 'new' treatments to improve patient outcomes have been reported from leading preoperative services in the USA.[47]

Other promising opportunities for improving patients' health status and perioperative outcomes require further research and development. These are new specific interventions pertaining to the perioperative period. Examples include:

- improved preoperative testing techniques (e.g. CPX testing)
- better perioperative pharmacological therapy
- preoperative exercise therapy
- preoperative transfusion medicine
- perioperative nutrition, diet and nutraceuticals
- obesity management
- novel uses of perioperative medication (e.g. anabolic steroids)
- immunological interventions
- preparation for convalescence.

There is also a requirement for better research and integration of knowledge. For example, comprehensive risk/benefit assessment requires improved knowledge of the 'natural history' of the patient's surgical disease (whether treated or not), and the effects of treatment on both survival and quality of life. This information then needs to be evaluated in partnership with the patient to enable genuinely patient-centred decision-making about appropriate patient care.

This is not just 'traditional' preoperative preparation being performed with improved quality, but a new scope of clinical practice – the preoperative component of perioperative medicine. These improvements in patient outcome can be achieved with greatest quality and efficiency by using a coordinated multi-disciplinary team approach, tailored to the needs of individual patients.

When evidence is not enough

As noted earlier, redesign of preoperative processes is an international phenomenon. This implies a general acceptance that it must be 'a good thing'. Clinicians with scientific training will seek evidence to advocate for and guide changes to the systems and processes that they are involved in. The evidence presented above, and from other sources, would appear to justify change. In particular, the economic justification would appear to be clear.[48] Such evidence may not be sufficient. Hospitals, like all human organisations, are political environments. Changing an organisation is a political activity, and scientific evidence is only one part of effecting change. Two case studies in which the author was peripherally involved are presented as examples.

1. In Australia, most specialist doctors are remunerated by fee-for-service payments in accordance with a schedule of fees (the Medical Benefits Schedule) that are negotiated annually between the federal government and doctors' industrial representatives. Since 1995, anaesthetists have been clinical leaders in driving the change in perioperative care systems in Australia, and have substantially changed their work practices as a result of these changes. In November 2006, the Departments of Treasury and Health agreed to changes in the fee for preoperative assessment

from $35 to a complexity-graded fee to over $150 per patient, establishing parity with sub-specialist physicians. Fees for postoperative consultations were also raised to parity. These changes happened because health bureaucrats recognised that clinical leadership had improved both patient care and the efficiency of the health system. The Treasury had been presented with a detailed economic analysis of the economic benefits of the perioperative system by the Australian Society of Anaesthetists. In addition to the evidence, however, there had been a sustained campaign of education, negotiation and lobbying of bureaucrats, parliamentarians and ministers for ten years prior to the decision. The evidence alone was not enough.

2. Hospitals in Australia are managed by State Departments of Health. In 2005, the Health Department in the largest state (New South Wales) convened a working party to define the best practice model for organisation of preoperative services. The Department anticipated some preconceived outcomes. The working party included a limited number of clinicians (nurses, anaesthetists, surgeons) as well as departmental officers. The clinicians on the working party brought their differing opinions, evidence and experience and laboriously negotiated with each other and the Departmental representatives. Additional clinicians were consulted. Finally, the group agreed on a general model of the preoperative process based on stated key principles, and recommended key performance indicators. This was published in a 'Pre-Procedure Preparation Toolkit', which was officially endorsed for general implementation by the Department.[49] Although evidence was used substantially during the deliberations of the working party, the success of the exercise was substantially due to the prolonged commitment and negotiation – a political process – involving the members of the working party. In this case, the result was generally endorsed by all as 'a good result'. It was, however, substantially different from outcomes that could have resulted otherwise. Again, the evidence alone was not enough.

These examples are presented to illustrate the general point that advocacy of change is a complex challenge. The scientific milieu has produced heavy emphasis on the need for evidence, and a disciplined, rigorous approach to analysing and evaluating evidence. This is very appropriate, where it is possible, in the world of clinical science. Hence clinician scientists must develop skills in gathering, analysing and using evidence.

By contrast, clinical process design and organisational management is far from an exact science. Clinicians wishing to manage perioperative systems must learn how to do so.[50] Evidence must be used where possible, and this requires the skills of clinician scientists. Over and above this, however, other skills – and the commitment of time, effort, and persistence – are necessary to be effective in achieving change.

REFERENCES

1. W. Runciman, A. Merry and M. Walton (2007). *Safety and Ethics in Healthcare: Getting it Right.* Aldershot: Ashgate Publishing.

2. M.T. Kluger, E.J. Tham, N.A. Coleman, W.B. Runciman and M.F.M. Bullock (2000). Inadequate pre-operative evaluation and preparation: a review of 197 reports from the Australian Incident Monitoring Study. *Anesthesia* **55**: 1173–8.

3. Such as 'Safety of Anaesthesia in Australia: A Review of Anaesthesia Related Mortality'. The Australian and New Zealand College of Anaesthetists, Melbourne 2002.

4. R.G. Borkowski, B.M Parker, B. Fitzsimmons and W.G. Maurer (2001). The incidence of cardiac related intraoperative quality indicators in ambulatory/same day surgery patients and inpatients after different preoperative evaluation processes. *Anesthesiology* **95**: A32.

5. M. Park, P. Markus, D. Matesic and J.T. Li (2006). Safety and effectiveness of a preoperative allergy clinic in decreasing vancomycin use in patients with a history of penicillin allergy. *Annals of Allergy, Asthma and Immunology* **97**: 681–7.

6. G.A. Caplan, A. Brown, P.J. Crowe, S-J. Yap and S. Noble (1998). Re-engineering the elective surgical service of a tertiary hospital: a historical controlled trial. *Medical Journal of Australia* **169**: 247–51

7. S.P. Fischer (1996). Development and effectiveness of an anesthesia pre-operative evaluation clinic in a teaching hospital. *Anesthesiology* **85**: 196–206.

8. R.K. Kerridge, A.L. Lee, E.M. Latchford, S.M. Beehan and K.M. Hillman (1995). The perioperative system: A new system for managing elective surgery patients. *Anaesthesia and Intensive Care* **23**: 591–6.

9. J.B. Pollard and L. Olson (1999). Early outpatient preoperative anesthesia assessment: Does it help to reduce operating room cancellations? *Anesthesia and Analgesia* **89**: 502–5.

10. W.A. Van Klei, K.G.M. Moons, C.L.G. Rutten, A. Schuurhuis, J.T.A. Knape, C.J. Kalkman and D.E. Grobbee (2002). The effect of outpatient preoperative evaluation of hospital inpatients on cancellation of surgery and length of hospital stay. *Anesthesia and Analgesia* **94**: 644–9.

11. M.B. Ferschl, A. Tung, B.J. Sweitzer, D. Huo and D.B. Glick (2005). Preoperative visits reduce operating room cancellations and delays. *Anesthesiology* **103**: 855–9.

12. D.J. Correll, A.M. Bader, M.W. Hull, C. Hsu, L.C. Tsen and D.L.Hepner. (2006). The value of preoperative clinic visits in identifying issues with potential impact on operating room efficiency. *Anesthesiology* **105**: 1254–9.

13. P. St. Jacques and M. Higgins (2004). Beyond cancellations: Decreased day of surgery delays from a dedicated preoperative clinic may provide cost savings. *Journal of Clinical Anesthesia* **16**: 478–9.

14. N.F. Holt, D.G. Silverman, R. Prasad, J. Dziura and K.J. Ruskin (2007). Preanesthesia clinics, information management, and operating room delays: Results of a survey of practicing anesthesiologists. *Anesthesia and Analgesia* **104**: 615–18.

15. M.D. Basson, T.W. Butler and H. Verma (2006). Predicting patient nonappearance for surgery as a scheduling strategy to optimize operating room utilization in veterans' administration hospital. *Anesthesiology* **104**: 826–34.

16. C. McIntosh, F. Dexter and R.H. Epstein (2006). The impact of service-specific staffing, case scheduling, turnovers, and first-case starts on anesthesia group and operating room productivity: A tutorial using data from an Australian hospital. *Anesthesia and Analgesia* **103**: 1499–516.

17. M.F. Roizen (2004). Preoperative evaluation. In R.D. Miller, ed. *Anaesthesia* (6th edn). Philadelphia: Churchill Livingstone: 927–97.

18. C.E. Klopfenstein, A. Forster and E. Van Gessel (2000). Anesthetic assessment in an outpatient consultation clinic reduces preoperative anxiety. *Canadian Journal of Anesthesia* **47**: 511–15.

19. K.L. Cantlay, S. Baker, A. Parry and G. Danjoux (2006). The impact of a consultant anaesthetist led pre-operative assessment clinic on patients undergoing major vascular surgery. *Anaesthesia* **61**: 234.

20. S. Armanious, D.T. Wong, E. Etchells, P. Higgins and F. Chung (2003). Successful implementation of perioperative beta-blockade utilizing a multi-disciplinary approach. *Canadian Journal of Anaesthesia* **50**: 131–6.

21. G. Kanter, N.R. Connelly and J. Fitzgerald (2006). A system and process redesign to improve perioperative antibiotic administration. *Anesthesia and Analgesia* **103**: 1517–21.

22. L. Wolfenden, J. Wiggers, J. Knight, E. Campbell, C. Rissel, R.K. Kerridge, A.D. Spigelman and K. Moore (2005). A programme for reducing smoking in preoperative surgical patients: Randomised controlled trial. *Anaesthesia* **60**: 172–9.

23. J. Munro, A. Booth and J. Nicholl (1997). Routine preoperative testing: a systematic review of the evidence. *Health Technology Assessment* **1**: 1–62.

24. M.A. Starsnic, D.M. Guarnieri and M.C. Norris (1997). Efficacy and financial benefit of an anaesthesiologist-directed university preadmission evaluation center. *Journal of Clinical Anesthesia* **9**: 299–305.

25. L.M. Power and N.M. Thackray (1999). Reduction of preoperative investigations with the introduction of an anaesthetist-led preoperative clinic. *Anaesthesia and Intensive Care* **27**: 481–8.

26. B.A. Finegan, S. Rashiq, F.A. McAlister and P. O'Connor (2005). Selective ordering of preoperative investigations by anesthesiologists reduces the number and costs of tests. *Canadian Journal of Anaesthesia* **52**: 575–80.

27. M. Roizen (2000). More preoperative assessment by physicians and less by laboratory tests. *New England Journal of Medicine* **342**: 204–5.

28. H. Kinley, C. Czoski-Murray, S. George, C. McCabe, J. Primrose, C. Reilly, R. Wood, P. Nicolson, C. Healy, S. Read, J. Norman, E. Janke, H. Alhameed, N. Fernandes and E. Thomas (2002). Effectiveness of appropriately trained nurses in preoperative assessment: randomised controlled equivalence/non-inferiority trial. *British Medical Journal* **325**: 1323.

29. R.K. Kerridge (2003). Effectiveness of trained nurses in preoperative assessment. *British Medical Journal* **326**: 600.

30. W.A. Van Klei, P.J. Hennis, J. Moen, C.J. Kalkman and K.G. Moons (2004). The accuracy of trained nurses in pre-operative health assessment: results of the OPEN study. *Anaesthesia* **59**: 971–8.

31. B.V.S. Murthy, S.P. Lake and A.C. Fisher (2008). Evaluation of a decision support system to predict preoperative investigations. *British Journal of Anaesthesia* **100**: 315–21.

32. L.C. Tsen, S. Segal, M. Pothier, L.H. Hartley and A. Bader (2002). The effect of alterations in a preoperative assessment clinic on reducing the number and improving the yield of cardiology consultations. *Anesthesia and Analgesia* **95**: 1563–8.

33. W.G. Maurer, R.G. Borkowski and B.M. Parker (2004). Quality and resource utilisation in managing preoperative evaluation. *Anesthesiology Clinics of North America* **22**: 155–75.

34. G.M. Edward, S.F. Das, S.G. Elkhuizen, P.J.M. Bakker, J.A.M. Hontelez, M.W. Hollman, B. Preckel and L.C. Lemaire (2008). Simulation to analyse planning difficulties at the preoperative assessment clinic. *British Journal of Anaesthesia* **100**: 195–202.

35. NHS Modernisation Agency (2003). *National Good Practice Guidance on Pre-operative Assessment for Inpatient Surgery. Operating and Pre-operative Assessment Programme.* London: Department of Health.

36. A. Bassett (2007). *Two steps forward, One step back.* Todmorden: Perigon Health Care Ltd.

37. D.L. Hepner, A.M. Bader, S. Hurwitz, M. Gustafson and L.C. Tsen (2004). Patient satisfaction with preoperative assessment in a preoperative assessment testing clinic. *Anesthesia and Analgesia* **98**: 1099–105.

38. G.M. Edward, J.C.J.M. de Haes, F.J. Oort, L.C. Lemaire, M.W. Hollman and B. Preckel (2008). Setting priorities for improving the preoperative assessment clinic: the patients' and professionals' perpective. *British Journal of Anaesthesia* **100**: 322–6.

39. B.V.S. Murthy (2006). Improving the patient's journey. The role of the pre-operative assessment team. *Bulletin of the Royal College of Anaesthetists* **37**: 1885–7.

40. E.P. Wittkugel and A.M. Varughese (2006). Pediatric preoperative evaluation: A new paradigm. *International Anesthesiology Clinics* **44**: 141–58.

41. G.M. Edward, L.C. Lemaire, B. Preckel, F.J. Oort, M.J.L. Bucx, M.W. Hollmann and J.C.J.M. de Haes (2007). Patient experience with the Preoperative Assessment Clinic (PEPAC): validation of an instrument to measure patient experiences. *British Journal of Anaesthesia* **99**: 666–72.

42. A. Cheung, B.A. Finegan, C. Torok-Both, N. Donnelly-Warner and J. Lucig (2007). A patient information booklet about anaesthesiology improves preoperative patient education. *Canadian Journal of Anaesthesia* **54**: 355–60.

43. E.G. VanDenKerkhof, D.H. Goldstein, W.C. Blaine and M.J. Rimmer (2005). A comparison of paper with electronic patient-completed questionnaires in a preoperative clinic. *Anesthesia and Analgesia* **101**: 1075–80.

44. D.L. Davenport, W.G. Henderson, S.F. Khuri and R.M. Mentzer (2005). Preoperative risk factors and surgical complexity are more predictive of costs than postoperative complications: a case study using the national surgical quality improvement program (NSQIP) database. *Annals of Surgery* **245**: 463–71.

45. S.J. Davies and R.J.T. Wilson (2004). Preoperative optimization of the high-risk surgical patient. *British Journal of Anaesthesia* **93**: 121–8.

46. D.A. Grimaldo, J.P. Wiener-Kronish, T. Jurson, T.E. Shaughnessy, J.R. Curtis and L.L. Liu (2001). A randomized, controlled trial of advance care planning discussions during preoperative evaluations. *Anesthesiology* **95**: 43–50.

47. A.K. Jaffer and F.A. Michota (eds) (2007). Proceedings of the 3rd Annual Perioperative Medicine Summit. *Cleveland Clinic Journal of Medicine* **74**: E-Supplement 1 (and preceding years).

48. G.L. Gibby (2002). How preoperative assessment programs can be justified financially to hospital administrators. *International Anesthesiology Clinics* **40**: 17–30.

49. Available free from the NSW Department of Health. Use of a general search engine (e.g. Google) and the term 'Pre-Procedure Preparation Toolkit' is suggested.

50. A.P. Harris and W.G. Zitzmann (1998). *Operating Room Management: Structure, Strategies and Economics*. St. Louis: Mosby Year-Book, Inc.

18 The challenge of implementing 'new' preoperative systems

Ross Kerridge

SUMMARY

This chapter will develop the concepts from the previous chapter, looking in more detail at:

- **changing approaches to perioperative care – the Australian experience**
- **practical considerations in developing new aspects of care**
- **how to monitor performance and activity in newly designed systems.**

INTRODUCTION

The last decade has seen a 'paradigm shift' in the organisation of preoperative assessment and preparation, towards a more structured and systematic approach to patient care. This change has been occurring internationally, and the 'new' model of perioperative patient management is continuing to evolve.

Despite the differences between different types of hospitals, a general or 'ideal' model can be described. The model is robust and can be appropriately adapted to the particular requirements and case-mix of different hospitals. While there are controversies about various details, the new model of preoperative preparation has generally been seen as providing improved patient outcomes and quality of care simultaneously with significant cost savings.

Comparing changes and innovations between hospitals, between health services, and especially internationally, is fraught with danger. There are always important differences affecting the factors that shape and drive change. Every hospital is different, sometimes in ways that are subtle and poorly recognised, even by those 'on the ground'. Inevitably, there is wide variation in the different systems that have been developed and implemented internationally. That said, there are common features and principles underlying these developments, and it is possible to conceptualise the key features of this 'new model of surgical care' as it continues to evolve internationally.

The following cannot be regarded as based on 'evidence', and thus is not referenced. It represents the author's personal summary of key issues noted from the literature (usually the 'grey' literature), from conference proceedings and discussions, from discussion with various centres involved in implementing perioperative systems, and direct observation during site visits to preoperative services in over seventy hospitals in Australia, New Zealand, Hong Kong, the UK, Scandinavia, Austria, the Netherlands, Canada and the USA. That said, most of the author's experience is in Australia. It is therefore appropriate to give some background to this setting.

The Australian healthcare system is highly fragmented, being split between state, federal, or private organisations, and funded by a mix of state, federal, private insurance, patient co-payments, veterans or compensation insurance. About 60% of all elective surgery, particularly simpler procedures, is performed in quasi-independent private institutions. Communication between healthcare professionals is variable in quality and reliability. Patients may attend multiple specialists and have procedures or investigations in a diverse range of settings, both public and private. Primary care practitioners and consulting specialists are less integrated with the health system than in the British NHS or similar systems. All these features exacerbate the challenges of global patient care, and particularly the challenge of optimising preoperative patient preparation.

It is notable that private healthcare providers are becoming more active in many countries that have been traditionally dominated by 'universal' public health systems. Thus the dysfunctional aspects of the Australian healthcare system may become more widespread.

The organisation of the hospital medical workforce is reasonably similar to the British system, with similar training and clinical roles. Australian surgeons and physicians are becoming highly subspecialised. Most Australian anaesthetists have a broad general medical experience before commencing specialist training.

While recognising the above differences between hospitals, health systems and countries, there are enough features in common to discuss the 'new' model. This chapter will review the features of this new model of preoperative care, and then discuss the challenges of implementing the model. The main focus will be on the preoperative components of the system.

The new model of the preoperative process

The common conceptual basis of the new preoperative system is to plan all stages of care of an elective surgery patient as a unified and integrated process. A cross-specialty and multi-disciplinary clinical service (the perioperative service) manages the assessment and preparation of all elective surgical admissions. When an operation is being planned, a hospital-based clinical service gathers information about the patient from the surgical team, from the patient (e.g. by interview or questionnaire), from the patient's GP and from other health providers. This is used to triage the patient to an appropriate level of preparation complexity, with selective use of outpatient clinic attendance prior to admission. Patients attending clinics are assessed by a multi-disciplinary team, predominantly nurses and anaesthetists. The perioperative service team then coordinates preparation until admission, including communication to relevant hospital care providers.

The key features of the process are:

- pre-admission patient preparation
- selective clinic review
- day of surgery admission
- centralised preoperative care
- 'hot bedding'
- planned hospital care and discharge
- elective surgery centrally organised and coordinated by a multi-disciplinary perioperative service
- ongoing service development and clinical process redesign 'driven' by the perioperative service.

The new preoperative process can be conceptualised graphically (see Figure 18.1). Comparison with Figure 17.2 (see page 321) makes clear the shift in emphasis away from in-hospital activity. Patient assessment and preparation commences at the time of booking, and patients do not enter hospital until ready for their procedure. Communication with all care providers is a major focus of activity. Care planning (particularly discharge planning) occurs proactively.

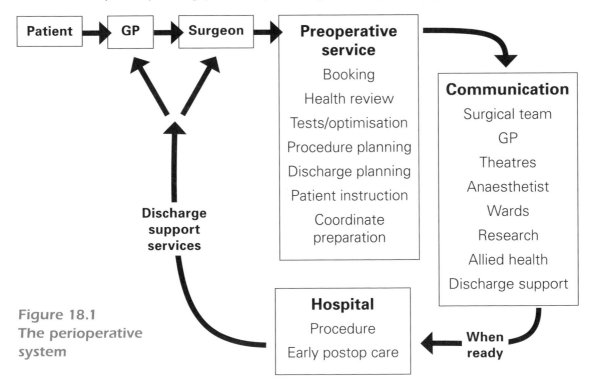

**Figure 18.1
The perioperative
system**

The preadmission assessment process can also be shown graphically (see Figure 18.2). Information about the patient gathered by questionnaire or from other sources is used to triage the patients into groups needing no clinic-based assessment, 'simple' clinic assessment, or multi-disciplinary assessment. Non-clinic patients are given preparation instructions (e.g. printed instructions by mail), and have any further necessary preparation managed by telephone (e.g. a call on the evening prior to admission). Some patients who attend for clinic assessment will be postponed pending further investigations or medical stabilisation. All patients are then admitted either as Day Only (DO) patients, Day of Surgery Admission (DOSA) or Inpatients (i.e. admitted on the day before surgery). With appropriate preparation, over 90% of admitted patients (i.e. excluding Day Only) can be managed as DOSA patients. This includes major vascular, neurosurgery, orthopaedic and cardiothoracic patients.

The new model of care represents a substantial clinical process redesign. The establishment of the perioperative service is both a result of this redesign, and a platform for ongoing redesign. Thus the functions of the perioperative service include both clinical service delivery, and ongoing driving of clinical process redesign.

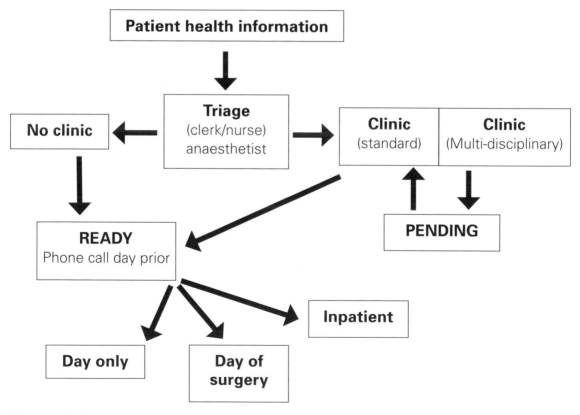

Figure 18.2
The preadmission assessment

Organisational considerations

The perioperative service is a clinical service. Therefore it will need the same organisational infrastructure as any other clinical service (see Box 18.1). As a new service working to deliver a new model of care, this infrastructure may take some time to develop. The function of the service will tend to be suboptimal until all the necessary infrastructure has been established. Local characteristics, such as numbers of patients, clinical complexity, financial drivers, workforce skills, space constraints, and intra-organisational politics will determine the particular organisational features of any perioperative service in any particular institutional setting

Box 18.1 Organisational infrastructure

- Staff – nurses, clerical, medical and allied health
- Budget
- Accommodation (clinic plus office area)
- Equipment
- Policy and procedures
- Medical clinician leader/director (generally an anaesthetist)
- Service manager (generally a nurse)
- Executive sponsor
- A place in the organisation chart

Staffing and leadership

As this is a clinical service, a service manager (generally with a theatre or surgical ward background) and a designated medical clinician leader/director are required. These roles are complementary. The function of the service, particularly in driving clinical process redesign, will be constrained until both positions are filled by clinicians with appropriate seniority and authority. The Medical Director will take clinical responsibility for policies and procedures and clinical decision-making, such as deciding on preoperative tests and investigations, and preoperative prescribing. An appropriate statement of position responsibilities for the medical director must be developed and agreed by the institution, in particular to clarify 'turf' issues with other medical clinicians. In the USA, the responsibility for ordering preoperative investigations has been a focus of this 'turf war'. This appears to have been less controversial elsewhere.

Workforce change

Workforce change is intrinsic in the new preoperative systems, and inevitably includes task transfer or substitution, transfer of skills, and extension of roles. Extension of nurses' roles into areas traditionally considered the domain of medical staff is both necessary and inevitable, but requires training and skill transfer. Many of the tasks involved in preoperative assessment, particularly information gathering and handling, are performed more effectively by 'clerical' staff than by nursing and medical staff. This involves extension and upgrading of traditional clerical roles to become 'para-clinical' staff.

For all staff, but for anaesthetists in particular, there is a 'philosophical' debate as to whether the process they are involved in is 'pre-anaesthetic' or 'preoperative' assessment and preparation. More broadly, this is a debate about whether the process (and those working in it) are aiming to provide a 'gatekeeper' or a 'roadmaker' function (see below).

Reconceptualising the decision framework

The 'new' model for preoperative assessment involves a change in clinical processes. It can also be thought of as representing a change in information flow and decision-making in preoperative preparation. As discussed in Chapter 17, the traditional model of care was based on relatively simple, linear information flow and decision-making. The new model is based on four separate sources of information feeding into decision-making in the preoperative process. These four areas are: (i) the procedure-specific information and procedural requirements, (ii) the patient's health status, (iii) the health system or hospital requirements and (iv) the patient's personal preferences and requirements. These areas all need to be considered during preoperative assessment to enable optimal preparation. A simple representation is shown in Figure 18.3.

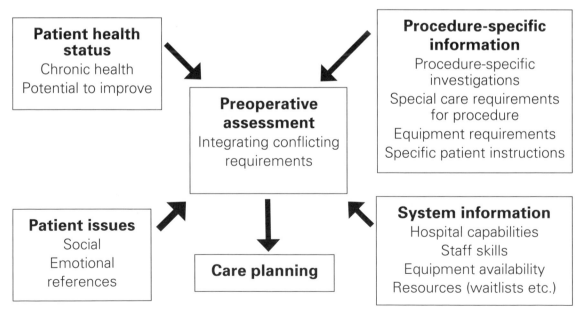

Figure 18.3
Perioperative information flow

The patient assessment process involves bringing together information in all these categories, integrating the information, identifying areas of conflict in requirements, and developing a plan to manage all the various demands from the different 'stakeholders' in the preoperative process. The various intersecting and conflicting demands can be integrated and developed into an overall strategic plan. This strategic plan can then be further developed into a detailed plan, which can then be used to manage the particular episode of care. This is shown in the more detailed graphic (see Figure 18.4). Note the flow of information and decision-making in the patient health stream. Information is gathered to enable triage. Some patients need to attend for clinic-based preparation. When this is completed, the patient's health is summarised in a Standard Health Profile. This information is integrated with surgical, system, and patient factors to make a perioperative assessment and plan. This is used to enable detailed planning for the episode of care.

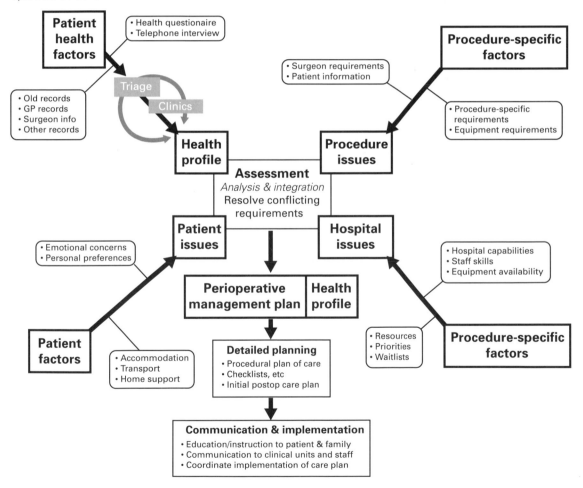

Figure 18.4
Perioperative process framework

In summary, 'new' preoperative assessment involves integrating the health status of the patient, the surgical requirements, the patient's personal requirements and preferences, and the system's requirements, to make an overall 'strategic', and then a detailed, plan of care.

Design and function of patient questionnaire

Despite the rising capability of information technology, most health systems internationally are characterised by poorly integrated health information, so that a patient-completed questionnaire to elicit health information is necessary to enable patient care planning and triage. At this stage most centres use paper-based systems, and this is likely to continue for some years. The following points primarily concern paper-based systems, although many points apply equally to electronic questionnaires.

The general purpose of the questionnaire is to enable appropriate triage. Thus detailed questions are unnecessary if they only apply to patients who will be further assessed in a face-to-face clinic. The questionnaire should not be considered as independent of the overall system. It must be *part* of a 'layered' *system* of patient assessment. This implies that the questionnaire is interpreted by trained staff who have the ability to contact the patient to clarify answers, can seek advice regarding interpretation from more senior clinicians, and will respond appropriately when the questionnaire fails to elicit the information required.

The questionnaire should be designed as a general patient health issues questionnaire. It should not be seen as 'just' a 'pre-anaesthetic' or a 'screening' questionnaire. Therefore it should include sections designed to elicit a general picture of the patient's health, to screen the patient for particular conditions that may affect perioperative management, particularly anaesthetic management, and to gather broader health and social information including domestic support and transport arrangements, to help patient management in the perioperative period and for discharge planning.

Questionnaire design should be guided by expert advice with regard to format and language. There is always tension between the size of the questionnaire and the detail requested of patients. A long well-designed and well-presented questionnaire is more acceptable to patients than a shorter poorly designed form that is generated by poor-quality photocopying. The rising availability of broadband internet and better information technology will enable better design of questionnaires, but similar expert advice will be required.

Duplicated, 'redundant' or overlapping questions, and a mixture of formats such as 'tick boxes' and open-ended questions without a fixed structure, are valuable to ensure comprehensive answers, and enable staff to develop a 'feel' for the patient while analysing the questionnaire in the absence of the patient. Even the quality of handwriting and spelling mistakes convey information about a patient. Some of this granularity of detail and non-lexical information may be lost by electronic systems.

Efforts to design questionnaires to identify all patients with potential airway problems have generally been unsuccessful, and there may be little to be gained by including such questions.

It is unlikely that anything can be done to change a patient's airway prior to surgery, although some warning may assist list scheduling and gathering difficult airway equipment in advance. Even after face-to-face assessment, it is impossible to predict all potentially difficult airways. Therefore anaesthetists must always be prepared to manage a patient with a difficult airway. The procedural anaesthetist must always examine the patient's airway immediately prior to induction and take appropriate steps to manage a predicted difficult intubation at that time. This will occasionally lead to delays in an elective surgery list while unexpected difficult airway management equipment is gathered, but this may be unavoidable.

Commitment of scarce resources to develop the questionnaire in different languages (e.g. immigrant minority group languages) may not always be appropriate. Pragmatically, most of the patients who are unable to comprehend the questionnaire will get help from their family or from their primary care doctor to complete it. The fact that a patient does not perform this task satisfactorily is, of itself, an indication that that patient should be brought to the preoperative clinic, at which time an interpreter should be used to assist assessment and preparation. This principle is equally applicable to a patient who speaks the local language. If the patient cannot comprehend and respond to the questionnaire appropriately, they may well not be able to follow written preoperative instructions. Clinic-based assessment and preparation may be indicated for these patients to identify the reason for difficulty in using written material (e.g. literacy, cognitive limitations, personal attitudes), and to ensure appropriate preparation within these constraints.

Development of questionnaires is a task that often becomes the focus of effort of a large range of hospital staff, all with strongly held but differing views on the various issues that are encountered. The development or improvement of the questionnaire involving a multi-disciplinary working party can be a useful strategy to engage all stakeholders in the process, and develop shared 'ownership' of the questionnaire. Beyond this, however, it may be inappropriate to use excessive staff time in prolonged efforts to develop the 'perfect' questionnaire. As noted earlier, the questionnaire must be seen as *part* of a 'layered' *system* of patient assessment. It may be better to accept an imperfect questionnaire, and devote more attention to developing the system within which the questionnaire functions.

Patient triage

Although all patients require early assessment and preparation, this does not mean that all patients require the same complexity of clinic-based preparation. Many patients can be appropriately prepared without clinic attendance. Patients should not be expected to waste their own time and resources on unnecessary clinic visits if these can be avoided by assessment by questionnaire, telephone, and by gathering patient information from the general practitioner or other healthcare providers, and past hospital records. Apart from resource issues, it is also frustrating for staff to waste time assessing patients in clinic unnecessarily.

For those patients who are required to attend the clinic, assessment may be of varying complexity. For some patients, assessment and preparation may be provided by a single trained nurse or other clinician, with assistance as required. Complex patients will require prolonged assessment by a multi-disciplinary team. Patients coming from geographically distant locations may be prepared by their GP, or by 'satellite' clinics, with distant supervision by the hospital-based service. A triage process is necessary to guide decision-making on these issues.

Triage will primarily consider patient health co-morbidities and the complexity of the planned procedure. Patient factors and social issues that may affect preoperative preparation or discharge planning must also be considered. The travel requirements imposed on patients by the preparation process may also be relevant. Systems for 'long-distance' preparation of patients are required, especially in tertiary referral and rural settings.

Triage decision-making can be assisted by guidelines. A set of guidelines based on two axes of complexity of surgery and patient health (e.g. ASA score) can be developed. An example is shown in Figure 18.5. These must always be regarded as guidelines to be used by trained, and experienced, staff working under supervision in a system. A clear process for 'escalating' triage decision-making to a more senior clinician should be established when triage guidelines are developed.

Operations ➡ Health score ⬇	Minor surgery		Intermediate surgery		Major surgery	
	Superficial surgery	Cataracts D&C Breast lump Wisdom teeth Removal of minor hardware	Laparoscopy Varicose veins Tonsillectomy Ing./Fem. hernia Arthroscopy Removal of major hardware Sinus surgery	Lumbar/cervical Distectomy Thyroidectomy Lap. chole. Minor vascular LSCS Pelvic floor Shoulder repair	TAH TURP	Total joints Cardiothoracis Bowel resection Major vascular Radical neck Dissection Nephrectomy Major ENT
1	E	E	D	C	B	A
2a	E	E	C	C	B	A
2b	E	D	C	B	A	A
3a	E	C	B	B	A	A
3b	D	B	A	A	A	A
4a	C	B	A	A	A	A
4b	B	A	A	A	A	A

Figure 18.5
Perioperative clinic triage guidelines

Perceptions of the appropriate level of triage of patients (i.e. what proportion need to be assessed face-to-face in the clinic) vary. In general, nurses advocate a high attendance, and anaesthetists a lower proportion. The appropriate proportion of patients who need to attend for face-to-face clinic assessment is dependent on the surgical case mix, the average level of co-morbidities and other complexities, and other local health service factors. In the author's experience, a well-functioning service will require 10% or less of day-stay patients and 25 to 35% of inpatients to attend for face-to-face preparation.

Ongoing development of shared protocols and guidelines, and continuing review of problems that are identified, is required to maintain the quality of the triage process. All triage processes have an unavoidable failure rate manifest as 'missed' patients and 'over-triage'. It is inevitable that there will be occasional delays and cancellations on the day of surgery, or unnecessary patient visits as a result. These 'failures' should be monitored as a Key Performance Indicator, and seen as a marker of the quality of the triage process. It must be accepted that they cannot be eliminated altogether. Development of trust and respect between clinicians to instill confidence in shared preoperative assessment has been problematical in some centres, but is fundamental to the ongoing function of a high-quality preoperative preparation service.

Clinical records

The patient's health status must be appropriately documented. Traditional hospital care commenced with a comprehensive record completed on admission. This was often duplicated by different health disciplines (i.e. nursing, medical, etc) working independently. In many centres, this is now less consistently performed. Records are often inconsistent in format, accessibility, legibility, terminology and comprehensiveness. They are also not multi-disciplinary in scope, thereby laying the ground for unnecessary rework and duplication of effort.

The patient's health status at the final stages of the pre-admission process should be documented in a consistent format that can be used by all health professionals caring for the patient. This standard approach should be applied to the whole perioperative system.

In order to address this standard during the pre-admission review, the multi-disciplinary team should develop an appropriately detailed summary statement of the patient's health status. This summary (a 'Standard Health Profile') should have the following characteristics:

- It should be compiled by the multi-disciplinary team, avoiding duplication of enquiry and avoiding the same question being asked multiple times.
- It should be usable for clinical patient care by all health professionals.
- It should be consistent in format (i.e. always look the same).
- The clinical terminology should be standardised where possible.
- It must be readily available at point of care.
- It must be legible.
- The information in the Profile must be reliable.
- The Profile must be validated ('signed off') by an authorised clinician when pre-admission preparation is finalised, and the patient is accepted as adequately prepared for admission.

The components of the Standard Health Profile should include the following:

- current active health problems or issues
- past health problems (including procedures and operations)
- allergies and sensitivities
- medications
- exercise tolerance
- normal activities and/or occupation
- social history and issues
- smoking, drug and alcohol use, etc
- relevant physical examination
- summary of investigations and results
- summary reports of consultations.

Apart from this summative record of the patient's overall health status and co-morbidities, the pre-procedural preparation process must result in other clinical records that include:

- a record of the patient's problem with regard to the planned procedure itself
- assessment with regard to the planned anaesthetic
- a 'perioperative' assessment integrating all the relevant issues pertaining to this particular procedure and episode of care; if necessary, this should include the rationale for resolving the various areas of conflicting requirements (i.e. risk balancing)
- a 'strategic' plan of care for this episode
- a record of discussions/instructions to the patient
- legal documentation of patient consent as jurisdictionally required.

These records lay the foundation for the various detailed care plans and records that will be used by the staff delivering the care.

The preoperative preparation area

The new model of preoperative care includes the development of a specialised preoperative preparation and holding area where all patients are admitted from home to hospital shortly before their procedure. Hence, patients do not go to the surgical ward until after their operation. Ideally, the area should be close to theatres (less transfer distance) or close to the hospital entrance (less travel time for patients on arrival). Pragmatically, this area is often developed in an area where there is available space. In hospitals that have a day surgery unit in close proximity to theatres, or where day-only patients are managed through 'main' theatres, Day Only and Day of Surgery Admission patients can be managed through the same area.

The separate preoperative area has not been implemented universally. The advantages of a central preoperative area include the following:

- All patients go to the same place preoperatively, hence allowing *simplified patient instruction.*
- A single geographical location creates simplified patient transfers.
- Staff are not distracted by postoperative patients, and can thus focus on the tasks of getting patients ready for their procedure, giving *improved coordination with theatres.*
- Centralisation of processes helps staff familiarity with tasks, builds skills, and fosters development of perioperative protocols, all leading to *better patient preparation.*
- It facilitates '*hot bedding*', whereby patients do not require a ward bed till the latter part of the morning, enabling the bed to be fully utilised overnight. This reduces the need for preoperative ward beds, and enables substantial financial savings.
- The centralised area can be a less threatening environment, which results in a *better patient experience.*
- Staff specialisation provides a platform that enables staff to facilitate change and further adapt their role (e.g. for clinical audit and research, etc).
- Patient exposure to the surgical ward environment is reduced, which may *reduce bacterial infections.*
- Centralisation enables *clarification of medical responsibility* for preoperative patient care policies and procedures.

Implementing the 'ideal' model – change management

Introducing a changed model of patient care, or making any other change in hospitals, involves all the 'usual' challenges of change management. This is becoming a sizeable body of knowledge and a new 'industry', with specialist practitioners available (at cost) to consult and manage the 'change process'. The health sector has its own particular challenges, and the complexity of change increases dramatically with the size of the system being changed. These are 'generic' issues concerning change management, and will not be dealt with further.

There are multiple strategies that are used to manage change and redesign. Many of these have been developed in the settings of other industries, and are used by management consulting groups as a framework for their work in the healthcare setting. Examples include Continuous Quality Improvement, Six Sigma, the Fifth Discipline, Lean Thinking, and Accelerated Implementation Methodology. It is unclear which if any of these methodologies work best in the healthcare setting. All external management experts bring new skills and knowledge, but these need to be used together with the existing workforce to adapt the methods for their own purposes.

All change management depends on ongoing work over a long time to be sustained. It also requires ongoing engagement at all levels of the organisation. This means the workers at the 'coal-face', the middle management, and the executive. In the healthcare setting, the 'coal-face' engagement should include both clinicians of all disciplines, and patients as active participants in redesign and change.

Common controversies encountered in changing preoperative systems

As discussed at the beginning of this chapter, despite the wide variation between hospitals, health systems, nations and cultures, a number of common themes or focal points of controversy and variation can be identified with regard to new systems of perioperative patient care. These are the issues that can be considered to be the particularly difficult challenges of implementing the new model of care.

All change is accompanied by controversy and disputation. Where there is a clear 'answer' or 'solution' this will usually become obvious reasonably promptly, although implementation may be delayed because of the cost or power implications of the proposed solution. If there is sustained controversy, it may be presumed that there is no 'right' answer. The best solution will vary between institutions and settings, and will be strongly influenced by local factors. Hence, although the same controversial issues may be encountered, a local debate must deal with the issue to develop an appropriate local solution. Some of the common controversial themes arising from the challenge of new preoperative care systems include the following:

- A shift from discipline-specific work practices to multi-disciplinary teamwork. The most obvious manifestation of this change is shared clinical records, and a breakdown of the traditional division of both clinical tasks and decision-making. Where this change is simple 'workforce substitution' (e.g. training nurses to perform tasks traditionally performed by medical staff), there may be cost savings, or evidence may be produced showing equivalence of care (but rarely both together). The real opportunity for improvement is in using the shift to multi-disciplinary teamwork as an opportunity for true process redesign. The question is not if worker A can substitute for worker B; rather we should first define what work needs to be done. This implies a labour-intensive process-mapping exercise, which must involve all stakeholders. The inevitable involvement of external facilitators, long committee meetings, and use of jargon can make engagement of clinicians problematic!

- Implementation of a multi-disciplinary model of care requires changes in supervision and responsibility – the traditional professional 'silos' dividing nurses, doctors and other health professionals must be broken down. Staff working within the preoperative service may be comfortable with this, if only because of a self-selection process. However, breakdown of professional silos may threaten the power structures of more senior management, and thus be resisted or sabotaged. For example, 'senior' medical, nurse, or clerical management may not accept 'their' junior staff being supervised by a different discipline.

- Staffing of the preoperative (perioperative) service has been a source of conflict in some hospitals. At initial stages of change, when only 'screening' preoperative assessment and basic preparation is undertaken, a 'simple' service with nurses working independently may be effective. As process redesign develops, a single-discipline service will become constrained in scope due to limited capacity and ability to interact with all health professionals involved in perioperative care. In order to achieve profound and ongoing clinical process change, both medical and nursing involvement in the service must occur. This should be augmented by other health professionals such as para-clinical staff, pharmacists, and allied health services.

● Leadership of the perioperative service is also controversial. Advanced nursing training provides skills and abilities in service management, so this position is most appropriately filled by a nurse (although allied health professionals and others have filled the role). A designated medical leader/director will be necessary as the function of the service expands to deal with more complex patients, takes a more active role in clinical decision-making and investigations, and initiates therapeutic interventions. While this role need not be discipline-specific, it is difficult to imagine any medical specialist other than an anaesthetist filling this role successfully.

● Preoperative processes can be based on 'generic' patients, or based on surgical sub-specialty. Traditional organisation of surgical care focuses on the specialised issues related to the particular operation the patient is having. In high-volume or low-variation specialities such as short day-stay procedures, cataracts or cardiac surgery this may be appropriate, but can lead to uncoordinated surgical 'empires' with unnecessarily different work practices within the same institution. Alternatively, all patients can be managed by a common system with expertise for most patients having most operations, backed up by highly specialised expertise on an 'as needs' basis for 'problem' cases. The latter model appears to offer the greatest potential for 'whole of hospital' system improvements, process flexibility, and efficiency of staff time. In both systems, active management is necessary to balance these conflicting advantages and disadvantages. A possible compromise can be a generic preoperative service with specialised clinical streams managed by designated staff.

● Appropriate standardisation. Any clinical system redesign programme (such as perioperative systems) will raise expectations of standardisation of clinical infrastructure (e.g. forms, terminology, workforce, work practices) as well as clinical care itself (e.g. standard clinical guidelines, protocols, etc). But at what level? In the same specialty, why should Doctor A treat her patients differently to Doctor B? In the same hospital, why should specialty X have a different fasting protocol to specialty Y? Why doesn't St Elsewhere's Hospital use the same paperwork as the Royal General? Why can't there be an agreed national definition of theatre start time, or funding standards? External imposition of standardisation, particularly in clinical care, can be unproductively divisive. Most of the benefits of standardisation can be achieved at the simple and basic level, and can be achieved 'under the radar' if more controversial areas of variation in practice are allowed to continue. In this area of controversy, change advocates frequently fall into the trap of trying to fix everything rather than 'just' 80%, and end up fixing nothing.

- The appropriate organisational role of the anaesthetist in supervising the preoperative patient care process continues to evolve. The process may presume that the anaesthetist must see every patient as an early preoperative consultation (as has been mandated in France). If the preoperative process includes a selective consultation system, then patients must be triaged to varying levels of preoperative care. This triaging can be based on a defined process that is designed, supervised and managed by anaesthetists. Alternatively, anaesthetists may be involved as 'passive' recipients, consulting when requested by others (such as the surgical team or advanced nurses) for occasional or complex cases. In situations where anaesthetists are seen as a technical service provider ('bag-squeezer'), are in relatively short supply, or if funding depends on time in theatre, the appropriateness of anaesthetists working in out-of-theatre settings will be challenged. The interest and enthusiasm of the local individuals and clinical specialty groups or disciplines is a major determinant of this development. This issue may become manifest as a 'political' turf war about whether the preoperative service should be surgeon-, nurse- or anaesthetist-led.

- The scope of the preoperative assessment service's involvement in patient care varies in 'depth'. Preoperative processes can be seen as limited to assessment – checking the quality of preparation performed by others (a 'gatekeeper'), or may be both assessment and preparation – actively involved in organising investigations, optimising the patient's health, and planning care (a 'roadmaker'). For all staff, but particularly nurses, a preparation rather than screening role implies a more active and ongoing involvement in patient care during the preoperative period. This may require ongoing attention to a particular 'problem patient' over days or weeks. Care processes need to be appropriately designed to ensure ongoing preoperative care, particularly to accommodate job-sharing or part-time work. Similarly, anaesthetists taking on the role of 'perioperative physician' must be prepared to provide a service that is not 'just' pre-anaesthetic assessment – they may need to become involved in explaining surgical procedures, discussing broader medical issues, and leading discussion of risk/benefits of anaesthesia and surgery. That said, enthusiasts may need to be restrained from becoming too involved in long-term patient care issues encountered incidentally which are better managed by their primary care provider. This can include opportunistic preventative healthcare, involvement in social issues, and investigation and treatment of hypertension, asthma, and other long-term conditions.

- The scope of the perioperative service/system also varies in 'breadth' or duration. When does the perioperative period start and finish? The perioperative period can be thought of as commencing at the time a decision is made that the patient should have an operation, and finishing when the patient has recovered to their stable postoperative health status. Ideally, the patient care should be an integrated sequence of steps that are planned and coordinated to produce optimal quality and efficiency of care. In reality, every hospital includes a collection of different groups jealously guarding their own 'empires', and subverting efforts to integrate patient care.

The 'big issues' and the 'little problems'

The shift towards a multi-disciplinary, team-based and protocolised perioperative model of patient care gives rise to ongoing 'big issues' and challenges associated with change in hospitals.

- Achieving the right balance in patient care between a 'sausage machine' (inappropriately rigid clinical protocols) and clinical freedom/anarchy.
- Maintaining staff satisfaction in a more 'disciplined' work environment.
- Achieving adequate levels of trust in the system of preoperative preparation so that (say) the procedural anaesthetist will accept assessment and preparation by a different anaesthetist or other health professional. This must be achieved while not developing an entire abdication of responsibility to others.
- Maintaining surgeons' 'sense of involvement' with managing patient care, and keeping the best features of the traditional hierarchical model of surgical care. Surgeons must not become surgical technicians.
- Recognising the skills and building the contribution of clerical (or 'para-clinical') staff in the perioperative team.
- Recognising the potential for skills- and task-transfer between different disciplines of health professionals, whilst accepting the important differences between them.
- Maintaining the momentum for change without underestimating the complexity and difficulty of achieving it.

There are also the myriad 'little problems'. These are the little issues that seem to recur ubiquitously, and become flashpoints for disputation or difficulties in managing change. Examples include legible completion of hospital forms, the process for obtaining documented consent, responsibility for writing up medication, timing of patient arrival on the day of surgery, patients arriving after commencement of surgical lists, administrators undervaluing clerical staff, managing 'standby' patients, arguments about paperwork, doctor/nurse issues, authorisation for test ordering, and ICU/HDU/Ward bed allocation problems. Despite their apparent 'triviality', these 'little' problems can become major stumbling blocks to implementation. Even with the help of highly paid external consultants, experts in 'change management', nothing can remove the tedious task of working through all the little challenges (and 'little victories') of process change.

Future developments

Existing 'high-functioning' comprehensive preoperative systems already include preparation for postoperative care and discharge. A logical development of this process would therefore be the integration of both the preoperative and postoperative phases of care into a multi-disciplinary perioperative service. This could be achieved by integration of the preoperative service with postoperative services such as the acute pain service. Extension of the preoperative service's role into involvement with non-elective patients (particularly complex sub-acute patients such as orthogeriatrics) would also be an appropriate development. The role of advanced practice nurses and anaesthetists in this model of care is yet to be defined. The potential exists for evolution into perioperative clinicians, building on skills and knowledge developed from current involvement in ICU/HDU, acute pain services, medical emergency teams, and preoperative assessment and preparation. Integration of this clinical service with the routine collection of outcome data provides the basis for integration of patient risk factors obtained preoperatively with patient outcomes, so that quality assurance, risk management and audit become internalised within the perioperative process.

Further development of preoperative assessment and preparation may also provide a platform for institutional risk management. Early assessment of the patient's health status and their perioperative risk can be used to make an appropriate decision as to whether the institution wishes to accept the risk of providing the proposed surgical or other procedure for the particular patient. In hospital settings providing 'free' surgical care, it may then become realistic to deny the patient surgery (such as a knee replacement) until the patient has lost weight or stopped smoking. Alternatively, high-risk patients may be diverted from surgical interventions at an early stage rather than after expectations have developed.

Around the world, medico-legal and general risk is being disseminated from individual practitioners to institutions. Adverse outcomes can no longer be blamed on a rogue practitioner. When a patient has an operation, it is not 'just' the surgeon providing the service – it is provided by the healthcare institution. By being 'proactive', the decision by the institution to provide a clinical procedure can be made at the time of booking the patient, rather than after the patient has been waiting in expectation of having surgery for some time. This is much more likely to be accepted by the patient, their family and the community. From an institutional or health system point of view, better systems for early preoperative assessment and preparation provide a better platform for managing the institution's, as well as the patient's, risk.

The development of better and more integrated systems and processes for preoperative assessment and preparation, and delivery of perioperative patient care will continue to evolve. While there will be ongoing differences, these general developments will result in systems and processes that will be better for the patient, better for the staff and ultimately better for the organisation delivering the care.

19 Audit and evaluation of a perioperative service

Ciaran Hurley

SUMMARY

- **What does evaluation mean?**
- **Why should perioperative services be evaluated?**
- **What should be evaluated?**
- **Designing a tool for evaluation of a service**
- **Ethical considerations.**

INTRODUCTION

The era of evidence-based healthcare is well and truly established and in this context it is important that service providers can demonstrate that they offer valuable returns for the investments that they receive, whether their funds are sourced from individuals, an acute care trust, primary care trust or from regional or national budgets. This chapter outlines some of the basic principles of evaluation with a focus on perioperative care services. To make some of the points relevant to readers' experience, a number of examples are used throughout the chapter to illustrate the application of the principles of evaluation; these are through the adherence with the National Institute for Health and Clinical Excellence (NICE) recommendations for preoperative investigations, the adherence with a target of universal preoperative assessment for surgical patients, the adherence with the RCN guideline for perioperative fasting, patient satisfaction in an ambulatory surgery department and identification of bottle-necks in the operating department's throughput of patients. These examples should allow the reader to make connections between some of the abstract principles of evaluation and the practical aspects of choosing a focus, design and method.

What does evaluation mean?

Commonly the word 'evaluation' relates to making a judgement or assessment. The technical application with which this chapter is concerned relates to approaches taken to assess the effect of a service or object. This assessment can take many forms. There are a number of forms of assessment, each with a distinct purpose, and the choice between them must be informed by the purpose of the assessment that is being carried out. The forms of evaluation are commonly known by the three terms *service evaluation*, *audit* and *research*. Service evaluation is used to identify the state of a service that is being offered and may be focused on a comparison of the reality with the recommendations of an advisory body such as NICE, or of a literature review. Audits seek to establish the compliance of a service with a standard that has been previously agreed. Research is concerned with the investigation of aspects of practice about which little is currently known or understood. A range of methods can be used to collect the data required for evaluation and the methods are not unique to any of the forms. Methods include survey, questionnaire, observation schedules, case studies and experiments of various types.

In their seminal book, Lincoln and Guba[1] coined the word *evaluand* to indicate the subject to be evaluated. Almost anything can be the subject of evaluation and in the context of organisations that provide service evaluands can be remarkably diverse. While almost anything can be the subject of evaluation it is important to bear in mind that the evaluation must have a purpose; evaluation for its own sake is a waste of resources, producing little benefit for the service provider, recipients the personnel delivering them.

Why should perioperative services be evaluated?

There are a number of reasons to evaluate perioperative services. I have already alluded to one of them, and that is to provide evidence that the service being provided meets the expectations of the people or organisations that provide the funds on which the service runs. The objective of evaluations motivated by finance is fairly crude; people putting up cash want evidence that it is used efficiently and that the service provides value for money.

Another group with expectations about a service may be the clients, patients or users; evaluation can identify patients' experiences and perceptions of the services provided and thus provide the basis for identifying targets for improvement and a framework for intervention. Possible motivations for such evaluation are complex. There is certainly an element of satisfaction in knowing that your clients enjoy the service they receive, but self-congratulation is hardly a laudable reason for undertaking evaluation. Providing patient groups, hospital management boards and those in primary care who purchase surgical services with evidence that the service provided meets the expectations of patients will make a difference in a climate where the *Choose and Book* system means patients exercise control and choice over the site at which they receive their treatment. Similarly, more patients might choose to have surgery in a hospital that can provide reliable evidence of the quality of their services, and under the *Payment by Results* scheme, more patients means more income for the hospital, something which the directors of a foundation hospital trust will want to see. Patient involvement groups can help to identify the correct focus for evaluation as well as advising on how to implement and sustain improvements to the services offered.

A third reason is to test the service provider's performance against targets set either internally or by external agencies such as NICE, the Department of Health, the National Health Service Executive and others. In some cases, such as the Essence of Care benchmarks, the targets and the methods of measuring them are quite simple. Others may be more complex, for example reducing the number of operations cancelled for non-clinical reasons; the causes of such cancellation are generally related to system or process failures. Problems that originate from system failures can be identified by an activity known as *process mapping*, in which people involved in the service gather to isolate the actual and potential problems and suggest possible solutions. Having identified the problems, a process of *service redesign* should aim to change the aspects of the system that are problematic. For this purpose a number of NHS organisations have set up *service redesign teams*, groups of people with experience and skills who support the process of change to ensure that it is effective and that the changes are maintained after the initial enthusiasm fades.

Reasons to evaluate perioperative services can be broadly categorised into those that justify financial outlay, those that demonstrate patient satisfaction and those that demonstrate the achievement of non-financial targets. In an organisational context, evaluation may be driven either by an external agency or by internal motivations and while external agencies often provide the basis of an assessment tool, it may need to be adapted in order to extract valid data from your organisation; internally motivated evaluation will almost certainly have many unique elements in its design.

What should be evaluated?

A number of aspects of perioperative practice that could be the subject of some kind of evaluation were listed in the introduction to this chapter. None of these aspects stand alone as a question of evaluation because they each lack focus, containing a number of potential questions: Why do deviations from the NICE recommended investigations occur and what are the financial and process costs? How many patients arrive for surgery without attending preoperative assessment services and what impact does this have on their care? For how long do patients fast before surgery and what is the incidence of the postoperative complications associated with fasting for too long? What elements of our service do patients like, not like and want to see improved? For how long do theatre personnel stand idle waiting for a patient to arrive at each stage of the perioperative journey? Are there patterns to the time and place at which personnel are waiting for a patient to arrive? All of these questions need to be further refined to identify the specific and singular problems that underlie the problem being evaluated.

Identifying these inherent questions represents one of the earliest and most important stages of the evaluative process: refining the question. Simply asking 'Are we meeting the

NICE recommendations?' will inevitably lead to the answer 'No', but experience and common sense suggest that there are often good reasons for deviating from recommended practices. Asking 'Do our staff ever stand idle?' will most probably be answered 'Yes', concluding the investigation. More pertinent questions may be 'Is there a pattern to the bottle-necks in the system?', 'What are the causes of the bottle-necks?' and 'Can the bottle-necks be overcome?'

Refining the questions in this way is important because it helps to identify the type of question to which the problem belongs. The list above contains two types of question; some are quantitative, having an answer that relies upon numerical data; others are qualitative and are answered according to the ways in which people or groups respond or interact with the evaluand.

Compliance with targets and personnel idle time are purely quantitative problems as the only way to answer the questions is to count things: the number of patients who have not attended preoperative services, the number of investigations that are not indicated by findings of an assessment and examination, the amount of time in which theatre personnel are not engaged in patient contact.

Patient satisfaction is a qualitative issue because it asks about aspects of service that patients liked and disliked, enjoyed or suffered. Some problems, such as fasting, have both qualitative and quantitative elements. While the duration of fasting is a simple measurement of time, it is equally possible to discover the patient's psychosocial response, which is qualitative in nature.

Already I have begun to outline an important aspect of the next section of this chapter which examines the design of the evaluation tool. The old adage that 'failure to plan means planning to fail' is as true in this context as any other, because failure to refine the question will very likely lead to choosing inappropriate methods of finding the answer. Refinement is therefore a vital part of the evaluation, demanding the investigator's attention at a very early stage.

Designing a tool for evaluation of a service

The following section is an overview of the process by which questions of evaluation can be answered. This is not a recipe that will guarantee desired results, merely a framework and one source of advice; some aspects of it may safely be ignored, others are essential; some aspects can be done in varying sequence while others are dependent on the outcome of previous stages. The vital elements are summarised in Table 19.1.

The critical review of literature before an investigation serves a number of purposes; it can identify an answer to the question and thus eliminate the need to spend resources on data collection and analysis; it can influence the questions asked by revealing new and important understanding of the evaluand and it can influence the methods of evaluation by identifying methods that have been successfully employed by others. Performing a literature review is not a matter of simply reading and summarising the published literature, however, and the skills of critical analysis and synthesis should be learned, fostered and supported in order to ensure that the findings of review are valid. Comprehensive advice regarding literature review is available from many sources; a handful are listed with the references to this chapter.[2,3,4]

Table 19.1 The stages of evaluation, their purpose and requirements

Stage of evaluation	Purpose of each stage	Requirements
Literature review	Identifying what is known about the evaluand in the literature and confirming the need to proceed with data collection	• Knowledge of and skill in the literature review method • Ability in critical reading • Ability to extract data from literature
Design	Plan and organise the collection and analysis of data	• Knowledge of the evaluand, from literature review and/or practical experience • Knowledge and/or experience of methods of evaluation
Analysis of data	Extract meaning from the data	• Ability to identify the method of analysis required by the nature of the data • Knowledge and skill to apply the method of analysis
Dissemination of findings	Sharing the findings with interested parties	• Basic IT skills • Access to the means of communication appropriate to the audience and the data

The design of any investigation is essential because it establishes the relationship between the three basic elements of any evaluation: the sample, tools and analysis. The sample, the source of raw data, may be a person or group, one or a number of objects or a set of data related to people or objects and should be capable of delivering the data that is required for the evaluation. The method of collecting the data should be appropriate to the type of data collected and should allow for storage and recall of the data for the purpose of analysis. Finally, the method of analysis must be suited to the type of data that has been collected. Failure to identify these relationships and to plan methods of evaluation that make congruent links between them can lead to invalid or unreliable findings.

The analysis of the data holds great significance for the overall validity and reliability of the findings of the evaluation. Quantitative data can be daunting for anyone without training in the use of statistics. There are written guides that can help an investigator decide what test is appropriate for the question and the type of data collected. It is advisable to seek advice as early as possible in the design process because a statistician will offer a range of advice: whether the data to be collected is amenable to statistical analysis, the best test to extract conclusions from the data, the sample size required for valid conclusions. Most organisations have access to the support of an audit department where people with expertise are available to help with all stages of evaluation, or a research department if the evaluation falls into that category.

Qualitative data are analysed in a very different way to quantitative data. The data generally takes the form of words, spoken or written, and the source of the data is people. Being notoriously unpredictable, people cannot be relied upon to fit into easy or simple categories and, to a certain extent, analysis requires a willingness to *go with the flow.*

If consistency in the type or presentation of the response is an important part of the evaluation, attention should be paid to the manner in which the data is collected; the researcher has little control over the responses in a self-administered questionnaire but a researcher-administered questionnaire provides an opportunity to answer queries, ensure that the respondent has understood the question and gives their response in a valid format. Qualitative analysis generally identifies themes in all or most of data and compares and contrasts the responses of the individuals in relation to each theme. A popular example of an approach to qualitative data analysis is the 'Framework' method detailed by Ritchie *et al.*[5,6]

A cautionary tale in evaluation design

A senior doctor wanted to know where and when patients were delayed in the process of being operated upon. He created a proforma, to be commenced when the department secretary telephoned the ward to request a patient be brought to the reception area. Each time a movement within the department was completed, the time was logged in the proforma; when the patient arrived in reception, when the support worker arrived to take the patient to the anaesthetic room, arrival in the anaesthetic room, arrival of the anaesthetist and so on. He thought he had planned everything to the letter, but on the day the investigation began a very significant problem became apparent. The many clocks in the department were not synchronised and differed, in some cases by as much as five minutes, resulting in data that was nonsensical. For instance, it appeared that some patients arrived in the anaesthetic room before they had left reception. It is clear that in this case the tools to collect the data (the clocks) were not fit for purpose; the proforma would have yielded the data the doctor required, the analysis was a matter of simple descriptive statistics, the sample of every patient was appropriate and the clocks were the only weak link in the whole project.

Ethical considerations

At face value it may seem that evaluation of perioperative services is unlikely to be ethically challenging; surely anything that aims to improve the services we offer is ethically justified? This section aims to demonstrate the potential for evaluation to breach the principles of ethics that are commonly accepted in western cultures.[7] The over-riding principle of ethical evaluation is the avoidance of unnecessary harm and disproportionate exploitation. If people are to be inconvenienced or put at risk as a result of the investigation a number of criteria must be met. To ensure good practice, investigations are subject to an approval and governance process and all investigations should be discussed with the administrator of the appropriate governance process. Service evaluation and audits are normally managed in-house by an internal department, research has a national governance process with local representation, and advice should be sought from the hospital's research and development department.

Good practice aims to minimise the risk of a range of potential problems including: inappropriate use of personal data and confidential information, conflict of interest between a patient's need for healthcare and the investigator's aims, creating conflict between employer and employee, and causing distress to people by asking them to recall unpleasant events from the past. Sometimes the subject of an evaluation is important enough to warrant a certain level of risk however, and where such risks are predictable, mechanisms are required to manage the consequences; if an audit of working practices results in criticism of an employer, the employees ought to be protected from subsequent bullying or harassment at work; if patients are being asked to recall events from the past, counselling services should be available to support those who find such recall distressing.

CONCLUSION

This chapter is not intended to be a 'how to...' guide to evaluating services. That would require a whole text of its own. Rather it outlines the basic principles that should be applied during the design stage, with reference to some common features of perioperative practice. The subject of the evaluation should be sufficiently focused to allow for precision in later stages of sampling, data collection and analysis. Once the focus is fixed, the investigator should identify the population that will provide the information required. This population may be people, objects or data; nonetheless it is essential to go to the source of the data, since any other source will bring data that is of little or no value to the project. The design of an evaluation should include the method by which the data is to be analysed to ensure that there is congruence between the question asked, the data collected and the means of analysis. Consideration should also be given in the design stages to the sources of dissemination of the findings and the audience to which the data will appeal. Finally, once the design is complete, it should be presented to a review body to ensure that the project meets the expected standards of ethics and design. Once the approval to proceed has been granted, the hard work begins! Good luck.

REFERENCES

1. Y. Lincoln and E. Guba (1985). *Naturalistic Inquiry.* Newbury Park CA: Sage Publications.

2. D.F. Polit (2006). *Essentials of Nursing Research: Methods, Application and Utilisation* (6th edn). London, Philadelphia PA: Lippincott, Williams and Wilkins.

3. C. Hart (1998). *Doing a Literature Review.* London: Sage Publications.

4. N. Burns and S.K. Grove (2005). *The Practice of Nursing Research: Conduct, Critique and Utilisation* (5th edn). St Louis MO: Elsevier Saunders.

5. J. Ritchie, L. Spencer and W. O'Connor (2003). Analysis: Practices, principles and process. In *Qualitative Research Practice*, ed. J. Ritchie and J. Lewis. London: Sage Publications.

6. J. Ritchie, L. Spencer and W. O'Connor (2003). Analysis: Carrying out qualitative analysis. In *Qualitative Research Practice*, ed. J. Ritchie and J. Lewis. London: Sage Publications.

7. T. L. Beauchamp and J. F. Childress (2001). *Principles of Biomedical Ethics* (5th edn). Oxford: Oxford University Press.

Chapter **20** Developing a competency framework for preoperative assessment

Hilary Walsgrove

SUMMARY

This chapter will cover:

- **the background to developing competencies for preoperative assessment**
- **standards of practice and levels of practice**
- **a competency-based framework for education, training and assessment**
- **the competency portfolio as a learning and assessment tool**
- **assessment of competence**
- **educational courses.**

Background

Preoperative assessment has developed as a service provided by a variety of members of the healthcare team, such as doctors, nurses and allied health professionals.[1] However, preoperative assessment services have tended to evolve within the United Kingdom in a rather ad hoc and haphazard fashion, often without clear structure, adequate finances and invariably as an 'add-on' to other surgical services. This has led to a lack of clarity around what constitutes best practice in preoperative assessment, a dearth of information relating to any minimum standards of practice for preoperative assessment and limited education and training packages for staff providing this vital service.

Against this general background, two key points emerge that need careful consideration if well-planned, effective and efficient services are to be developed that meet the needs of patients, as well as being in line with the organisation providing the services. First, the development of clear, good practice guidelines for preoperative assessment is necessary, such as those produced through work carried out by the NHS Modernisation Agency (NHSMA), which were published by the Department of Health.[2,3] Secondly, a robust, comprehensive education and training programme needs to be developed for staff involved in preoperative assessment, if best practice is to be established and maintained.

The purpose of preoperative assessment

Preoperative assessment is not only about determining the medical fitness of patients for surgery.[4] It should also involve a two-way consultation between patient and preoperative assessor whereby the patient is assessed for physical, psychological and social suitability to have surgery performed.[5] This provides the healthcare team with relevant information about the patient prior to admission. Also, it should be an opportunity for the patient to gather information about pending surgery and its implications. Some main aims for preoperative assessment, which feature in current literature, are as follows:

- to minimise patient risk[2,3,6,7]
- to identify patient suitability/fitness for surgery/anaesthetic[2,3,6,7]
- to provide information for informed choices[1,6,8]
- to facilitate better utilisation of theatre/ward resources[2,3,6]
- to reduce fears and anxieties for patient[2,3,6,7,8]
- to improve surgical patients' hospital experience.[2,3,9]

Standards of practice for preoperative assessment

Standards of practice for preoperative assessment are likely to vary according to local requirements and the specific specialist areas involved.[8] However, the standards are likely to fall into the following broad categories:

- management of clinics/patient appointments
- patient assessment for surgery and anaesthesia
- information-giving and consent for surgery and anaesthesia
- patient admission and discharge planning.

If these categories are looked at in more detail, the sort of aspects that emerge might be as follows.

Minimum standards of practice within the category of 'Management of clinics/patient appointments' would include aspects such as:

- ensuring that patients are seen promptly, within 10 minutes of their allocated appointment time
- making sure the appointment runs to time and patients aren't kept waiting to see other members of staff
- making sure that communication channels between all relevant departments are good, enabling the patient's journey to run smoothly

- ensuring patients have all necessary details relating to their admission, contact details for enquiries and so on
- making sure patients are preoperatively assessed at least seven days prior to their admission for surgery
- ensuring patients are treated with dignity and respect and offered appropriate reassurance and support by the preoperative assessor.

Within the category of 'Patient assessment for surgery and anaesthesia', minimum standards of practice should include elements such as:

- checking the patient's current health and social status, in relation to suitability for surgery within the allocated environment (e.g. day surgery, inpatient facility)
- checking patient's suitability for planned surgery
- carrying out a relevant patient assessment including medical, surgical, anaesthetic, nursing, social and psychological issues
- carrying out all relevant vital signs and preoperative investigations and checking and appropriately actioning the results of these tests
- carrying out physical examination relevant to the impending surgery and anaesthetic
- documenting in full all of the above points, making appropriate referrals based on the information gathered and acting on the results of the assessment carried out
- dealing with any problems identified during patient assessment appropriately and in a timely and efficient manner.

Within the category of 'Information-giving/Consent for surgery and anaesthesia', minimum standards that apply should include:

- provision of verbal and written information to the patient and/or carer pertaining to their admission to hospital, anaesthetic, surgical procedure, pre- and postoperative care and discharge arrangements required
- providing patients with adequate information and checking their understanding in relation to being able to give their fully informed consent for both anaesthetic and surgery[10,11]
- giving patients the opportunity to ask questions and voice concerns about their pending admission for surgery.

Once standards of practice for preoperative assessment have been formulated and agreed within the local area, which are also in line with national guidance,[12] they can provide a baseline for acceptable performance for staff working within preoperative assessment[13] and can act as a benchmark for best practice.[14] From the perspective of the organisation, standards of practice help protect patient safety as well as safeguarding the organisation's liability.[15]

In order to meet the aims of preoperative assessment and to run a preoperative assessment service that is characterised by acceptable and agreed standards of practice, a relevant programme of education, training and assessment should be developed for all staff involved in the preoperative assessment of patients. Currently there is no national educational programme for preoperative assessment across the United Kingdom and therefore different areas have set up their own programmes, depending on local requirements.[4,7,16] Such programmes range from short, in-house training involving mainly observation of others' practice and sometimes some theoretical sessions up to first degree and Masters programmes for advanced nursing practice, which include history-taking and physical examination skills.[4,17] There are also courses provided by commercial companies as well, such as MandK, whose course provides an introduction to preoperative assessment and assists in offering evidence-based care to improve patient outcomes.[18]

Levels of practice for preoperative assessment

Before a framework of education can be formulated, it is important to review what staff are actually doing at present. This will highlight that individuals work at different levels of practice within different preoperative assessment structures. Staff working at different levels of practice can all make a valuable contribution to patient care and this should be inherent within any programme that is set up to support learning. What is important is that individuals are working safely and effectively within their own level of competence and not beyond their limitations.[19] There must be a clear and transparent outline of the roles and responsibilities of the different members of the preoperative assessment team. This will enable an educational programme to be developed based on the knowledge and skills required for safe and effective practice. This should then meet the varied individuals' needs within the context of the preoperative assessment team and meet the requirements of the organisation they work for.

Due to wide-ranging variation across the United Kingdom in relation to the structure of preoperative assessment services, there is no single particular model to use as a template for the 'ideal preoperative assessment service'. However, where a service is provided by an integrated team of individual healthcare workers, the level at which these individuals work is likely to range through healthcare assistant, registered nurse or allied health professional, registered nurse or allied health professional with advanced knowledge and skills, such as advanced nurse practitioner or surgical care practitioner, junior doctor, junior and consultant anaesthetist.

Benner's (1984)[20] levels of skills acquisition model is one model that can be used as a structured framework for identifying levels of practice for healthcare professionals working in preoperative assessment. This model has been used extensively within nursing[21,22,23,24] and, as many staff involved with preoperative assessment are nurses, this tool is ideal to use within this area.

Benner's 'Novice to Expert' model[20] was used as a basis for a competency framework for preoperative assessment that was developed within an acute hospital trust in the South of England. It fitted well with the development of skills and knowledge for the preoperative assessment nurses involved. Benner's levels of practice as applied to this particular organisation are outlined in Box 20.1. These levels of practice suited this particular hospital Trust but may not be appropriate in other organisations with preoperative assessment services that are structured differently, but they could be adapted to suit individual requirements. The model provides standard level descriptors that are used for the education programme that has subsequently been devised. The level descriptors are the definition of achievement against the identified standard: 'novice', 'advanced beginner', 'competent', 'proficient' and 'expert'. Within this particular Trust, levels 1 to 3, which loosely equate to Benner's 'novice', 'advanced beginner' and 'competent', relate to the expected knowledge and skills of the Band 5[25] preoperative assessment nurses, depending on what level they are at within their own personal career structure. They can move along the continuum as they progress through their personal and professional development. Level 4 preoperative nurses tend to be Band 5 or 6 nurses[25] with advanced nursing skills, such as physical examination and history taking and student advanced nurse practitioners. Level 5 nurses are usually qualified advanced nurse practitioners, usually working at Band 7.[25]. The level 4 and 5 nurses would loosely equate to Benner's 'proficient' and 'expert' levels.

Box 20.1 Levels of practice for preoperative assessment

There are five levels of practice for registered nurses working within preoperative assessment (POA), which are based on Benner's (1984) 'Novice to Expert' model.

Level 1: Novice
A registered nurse who has been qualified for one year or less and has been working within a surgical environment or a registered nurse who has been working within a different specialist area and has minimal or no surgical experience.

Level 2: Advanced Beginner
A registered nurse who has completed the preoperative assessment competency portfolio and has been assessed as competent. Once competent, the nurse can see a patient in an unsupervised capacity, within a joint nurse/junior doctor clinic.

Level 3: Competent
As for level 2. In addition, the nurse will have successfully completed the preoperative and planning unit of learning. The nurse also takes on some additional responsibilities within own speciality area.

Level 4: Proficient
As for levels 2 and 3. In addition, the nurse will have successfully completed physical examination and health assessment unit of learning. This nurse will conduct nurse-led POA clinics without doctor involvement.

Level 5: Expert
As for levels 2 to 4. In addition this nurse will be a qualified nurse practitioner who has completed an RCN-accredited nurse practitioner programme.

Although these levels were identified within the framework, it is important to point out that these are considered to be flexible descriptors. The preoperative assessment nurses are able to move between levels interchangeably depending on their practice at the time and this ensures that the framework takes into account individuals involved at different levels of training and education. As the nurses progress in terms of professional development and confidence and competence in practice for preoperative assessment, they can move through the competencies at increasingly higher levels of achievement within the framework (from levels 1 to 5).

With standards of practice for preoperative assessment and the levels of practice established that staff are either working at or working towards, it is possible to devise a suitable education, training and assessment programme. In the case of nurses, who tend to make up the majority of preoperative assessors, there is a general perception that they should be 'experienced', but this is not clearly elaborated upon within current available literature. As it is likely that preoperative assessment constitutes adjustments to the nurse's scope of practice,[19] if the role is to be undertaken effectively, they should have sound knowledge of anaesthesia and the surgical speciality involved, as well as well-developed assessment skills.[1] Alongside this, competencies can be identified that meet with the standards of best practice within that specific preoperative assessment service.

Competence for preoperative assessment

Competence attracts different definitions depending on the context within which it is used.[26] Competence may be defined within a professional context and is the broad ability with which a professional person is able to practise to required standards in a range of situations. Competencies are the various aspects performed to the predetermined standard, which combine to create professional competence in a defined role.[27] For the purpose of a preoperative assessment competency framework, Eraut's (1994)[26] notion of competence and competency would be an appropriate approach to adopt. Competence is a generic notion that refers to a person's overall capacity, while competency refers to a specific capability. Competencies consist of knowledge and skills combined with attitudes and values required in a particular context to perform to a prescribed standard,[28] which in this case is preoperative assessment. Trust, caring, communication skills, knowledge and adaptability are identifiable attributes of competence, together with emotions and values.[28,29,30] The competency approach to training, job selection, appraisal and development is advocated as a strategy for helping to deliver quality, cost-effective healthcare.[31,32] It is important from an organisational perspective for competence of healthcare staff to be continuously identified, monitored and assessed if safe and effective practice is to be maintained.[28]

With the above issues in mind, it is possible to see that overall competence is dependent on the level of every specified competency. This fits well with the idea of staff working at different levels of practice, which has been discussed earlier in this chapter. A holistic approach to competence, incorporating specified work tasks and roles as well as the concepts of knowledge and understanding drawing on Benner's[20] levels of skills acquisition, is an appropriate starting point for considering the development of a competency framework for preoperative assessment that is based on identified standards of care.[31,33,34]

Developing a competency framework

The development of a competency-based approach to training, education and assessment for preoperative assessment can help to safeguard the interests of patients, the practitioner and the organisation. It promotes the identification of best practice from a sound evidence base and allows practice to be advanced in a safe and supportive manner. It promotes professional and personal development, enabling practitioners to demonstrate advancing practice from novice to expert, and increasing personal awareness to recognise competence as well as limitations of practice. It also encourages self-reflection and peer review and contributes towards professional profiling. It has been suggested that a practitioner's self-recognition of their own level of competence is essential in maintaining high standards of care.[28]

A competency-based framework for education, training and assessment for preoperative assessment

This section will provide an overview of the competency-based framework of education, training and assessment that was developed within a particular hospital Trust. It is likely that numerous different models exist that would be equally appropriate to other organisations. However, this particular framework has been introduced and is now an established and well-evaluated local initiative within preoperative assessment that meets the requirements of this hospital Trust. The two main components of the programme are an in-house competency portfolio and a number of educational courses offered by the local university for post-registration healthcare professionals. It seems reasonable that other preoperative assessment services could draw on the experiences of this particular Trust in order to provide a robust and effective process for their own staff. In fact, this has proved to be the case, as publicity around the framework generated interest from other preoperative assessment services, which have used the package as a basis for their own areas.

Standards and levels of practice

Prior to devising the preoperative assessment programme at the Trust, a number of standards of practice were identified as a baseline, through work undertaken by the preoperative assessment group, led by the Trust's preoperative assessment lead nurse and comprising representatives from all surgical inpatient wards, day case and short-stay unit, all preoperative assessment clinics and main and day theatres. Once this baseline of standards had been devised, an audit of current practice across the Trust was carried out using these standards. The standards focused on a number of key areas, namely management of clinics, patient assessment, information-giving and staff education. Data from the audit demonstrated that improvements could be made in all of these key areas and it was agreed that the formulation of a relevant preoperative assessment education, training and assessment programme would be a tool to enable improvements to be made, in order to develop and maintain high standards of practice and promote high-quality patient care. The audit was also instrumental in highlighting the different levels of practice that staff were working at and helped to highlight and shape the levels of practice that form an inherent part of the programme.

Preoperative assessment competency portfolio

The competencies within the preoperative assessment portfolio were compiled in line with the National Heath Service Modernisation Agency's guidance for preoperative assessment,[2,3,12] local and regional guidelines and standards and evidence gained from current literature relating to preoperative assessment practice. They give the preoperative assessment nurses, their employers and education providers with standards to work towards in order to achieve quality care and consistency within preoperative assessment. Although this is currently a local initiative, it is being rolled out across the region and is being used as the gold standard for preoperative assessment education, training and assessment within other local Trusts, thus increasing consistency and parity of practice at a wider level.

In addition, an analysis of the nurse's role in preoperative assessment identified a number of components, which closely match those that are inherent within the portfolio outlined here. These components were: administrative function, physical assessment (medical and nursing history), psychological and social assessment, decision making, interventions (referral, counselling, ordering and performing tests and investigations).[35] An analysis such as this has helped to strengthen the evidence base for development of both standards of practice as well as the competencies required to meet those standards, within the Trust identified here.

Currently the portfolio is available for registered nurses working within preoperative assessment, as it is nurses who predominantly make up the workforce within preoperative assessment at this particular Trust. However, the competencies could easily be adapted to meet the requirements of other healthcare professionals undertaking preoperative assessment.

A set of competencies for each level of practice are categorised into a number of sections that make up the competency portfolio (see Table 20.1). The competency sections are not presented in any particular order of priority, as each section should be considered equally important in terms of providing a service that adequately meets patient and organisational need. Each individual section starts with a broad competency statement, followed by a set of specific competencies designed to enable the nurse to achieve the overall competence. The competency statements identify the knowledge, skills and attitudes needed to perform within different elements of preoperative assessment.[36]

Table 20.1 The competency portfolio

Section number	Title of section	Level of practice
1	Knowledge and skills for patient appointments/clinic management	1 to 5
2	Interpersonal skills	1 to 5
3	Patient consultation and information-giving skills	1 to 5
4	Teaching and assessing skills	3 to 5
5	Maintenance of standards of practice	3 to 5
6	History taking	4 and 5
7	Physical examination	4 and 5
8	Informed consent (written)	4 and 5
9	Lead POA role for Trust	5
10	POA service delivery	5
11	Advanced practice	5

The competencies within the portfolio

Section 1: Knowledge and skills for patient appointments/clinic management

The competency statement for this section of the portfolio is that: 'The nurse is able to work without supervision, maintaining a smooth running, systematic and well-organised clinic that meets the needs of the patient, staff and the service, in line with the guidelines and standards for practice for preoperative assessment'.

This section involves the preoperative assessor using a systematic approach to preoperative assessment appointments and ensuring that all aspects of the process are carried out and lead to a satisfactory outcome for both patient and assessor. The assessor requires good knowledge and understanding of the patient's surgical journey and who and what is involved in the various stages of that journey. They need to be able to work effectively as a team member who is fully aware of their own role responsibilities and the responsibilities of other members of the team and be able to access the right individuals to liaise with in relation to communicating information about individual patients. This is likely to include admissions staff, the admitting ward/department, anaesthetic department and anyone that the assessor may need to refer the patient to. In addition to ensuring that appointments run smoothly, the assessor needs to be aware of time management issues, such as keeping to appointment times and being mindful of keeping patients waiting for long periods of time.

Section 2: Interpersonal skills

The competency statement reads: 'The nurse has good interpersonal skills during interactions with patients/carers in the preoperative assessment appointment.'

The importance of good communication skills for preoperative assessment cannot be overlooked as it is key to building a therapeutic relationship with the patient, which will help them to travel along their surgical journey. Qualities such as empathy and caring should be evident. The preoperative assessor needs to convey to the patient a level of self-assurance that demonstrates confidence in their role, not showing any undue hesitation, confusion or embarrassment. The assessor should encourage the patient to be an active participant in the preoperative assessment process, to encourage interaction with patient and carer, encouraging them to express their feelings and thoughts, helping the patient to articulate fears and anxieties, to voice any concerns or queries about their pending admission and to ask appropriate questions. The assessor needs to be able to convey information to the patient so that they have a good understanding of what is going to be happening to them and to use language that the patient will understand.

Section 3: Patient consultation and information-giving skills

The competency statement for this section reads: 'The preoperative assessment nurse confidently and competently conducts a patient consultation within a framework that includes the following elements: opening the consultation, patient assessment, information giving, closing the consultation, and team work.'

This section of the portfolio involves the content of the preoperative assessment appointment undertaken by the preoperative assessor, considering each individual appointment as a whole patient consultation. Opening the consultation is important, as it sets the scene for how the rest of the appointment will run and is the starting point for building a good relationship and partnership with the patient in a short space of time. Included within this section is assessment of the patient from a physical, psychological and social perspective, building up a picture of the patient that will help in planning their care and treatment during admission for surgery and planning for their discharge home and recovery following surgery. As part of the patient's preoperative assessment appointment, the preoperative assessor will provide the patient with information about their pending admission and what to expect following surgery, helping them to make informed choices about the surgery, as well as the anaesthetic. Good closure of the consultation is also key to the process, ensuring that the patient is fully aware of what to expect and that preoperative assessor and patient both have all the information required to enable the best possible outcome. The preoperative assessor does not work in isolation but as part of a team, and therefore team-work is an essential element of the process.

Section 4: Teaching and assessing skills

The competency statement reads: 'The level 3 nurse assumes a teaching and assessing role within preoperative assessment and acts as a mentor, providing support, guidance and advice to level 1 and 2 nurses.'

Once the preoperative assessor has gained experience within their role and is competent and confident in their abilities as a preoperative assessor, they need to be able to help maintain high standards of practice and high-quality patient care. This can be partly realised through teaching and assessing junior members of staff using the competency portfolio as guidance. The preoperative assessor needs to develop good teaching skills, to be able to act as an effective mentor and to be able to assess competence of junior staff.

Section 5: Maintenance of standards of practice

The competency statement reads: 'The nurse will be responsible for ensuring that standards of practice for preoperative assessment are maintained.'

The preoperative assessor needs to be fully aware of the standards of practice for the POA service and must ensure that high standards are maintained at all times. They should ensure that they have good knowledge and understanding of up-to-date research and developments relating to preoperative assessment generally and within their specialist area of practice.

Level 4 preoperative assessors are expected to meet the competencies numbered from 1 to 5 and in addition will meet further competencies, which are detailed within Sections 6 to 8 of the portfolio.

Section 6: History taking

The competency statement reads: 'The nurse confidently and competently obtains a comprehensive and accurate health history from the patient and/or carer.'

The preoperative assessor should be able to obtain an accurate account of the patient's health history, distinguishing between relevant and irrelevant information and use this information to guide the physical examination of the patient. They should be able to identify the reason for patient admission, their presenting problem/s and the planned course of action. Accurate and comprehensive documentation of both the patient's health history and physical examination is an essential aspect of the preoperative assessor's role.

Section 7: Physical examination skills

The competency statement reads: 'The nurse will be able to confidently and competently physically examine a patient in relation to assessing their fitness for surgery and anaesthetic.'

The preoperative assessor needs to be able to carry out an appropriate physical examination of the patient, in order to ascertain their fitness for surgery and anaesthetic. The preoperative assessor should be able to demonstrate an ability to distinguish between significant and nonsignificant findings, in relation to the examination. They must have good knowledge of the protocols regarding preoperative testing and their ordering and be able to act on results. They will be able to request and/or perform relevant investigations, based on patient assessment and examination, in accordance with guidelines.

Section 8: Informed consent (written)

The competency statement reads: 'The nurse will obtain the patient's informed consent for operation in writing and document this accurately on the consent form.'

If the preoperative assessor is to take on responsibility for obtaining written consent for surgery and/or anaesthetic, they need to have a good working knowledge of relevant anaesthetic and surgical procedures, risks and benefits, contra-indications and what actions need to take place. They have to be able to provide adequate, accurate information for patients to be able to make informed decisions about their operation and anaesthetic. Documentation of the information given to the patient and use of the appropriate forms is essential, in relation to obtaining written consent.

At level 5, the preoperative assessor is likely to have met all the competencies from all the previous sections and, in addition, will assume a leadership role within preoperative assessment.

Section 9: Lead preoperative assessment role for the Trust

The competency statement reads: 'To act as a lead nurse for the Trust.'

At this level, the preoperative assessor assumes a wider remit with regard to preoperative assessment. They will actively participate in local and regional activities and act in a leadership role for preoperative assessment within the organisation.

Section 10: Preoperative assessment service developments

The competency statement reads: 'The nurse is able to act as a key player in initiating, taking forward and promoting preoperative assessment service developments at local and regional levels.'

At this level, the preoperative assessor will be proactive in identifying and taking forward developments in preoperative assessment. This will include areas such as audit, research and development, and key aspects of any change processes.

Section 11: Advanced practice

The competency statement reads: 'The nurse works at an advanced level of practice and is involved at a strategic level with clinical, managerial, education, research and practice development aspects of preoperative assessment.'

This will involve areas such as autonomy and accountability at an advanced level of practice and consideration of legal, ethical and professional issues relating to the advancement of practitioners' roles. They are able to work as an autonomous practitioner within preoperative assessment but are also part of the multi-disciplinary team.

Each section contains activities that are required in order to enable the nurse to achieve the competencies identified and the evidence that they need to gather in order to demonstrate that the competencies have been successfully achieved. All preoperative assessment nurses are expected to meet all the competencies outlined within sections 1 to 3 of the portfolio. As the nurse progresses in relation to their level of practice, they are able to build on these initial competencies, depending on which level they have reached or is progressing towards. As the nurse moves from levels 1 to 5, they are expected to meet more competencies, in accordance with that particular level of practice.

The portfolio as a learning tool and an assessment tool

Due to the progressive nature of the preoperative assessment portfolio, it is used as both a learning tool and as an assessment tool. As a learning tool, it is used to help guide staff who are new to preoperative assessment. It enables them to identify the knowledge and skills required to practise within preoperative assessment and provides them with a structured plan for working towards the development of their knowledge and skills. Once they have worked through the portfolio, through self-directed learning, supervised practice and observed practice, they can be assessed as competent to practise at whichever level of practice they fit.

For more experienced preoperative assessment staff, the portfolio can be used as a tool to reflect on their current practice and to guide them in advancing their practice within preoperative assessment. As it is likely that this group of staff will be supervising and teaching more junior members of the team, they can use the portfolio to help with teaching and assessing junior staff. The portfolio is also useful in terms of identifying personal and professional development opportunities and achievements from a career planning and appraisal viewpoint.

Assessment of the competencies

Once the portfolio has been completed and reviewed by the preoperative assessment lead nurse or another senior member of preoperative assessment staff, the nurse is ready to be assessed in practice by one of these senior members of staff. Prior to completion of the final practice-based assessment, the nurse is encouraged to use the portfolio in a reflective manner, and to consider their own skills and knowledge and the extent to which they feel they are able to meet the specified competencies and at what level (levels 1 to 5), thus using the portfolio as a form of self-assessment.[37] Having assessed their performance against the specified competencies, it is possible to establish a 'strengths versus opportunities' ratio that can be used to highlight competence or identify opportunities for further development.[38]

The final assessment involves the nurse being observed in practice by a senior member of preoperative assessment staff, who has previously undergone assessment through this portfolio process. An assessment form is used, which enables the assessor to check whether the nurse has achieved each of the specified competencies required within a particular level of practice. This element of peer review strengthens the initial self-assessment process and facilitates the provision of constructive feedback to the nurse.[39] Constructive feedback is considered to be an essential step in developing skills and in improving practice.[40] Although not currently incorporated within the framework outlined here, it would be useful to consider patient feedback as part of the competency assessment for preoperative assessors.[41] The interaction between the assessor and the patient and/or carer is so vital to the patient's overall experience of their surgical journey and should not be overlooked.

Other competency frameworks have been developed across the United Kingdom, which are designed to meet the needs of the organisations they serve and have been developed very much as locally based initiatives. One example is of a competency package for all new preoperative assessment nurses, that covers assessment of competencies for anaesthetic assessment forms, electrocardiograph recording and reading, lung function testing, blood pressure monitoring and referrals. Another framework describes three essential components for the preparation of preoperative assessment nurses, using a medically orientated approach, namely undertaking masters-level modules in anatomy, physical examination and test ordering, having a senior doctor as a clinical mentor and being required to maintain a learning log book as evidence of developing skills.[35]

Other competency frameworks have been developed from a much wider perspective involving the Department of Health and various professional organisations and are designed to fit with nationally based education and training programmes. A training guide published by the Royal College of Anaesthetists[42] outlines the training and assessment required for different levels of anaesthetic trainees, which leads them to a certificate of completion of training in anaesthesia. This is a competency-based training and assessment tool used as part of the anaesthetist's overall anaesthetic training programme, which includes competencies for preoperative assessment.

The Surgical Care Practitioner programme was developed as part of a national initiative by the Department of Health, in conjunction with professional bodies, including the Royal College of Surgeons of England and Association of Operating Department Practitioners.[43] It is aimed at nurses and other healthcare professionals who are working at or towards senior/specialist and/or advanced practitioner levels 6 and 7 of the Agenda for Change banding scale.[25] It requires the trainee surgical care practitioner to demonstrate competence in both core and speciality elements, including elements inherent within preoperative assessment. Two levels of competence are utilised within this programme, and the trainee practitioner maintains a portfolio of evidence which provides a record of progress that informs the assessment process and its outcome.

The Department of Health and NHS Modernisation Agency worked with a number of professional bodies, including the Royal College of Anaesthetists, in the production of the Anaesthetic Practitioner Curriculum Framework.[44] This is a programme delivered at post-graduate diploma level. Within this framework, communication, practical procedural and clinical examination skills are identified to meet the requirements of the programme. This includes a framework of competencies that the Royal College of Anaesthetists use for the clinical teaching of the anaesthetic practitioner student. Amongst these competencies are a number of core competencies that relate to preoperative assessment. A selection of these competencies can be found in Box 20.2.

Box 20.2 Anaesthetic practitioner curriculum framework

(Selection of competencies within programme)

1. The anaesthetic practitioner shows an understanding of the principles underlying the preparation of the patient for surgery:

- Knows the ASA classification and other scoring systems such as Glasgow Coma Scale
- Explains the implications for anaesthesia of common operations
- Explains the implications for anaesthesia of common medical conditions
- Explains the importance of the patient's anaesthetic history
- Describes the relevant protocols and guidelines relating to preparation of patients for anaesthesia and surgery

---

Another example of a national framework has been produced by NHS Education for Scotland for the role of anaesthetic assistant.[44] They have developed a portfolio of core competencies for anaesthetic assistants. These competencies are used as a benchmark for training and education courses; for practitioners to check their existing levels of competence and to use as a portfolio of evidence for continuous professional development. These competencies relate closely to the NHS Knowledge and Skills Framework.[25] Within the portfolio are core themes, including patient care and communication. In addition, there are general core competencies, such as preparation of patients for theatre and airway management. Again, the competencies cover numerous aspects of preoperative assessment.

By reviewing the available competency frameworks, such as those identified above, it is possible to build a picture of what competencies are required for preoperative assessment and what the standards of practice should be. This is based on available examples of best practice and a sound evidence base, in addition to recognition of consultations with experts within the field of practice under consideration, namely, within the context of preoperative assessment.

Educational courses for preoperative assessment

Since the 1990s, higher education institutions and health service providers in the United Kingdom have been encouraged to work more closely together in order to provide relevant educational programmes that enable fitness for practice and purpose on registration.[45] This theme has filtered into post-registration education as well and certainly influenced decisions in terms of designing units of learning at the local university that were applicable to preoperative assessment practice. The preoperative assessment lead nurse at the hospital Trust under consideration worked at the local university as well as within the hospital Trust. This was valuable in creating a link between academia and service provision and in ensuring that relevant units of learning were designed and delivered in line with the reality of practice within preoperative assessment. In conjunction with the competency portfolio, it was decided that preoperative assessment nurses would enhance their practice further through attendance at formal educational courses.

The first unit of learning is *preoperative assessment and planning* which covers the main elements of preoperative assessment, such as the aims of preoperative assessment, assessment strategies, information-giving, informed consent, physical examination and history taking, operating theatre experience, admission and discharge planning and preoperative investigations. it also covers the wider picture of preoperative assessment to enable nurses to see preoperative assessment within the broader context of surgical services, locally, nationally and globally. Attendance at the university provides an opportunity for preoperative assessment nurses from across the region to get together within a supportive environment. Students find this extremely valuable from the point of view of structured time for group reflection, sharing practice, discussing difficulties and other general networking issues. It has been suggested that reflecting on practice can help to maintain or improve the quality of patient care by encouraging self-awareness and critical appraisal.[46]

The second unit of learning, *Health Assessment and Physical Examination*, is more practical and enables students to develop physical examination, history taking and clinical decision-making skills. This unit of learning is appropriate for those preoperative assessment nurses or other healthcare professionals who are working towards more autonomous preoperative assessment roles and running practitioner-led preoperative assessment services. For those preoperative assessment nurses wishing to further their education and to take on higher level or leadership roles within preoperative assessment, the university also offers a Royal College of Nursing-approved Nurse Practitioner programme.[47]

Current thinking within nurse education aims at alleviating the theory-practice gap that is said to exist.[48] The combination of the preoperative assessment competency portfolio and the education provided by the local university appears to be a step in the right direction in terms of enabling staff to balance the theory and practice aspects needed for gaining knowledge, skills and understanding for preoperative assessment, at least at this local level.

Over the last few years, universities and other educational organisations, as well as commercial companies, have developed a variety of different courses to provide both the theory and practice of preoperative assessment knowledge and skills. An interactive electronic learning tool was developed in 2002 by Southampton University and the NHS Modernisation Agency[7] and provides a good educational tool to support learning around preoperative assessment. This focuses on learning around three cases studies and covers areas such as anaesthetic concerns, history taking, physical examination, investigations and care planning.

Conclusion

This chapter has provided an insight into an education, training and assessment programme for nurses working at specified levels of practice within preoperative assessment that has successfully been introduced within one particular hospital Trust. This programme provides a model for supporting the education, training and assessment of preoperative assessment nurses at this particular Trust. Although this is very much a local initiative, it may well be worthy of consideration in planning and implementing preoperative assessment programmes elsewhere.

References

1. D. Casey (2003). The effectiveness of nurse-led surgical pre-assessment clinics. *Professional Nurse* **18**(12): 685–7.

2. Department of Health (2002). *NHS Modernisation Agency: National Good Practice Guidance on Pre-operative Assessment for Day Surgery.* London: The Stationery Office.

3. Department of Health (2003). *NHS Modernisation Agency: Operating Theatre and Pre-operative Assessment Programme.* London: The Stationery Office.

4. L. Wadsworth, A. Smith and H. Waterman (2002). The Nurse Practitioner's role in day case pre-operative assessment. *Nursing Standard* **16**(47): 41–4.

5. L. Markenday and H. Platzer (1994). Brief encounters. *Nursing Times* **90**(7): 38–42.

6. Association of Anaesthetists of Great Britain and Ireland (2001). *Pre-operative Assessment: The Role of the Anaesthetist.* London: AAGBI.

7. E. Janke, V. Chalk and H. Kinley. *Pre-operative Assessment: Setting a standard through learning.* (Southampton: University of Southampton, 2002).

8. H. Walsgrove (2004). Piloting a nurse-led gynaecology pre-operative assessment clinic. *Nursing Times* **100**(3): 38–41.

9. V. Newton (1996). Care in pre-admission clinics. *Nursing Times* **92**(1): 27–8.

10. Department of Health (2001). *Good Practice in Consent Implementation Guide.* London: Department of Health.

11. B. Dimond (2003). *Legal Aspects of Consent.* Dinton: Mark Allen Publishing.

12. Department of Health (2003). *NHS Modernisation Agency: National Good Practice Guidance on Pre-operative Assessment for Inpatient Surgery.* London: The Stationery Office.

13. R.W. Redman, C.B. Lenburg and P.H. Walker (1999). Competency assessment: methods for development and implementation in nursing education. *Journal of Nursing Issues* (online). 30 September. Available from http://www.nursing-world.org/ojin/topic10/tpc10_3.htm (accessed 10.6.2006).

14. A. Graham (2005). The development of a competency assessment for vacuum assisted closure therapy. *Nurse Education in Practice* **5**(3): 144–51.

15. H. Walsgrove (2006). Putting education into practice for pre-operative patient assessment. *Nursing Standard* **20**(47): 35–9.

16. R. Watson (2002). Clinical competence: Starship Enterprise or straitjacket? *Nurse Education Today* **22**: 476–80.

17. Bournemouth University (2007). *Nurse Practitioner Masters Programme Handbook.* Bournemouth University.

18. M&K Update. Courses: Pre-operative Assessment. Available from http://www.mkupdate.co.uk/coursedetails (accessed 16.11.2006).

19. Nursing and Midwifery Council (NMC) (2004). *Code of Professional Conduct.* London: NMC.

20. P. Benner (1984). *From Novice to Expert: Excellence and Power in Clinical Nursing Practice.* Menlo Park, California: Addison-Wesley.

21. B.S. Barnum and K.M. Kerfoot (1995). *The Nurse As Executive* (4th edn). Maryland: Aspen Publishers.

22. M.J. Nicol, A. Fox-Hiley, C.J. Bavin and R. Sheng (1996). Assessment of clinical and communication skills: operationalizing Benner's model. *Nurse Education Today* **16**(3): 175–9.

23. E.P. Gatley (1992). From novice to expert: The use of intuitive knowledge as a basis for District Nurse education. *Nurse Education Today* **12**(2): 81–7.

24. M.L. Pullen (2003). Developing clinical leadership skills in student nurses. *Nurse Education Today* **23**(1): 34–9.

25. Department of Health (2004). *Agenda for Change: Final Agreement.* London: Deptartment of Health.

26. M. Eraut (1994). *Developing Professional Knowledge and Competence.* London: The Farmer Press.

27. C.C. Stuart (2003). *Assessment, Supervision and Support in Clinical Practice.* London: Churchill Livingstone.

28. R. Meretoja, H. Leino-Kilpi and A.M. Kaira (2004). Comparison of nurse competence in different hospital work environments. *Journal of Nursing Management* **12**(5): 329–36.

29. E.A. Girot (1993). Assessment of competence in clinical practice – phenomenological approach. *Journal of Advanced Nursing* **18**: 114–19.

30. P.L. Ramiruti and A. Barnard (2001). New nurse graduates' understanding of competence. *International Nursing Review* **48**: 47–57.

31. K. Manley and B. Garbett (2000). Paying Peter and Paul: reconciling concepts of expertise with competency for clinical career structure. *Journal of Clinical Nursing* **9**: 347–59.

32. R. Meretoja, E. Eriksson and H. Leino-Kilpi (2002). Indicators for competent nursing practice. *Journal of Nursing Management* **10**(2): 95–102.

33. M.J. Watkins (2000). Competency for nursing practice. *Journal of Clinical Nursing* **9**: 338–46.

34. S. Redfern, I. Norman, L. Calman, R. Watson and T. Murrells (2002). Assessing competence to practise in nursing: a review of the literature. *Research Papers in Education* **17**: 51–77.

35. H. Kinley, C. Czoski-Murray, S. George, C. McCabe, J. Primrose and C. Reilley (2001). Extended scope of nursing practice: A multi-centred randomised controlled trial of appropriately trained nurses and pre-registration house officers in pre-operative assessment in elective general surgery. *Health Technology Assessment* **5**: 20.

36. M. Fearon (1998). Assessment and measurement of competence in practice. *Nursing Standard* **12**(22): 18–24.

37. F.M. Quinn (2000). *Principles and Practice of Nurse Education* (4th edn). Cheltenham: Stanley Thornes.

38. D. King (2005). Development of core competencies for infection prevention and control. *Nursing Standard* **19**(41): 50–4.

39. N. Gopee (2000). The role of peer assessment and peer review in nursing. *British Journal of Nursing* **10**(2): 115–21.

40. C.M. Knight, P. Moule and Z. Desbottes (2000). The grid that bridges the gap. *Nurse Education Today* **20**(2): 116–22.

41. J. Carnie (2002). Patient feedback on the anaesthetist's performance during a pre-operative visit. *Anaesthesia* **57**(7): 697–701.

42. Royal College of Anaesthetists (2007). *The Certificate of Completion of Training in Anaesthesia III.* London: RCoA.

43. Department of Health (2006). *The Curriculum Framework for the Surgical Care Practitioner.* London: Department of Health.

44. Department of Health/Modernisation Agency (2005). *Anaesthesia Practitioner Curriculum Framework.* London: Department of Health.

45. Department of Health (2001). *Working Together, Learning Together.* London: The Stationery Office.

46. N. Chambers (1999). Close encounters: the use of critical reflective analysis as an evaluation tool in teaching and learning. *Journal of Advanced Nursing* **29**(4): 950–7.

47. Royal College of Nursing (2002). *Nurse Practitioners: An RCN Guide to the Nurse Practitioner Role, Competencies and Programme Accreditation.* London: Royal College of Nursing.

48. M. Williams (2003). Assessment of portfolios in professional education. *Nursing Standard* **18**(8): 33–7.

21 Developing protocol and guidance to support assessment services

Paul Knight
Liz Kenny

SUMMARY

This chapter will describe:

- **definitions of guidelines and protocols**
- **approach to development of perioperative guidelines**
- **practical considerations in reviewing existing guidelines and protocols**
- **a case study from the UK NHS.**

INTRODUCTION

Like it or not, guidelines and protocols are becoming an increasing part of modern life in general and healthcare in particular. But one must be aware right from the start of the difference between guidelines and protocols, a distinction not lost on politicians and lawyers in other walks of life. In the Scott Enquiry on export of defence equipment to Iraq, Lady Thatcher[1] demonstrates an awareness of the real scope of guidelines when she states: 'They are what they say, guidelines, they are not the law. They are guidelines.'

In this chapter we will discuss the difference between clinical guidelines and clinical protocols, how they work harmoniously in the healthcare arena, and the legal aspects of working with clinical protocols and clinical guidelines. We will show the reader how integrated care pathways (ICPs) use and promote the use of clinical guidelines and clinical protocols for the benefit for patients. The use of clinical protocols and guidelines is paramount in the preoperative assessment (POA) specialism if nurses are to be equipped to work in nurse-led clinics so we will be discussing the sort of guidance needed in POA and the considerations involved.

Finally, the authors will discuss how they and their team members managed the successful development of POA clinical protocols and clinical guidance in their hospital.

Clinical protocols and clinical guidelines: What are they and why do we need them?

There are various dictionary definitions of the term 'protocol'; however, definitions related to 'clinical protocols' are as follows:

- 'the plan for a course of medical treatment or scientific experiment'[2]

or

- 'a document that describes the objective(s), design, methodology, statistical considerations, and organization of a trial. The protocol usually also gives the background and rationale for the trial'[3]

Clinical protocols are also described as an agreed framework, outlining care to be provided to patients in a designated area of practice.[4] They are rigid statements, allowing little or no flexibility or variation, setting out a precise sequence of activities that need to be adhered to when managing an identified clinical condition.[5]

Clinical protocols are commonly used in clinical trials, such as drug trials, allowing a plan of action to be documented and agreed upon on the basis of best available evidence by a designated group of professionals. Clinical protocols are frequently designed to be concise reference documents, allowing professionals to access quickly agreed methods of action/ treatment. In a large organisation clinical protocols can be used to review and improve service quality, providing evidence of actions that the organisation has taken to assure services.[6]

The NHS Modernisation Agency and National Institute for Health and Clinical Excellence (NICE) promote protocol-based care to give staff greater opportunities to work in new ways and to make the best use of their skills, knowledge and expertise.[7] The government bodies say that clinical protocols address the key questions of what should be done, where, when and by whom, maximising the contribution of the multi-disciplinary team (MDT) to patient care. Clinical protocols can assist in removing barriers that only allow doctors or nurses to perform particular types of care.[7] Some would argue that the 'removal of barriers' justifies the previously quoted anxiety regarding the breaking down of professional practice, as clinical protocols allow unskilled staff to perform tasks that were previously performed by highly skilled and educated staff. However, clinical protocols and guidelines are a reflection of a changing workforce, in which the numbers of highly skilled and educated staff are diminishing, while the workload is rapidly increasing. Therefore, clinical protocols are necessary to support the workers who are increasingly filling these gaps (see Box 21.1). An example of clinical guidance on the development of clinical protocols is the European Medicine Agency guidelines for good clinical practice,[3] which define how protocols should be written and followed to ensure international standards are achieved.

Unfortunately, clinical protocols can be perceived as de-personalising care, as they can break down professional practice into chunks of activities. Clinical protocols have been described as negatively affecting individual care management by restricting clinical discretion and by increasing workload as they need regular review. Eventually, they may impact on the need for qualified staff in a variety of care settings.[4] Compliance with protocols can be problematic and dissemination needs to be effective.

However, clinical protocols can also have a positive effect as their development can permit staff to feel justified or confident in providing care that was previously seen as an inefficient use of resources[6] such as certain drug therapies. Clinical protocols can provide a framework for a complex, specialised sequence of activities and can ensure consensus within a team, contributing towards facilitating change.[4]

Box 21.1 The benefits of working with protocols to extend a nurse's role[8]

The NHS Modernisation Agency discussed how the redesign of a nurse's role into that of a 'perioperative specialist practitioner' (PSP) benefits the patient and the surgery and anaesthetic division. The aim is to help reduce waiting lists for inpatient and day surgery by allowing a speeding up of care delivery whilst simultaneously the patients benefit from having dedicated one-to-one care from the PSP. The PSP is able to perform a range of diagnostic and procedural tasks, including many tasks previously carried out by pre-registration house officers and senior house officers, by using rigorous protocols that clearly state what the PSP can do, when and where. The PSP is supported legally to practise beyond the original role boundaries.

Guidelines are commonly described as 'a general rule, principle, or piece of advice'[9] However, clinical guidelines are defined as: 'Systematically developed statements to assist practitioner and patient decisions about appropriate health care for specific clinical circumstances.'[10]

Clinical guidelines are collated summaries of the current best available evidence regarding clinical efficacy and cost-effectiveness of aspects of healthcare provided to individuals and the general public and the use of technology and interventional procedures in primary and secondary practice. Clinical guidelines are more common than clinical protocols and are intended to help guide an already very busy health professional to provide the most suitable evidence-based care. They don't replace the health professional's existing knowledge and skills to make decisions based in individual cases and circumstances. National clinical guidelines aim to ensure that care is consistent and therefore lessen the chance of individual patients being affected by the 'postcode lottery' effect if a patient needs a particular, expensive form of treatment.

Clinical guidelines are used by large organisations to develop standards in healthcare and therefore should be of good quality to allow practitioners to be confident when using them.[5] They can be used nationally or can be adapted for local use with the inclusion of operational information.[10] Clinical guidelines can be used to assist in the assessment of individual health professionals and can also be used as a tool to assist with the ongoing education and training of individuals or groups of healthcare professionals.[11]

Clinical guidelines are devised by multi-disciplinary groups with the intention of improving the quality of care. There are national and international organisations providing clinical guidance and assistance, such as NICE, Appraisal of Guidelines Research and Evaluation (AGREE), Guidelines International Network (GIN) and the Scottish Intercollegiate Guidelines Network (SIGN) which are used in all areas of healthcare practice, encompassing the professional practice of healthcare professionals and the care they are expected to provide to patients/carers. For example, UK-based nurses are governed by the Nursing and Midwifery Council (NMC) and their unions, such as the Royal College of Nursing (RCN), who provide clinical guidelines on subjects such as wound care, record keeping and fitness to practice. NICE[12] have recently released an updated 'Guidelines Manual' offering advice to its guideline developers on the processes that should be undertaken in the production of guidance. The AGREE Instrument[13] was designed by an international collaboration of researchers and policy makers to improve the quality and effectiveness of clinical practice guidelines in any disease area, including those for diagnosis, health promotion, treatment or interventions. AGREE promote use of the instrument to provide a framework for assessing the quality of clinical practice guidelines developed by local, regional, national or international groups or affiliated governmental organisations.

NICE[11] describe their clinical guidelines as 'recommendations on the appropriate treatment and care of people with specific diseases and conditions within the NHS'. The GIN website[14] states that their aim is to promote clinical guidelines through supporting international collaboration of large organisations. It has a database of thousands of guidelines that members can access to review existing international guidelines. SIGN[15] aim to improve the quality of healthcare for patients by reducing variation in practice and outcome. They do this through the development and dissemination of national clinical guidelines, containing recommendations for effective practice that are based on current evidence.

Box 21.2 Five key reasons for choosing an area in which to develop clinical guidelines[16]

1. Where there is excessive morbidity, disability or mortality

2. Where treatment offers good potential for reducing moridity, disability or mortality

3. Where there is wide countrywide variation in clinical practice

4. Where resources involved are resource intensive – either high volume and low cost or low volume and high cost

5. Where boundary issues are involved, across sector and across professional boundaries.

Five key reasons for choosing an area in which to develop clinical guidelines[16] have been identified in Box 21.2. However, guidelines that have cost-reduction at the heart of their rationale or pay no attention to the level of resources required may not always be an appropriate basis on which a health professional can be expected to make a clinical decision. But they can be used as a tool to help the healthcare professional to make a decision according to the best available evidence.[5]

Clinical guidelines that impact the POA specialism are the NICE guidelines[17] regarding the use of routine preoperative tests for patients having elective surgery. The clinical guidelines offer advice on which tests are relevant, depending on the health status of the individual patient and type of planned surgical procedure. Evidence was collected to examine the implications of ordering or omitting preoperative tests such as blood tests, X-rays and ECGs, from patients who were apparently healthy. The outcome was to offer guidance to reduce the number of tests performed following the preoperative assessment of healthy patients. Clinical guidelines produced by the NHS Modernisation Agency[18,19] offer guidance regarding the who, where, what, when and how of setting up preoperative assessment services for inpatients and day surgery.

Clinical protocols and clinical guidelines can be integrated to operate together. Protocols can be a functional part of a clinical guideline or integrated care pathway (ICP), advising on topics such as administration of IV medication, or X-ray procedures.

Legal aspects of guidelines and protocols

The law does not distinguish between definitions of clinical protocols and clinical guidance, or any other statements of clinical guidance, as they share the same general meaning as statements of advice to healthcare professionals on how to proceed in particular circumstances.[20]

Clinical guidelines can be used in a court of law as evidence of accepted and customary standards of care by the defendant or prosecution during trials examining claims of negligence. They can demonstrate if a healthcare professional has deviated from or adhered to an accepted standard of practice, providing the courts with a benchmark by which to evaluate clinical judgement, but they do not actually set legal standards for clinical care.[21] However, clinical guidelines are unlikely to be accepted as a 'gold standard' of care as the specific details of individual case circumstances will also need to be taken into account.[22] The Bolam test is a standard test of negligence, allowing a court to measure the defendant's actions against that of an average person. But because healthcare professionals have more than average abilities, the court measures them against the experts in their fields of expertise. Therefore, it is the testimony of an expert witness that the courts draw on to establish accepted and proper practice in specific individual cases, not the standards within a set of guidelines.[22]

The authors of clinical guidelines do not have a standardised duty of care; ultimately it is the responsibility of the healthcare professional using the guidelines to be aware of this when they choose to utilise the guidance.[22] There are known cases where the judge has considered the guideline development process;[23] therefore documentation of discussions and meetings is essential to provide evidence of the consultation process between the healthcare professionals involved. The courts will consider whether the clinical guidelines are reasonable, so it is important that they reflect the opinions of a responsible body of healthcare professionals, even if there is another group of healthcare professionals who consider a different method of treatment/care is equally reasonable.[23]

In 1997, clinical guidelines were predicted to improve the quality of record keeping and communication between staff and patients[23] as, in the case of Integrated Care Pathways, the processes of individual care would be signed for when completed and any variance from the norm documented for all the healthcare professionals involved to comment or act upon. Poor communication within the NHS caused 9% of complaints from patients in 2005/6. Of the 95,047 complaints, 8,962 were related to written and oral communication/information given to patients.[24] It was the same percentage in 2002/3,[25] which could be interpreted as reassuring as there has been no increase but can also be noted as disappointing as there has been no reduction either. It is vital for healthcare professionals to be aware that all documentation can be used in a court of law as evidence in negligence cases; therefore it is important to document care given, protocols and guidance used and any variance from the predicted pathway of care.

Making effective guidelines

Effective guidelines are embedded in practice and their use is sustained by their being a helpful tool for the clinical teams that are using them. It is all too easy to generate guidance which, although well researched, has no chance of implementation in the areas that it is designed for. Guidelines must be relevant enough to be 'owned' by those people using them.[6]

Schwartz *et al.*[1] argue that good guidelines need to be judged against the following criteria:

- Face credibility: This describes the credibility of the authors/organisation behind the guidelines in the eyes of the target group. For a national guideline, it is important that the organisation(s) producing them be respected by the target audience. For example, an audience of anaesthetists is more likely to take note of fasting guidance from the Royal College of Nursing[26] because there has been involvement and endorsement by the Royal College of Anaesthetists. (And nurses are more likely to take note of the guidance since it is endorsed by their college.) For a local guideline, the group working on the guideline needs credibility amongst all parts of the target audience.

- Validity: Guidelines can be seen to be valid if their adoption results in better outcomes. This is an argument for audit of guideline adoption, and reminds us that new ways of working are often evaluated well with a Plan, Do, Study, Act (PDSA) cycle, where a new change is planned and implemented, evaluated and then modified or discarded as appropriate. In many circumstances, the validity initially comes from clear evaluation of all (not selected) evidence. Systematic review is a tool used to evaluate and summarise evidence from the literature.[27] Criteria are outlined prospectively that are used to identify relevant studies, while rejecting those with poor methodology. This reduces one aspect of bias that is possible in a conventional review, but authors must still be aware of the potential for unregistered negative trials and of the potential for duplication of positive data in several trials. Once the guideline writers have evaluated the quality of the evidence, they should in turn make clear to the audience the basis for their recommendations. Harbour and Miller, on behalf of SIGN,[28] advocate a system of grades of recommendation for guidelines depending on the evidence base available. The availability of good-quality evidence can be particularly challenging in the field of preoperative assessment, where there is often a paucity of good-quality evidence on exactly what to do (note that the NICE guidance on preoperative tests, for example,[17] is based mainly on level IV evidence, expert opinion).

- Reproducibility: Since valid guidelines should be developed with robust evaluation of all available evidence, the users of guidelines have an expectation that different organisations should come up with similar guidelines. Where two organisations publish different guidance there is potential for a loss of faith in the guideline process. It was heartening to see that the British Hypertension Society and NICE produced common guidance on management of hypertension in 2006,[29] after a period of two years when guidance had not been seen to be entirely consistent between the two bodies. One of the best examples of this in the field of preoperative assessment is in the area of planning surgery for patients on warfarin, where there are many local guidelines available, and where close scrutiny reveals slightly differing approaches to the problem.[30-32]

- Representativeness: People developing guidelines are trusted to produce objective guidance that is free of vested interests. They need to be representative of the groups who are expected to follow such guidance, and be seen as people who are well practised in dealing with the everyday challenges of delivery of care.

- Clinical applicability and flexibility: Rigid guidance that takes no account of local circumstances is less likely to succeed than a more pragmatic approach that takes account of how best to use local resources. Sometimes the best solution nationally may not apply where there are unusual local circumstances.

- Clarity and reliability: It is essential that the messages intended by the authors are conveyed to the guideline users without ambiguity, and that the guideline is clear, readable and easy to follow.

- Transparency: It should be clear how and why the conclusions of the guideline have been reached.

- Scheduled review: The ongoing care of clinical guidelines and clinical protocols is the same; they need regular reviews as promoted by the AGREE instrument, which states that all clinical guidelines should have agreed procedures for updating. This is important as it encourages the developers to investigate whether new evidence regarding treatment and new clinical techniques have become available, reinforcing the strength of the clinical guideline. Such a guideline review offers the opportunity to evaluate implementation of the guideline. Following the decision to use a clinical guideline, the date recommended for update of the clinical guideline should be noted, as it may be due for review and the time and effort for all involved in implementation may be wasted if the updated version is going to change practice again.[6] Some guidelines and protocols may be dependent on the number of existing healthcare professionals available. If this, or the availability of equipment and resources changes, then the clinical guidelines or protocols will need updating to ensure that they remain safe.[22]

The final challenge – getting guidelines into practice and the role of ICPs

If guidelines are developed with these recommendations in mind, there is a chance that they will come to be respected and 'owned' by all healthcare professionals making use of them. This is possibly the biggest challenge, to produce guidelines that are used in practice and affect outcomes. The first step has just been described: to make guidelines in such ways that people really *want* to use them. But even the best guidelines can be left on the shelf if the use of the guidelines is not embedded in practice. This is where ICPs come in.

Lady Thatcher's opening quote reminds us that use (or otherwise) of guidelines is now endemic through the whole of society to aid decision-making in complex areas. In industry the pioneers of mass production realised early on that a consistent process was important in producing a top-quality product for the cheapest price. 'Industrial engineering' started appearing as an academic pursuit in the late 18th century and revolutionised the way that manual workers worked to improve overall efficiency by laying out maps of the optimal processes that then had to be followed.[33]

More technical tasks proved to be more difficult to prescribe for, considering both the need for complex decision-making and the perceived challenge to the autonomy of a professional workforce. However, even within healthcare Frank Gilbreth was able to influence the more efficient functioning of the surgical team by advocating that the scrub nurse act as 'caddy' to the surgeon by passing instruments required on demand![34]

The fields of process mapping and the use of standard operating procedures began to influence more complex areas in industry through the 20th century, but healthcare seemed to lag behind until the 1980s. Some clinicians in the USA developed pathways as a means of demonstrating cost effective care and measurable outcomes to insurers, and interest in these concepts spread across the Atlantic over the next decade.[35]

The preceding paragraphs have described how processes can be developed that embed guidelines and best practice into the routine, whether in industry or in healthcare. But healthcare is a complex area, and there may sometimes be valid reasons to deviate from the prescribed pathway. For example, it is probably quite rational in general that a patient be mobilised on the first postoperative day after a total hip replacement, but it is equally rational that this should not take place if a patient is profoundly hypotensive. Crucially an ICP records such deviations from planned care as variances, and these variances can be audited.

If audit reveals that variances occur frequently, there is an opportunity to study the variances in more detail to determine whether any changes to staff training, resources or the pathway itself are required to improve the service, or whether the presence of a variance might simply be a marker of responsible health professionals making sound judgements rather than simply following a rule book.

In their short history, ICPs have had many definitions and many advocates. Venture Training and Consultancy, a company specialising in ICP support and development, produced this definition in 2002:

> An ICP is a document that describes the process for a discrete element of service. It sets out anticipated, evidence based, best practice and outcomes that are locally agreed and that reflect a patient centred, multi-disciplinary, multi-agency approach. The ICP document is structured around the unique ICP Variance Tracking tool. When used with a patient/client, the ICP document becomes all or part of the contemporaneous patient/clinical record, where both completed activities and outcomes, and variations between planned and actual activities and outcomes, are recorded at the point of delivery.[35]

This definition reminds us that ICPs incorporate and encourage adherence to protocols and guidelines of best practice. They become a means of clinical record keeping that not only makes records more structured and accessible to the multi-disciplinary team, but also has a built-in audit tool to evaluate compliance with the planned process of care.

One of the characteristics of POA is that it does need to be tailored to the needs of the client. Undoubtedly there are common elements to any POA, in terms of the questions asked and the physiological observations made, but clearly guidelines have to help the professionals to extract the correct information, deliver the appropriate advice and document it clearly. Examples in POA practice will be discussed later.

The POA healthcare professional has many roles, and guidance is needed to aid assessment and optimisation of fitness, health promotion, information giving and planning for the perioperative period. Each of these areas encompasses a multitude of guidelines, so the challenge in producing the sheer quantity of guidance cannot be underestimated.

How POA clinical protocols and clinical guidelines were developed in Halifax

Earlier in this chapter we discussed the possible reasons why guidelines might be developed. In this case guidelines were required to support a significant reform of the preoperative assessment process, moving from a somewhat inconsistent process run with junior doctors and ward nurses to one where dedicated preoperative assessment nurses would work with sessional consultant anaesthetic support to provide a more consistent process. It was anticipated that such a process would reduce on day cancellations, improve patient optimisation for surgery, reduce the time taken for anaesthetic and surgical assessments on arrival and therefore facilitate same day admission. Happily it has achieved these aims.

Since there was a wholesale change in process, we had a unique opportunity to develop paperwork that fitted into our new process, and to design documentation that automatically referred to other guidance, such that any guidelines that we make are automatically embedded in practice.

Having a number of integrated care pathways already in existence in our organisation, it was logical to use this as a tool, using the preoperative section of a total hip replacement pathway as a starting point. This had the added advantage that the broad appearance and function of the document would be familiar to nursing and medical staff.

The Calderdale and Huddersfield POA ICP (see Appendix, pages 395–406) works with some accompanying notes that describe actions to be taken in response to information obtained from patient or notes. The POA ICP was designed to accommodate the multi-disciplinary team (MDT) who would use the pathway in the POA unit and on admission. It was divided into sections for ease of reference; a quick referral sheet was developed for use by the nursing staff that combined demographic details with a short medical/surgical history and social history. A section is then allocated for the POA nurse to identify MDT members the patient has been referred to such as occupational therapist, physiotherapist, social services or the dietician. The ICP also includes a section containing a list of health conditions with a tick box history sheet, which, at a glance, identifies the health conditions of the patient (see Figure 21.1, page 390). If a problem is identified, a tick would appear in the 'yes' box and this is flagged as a variance on a variance list (see Figure 21.2, page 390).

The problem is expanded on in line with a guideline and an action to be taken is documented in the light of this information.

So in the Halifax POA ICP, a completely healthy person will have no variances listed in the variance box that follows the medical history tick list.

This means that for the medical assessment parts of the pathway (but not the investigations done or information given parts) a variance demonstrates a deviation of the patient from the norm, rather than a deviation from the planned pathway of care. This approach is probably not for the ICP purists, but is a pragmatic approach based on the fact that POA patients have a variety of co-morbidities and no two patients are the same. Since these variances can easily be compared with the guidelines that are structured around the ICP, we believe that we still have the ability to compare the care that should be planned, with that actually delivered. This system of care facilitates variance tracking and audit.

By performing POA early in the surgical journey, we are able to ensure that only fit patients are on surgical waiting lists and comply with the UK Government commitment on surgical waiting times. The timing of the patient's POA appointment had an impact on the design of the POA ICP. We arranged for the appointment to take place soon after the decision to operate was made; therefore a further assessment is necessary before the patient is admitted for surgery. A telephone assessment was incorporated within the ICP, and this takes place up to four weeks prior to admission to ensure there have been no changes to the patient's health since the initial assessment. The POA appointment is also an appropriate time to arrange preoperative tests or special admission arrangements, so a check list was developed to allow the POA nurse to identify, at the original POA appointment, any preoperative preparation required, which could then be referred to at the later telephone assessment.

The accompanying notes and POA ICP incorporate health promotion as information regarding smoking, alcohol intake and illicit drug use is not only requested from all patients but it is also acted upon. The guidelines advise accordingly, regarding excessive use of alcohol, smoking cessation and weight loss. Further assistance is offered in the form of referrals to health specialists such as dieticians and smoking cessation and documented in the POA ICP so each MDT member in contact with the patient is aware of previous discussions and can follow up to review the referrals.

The POA ICP has an MDT section for the anaesthetists to document actions about patients reviewed in the anaesthesia clinic. There are two anaesthetic clinics a week, attended by patients referred to the clinic by the POA nurses due to surgery type (for example, major vascular or abdominal surgery) or uncontrolled or undiagnosed health conditions. Following these appointments, the consultant commonly dictates a letter which is later filed within this section. The anaesthetists also review the ICPs of patients where the POA nurses have concerns, such as patients with complicated but controlled medical histories or unusual diseases. The anaesthetists review all abnormal ECGs and blood tests; therefore a tick box was incorporated to allow the doctors to quickly note if the test was abnormal and needed action. Again, if a letter is generated to a GP, then a copy of it is placed in this section for the MDT, promoting communication between all concerned parties. The MDT section is also used by the POA nurses in the event that a patient is deemed unfit for surgery. The continuing activities that assist the nurses to ensure the patient is eventually safely admitted for planned surgery are documented here.

The POA ICP continues to evolve. For example, originally a smaller variance list was used which did not accommodate the amount of information each health condition required, even if the patient didn't have a complicated health history. This was made twice the size by the ICP facilitator. Also, the brief information regarding surgical and medical history for the ward nurses was originally on separate pages but these were time-consuming to complete and refer to, so the information is now combined in one box on the same page.

This continued evolution of the ICP has been informed by surveys of the POA ICP to assess how various members of the MDT feel about the documentation. Audits have been performed to assess completion of the ICP by the POA MDT and feedback given to the team in order to improve performance and further modify the document. The POA ICP has been used to audit preoperative testing, providing evidence that assists the team in identifying how to reduce costs and identify sections of the accompanying notes in need of updating. Evaluation of the effect of adherence to the guidance has been performed from the perspective of patients and from the perspective of ward nurses and allied health professionals, surgeons, and anaesthetists, and has produced evidence of the resulting improvements in patient preparation and reduced operative cancellations.

Figure 21.3 Example of medical condition list

MEDICAL HISTORY		YES*	NO			YES*	NO
1	Hypertension	√		21	Kidney/Urinary problems		✓
2	Chest Pain/Angina	√		22	Bowel problems		✓
3	Palpitations/Syncope/Fainting		✓	23	L.M.P _____ (Women Only)	N/A	
4	MI		✓		Is there possibility of pregnancy?		
5	Heart Disease	√		24	Diabetes		✓
6	Breathlessness	√		25	Thyroid	√	
7	Chest Diseases		✓	26	Unintentional weight loss		
8	Sleep Apnoea / Snoring		✓	27	Leg Ulcers / Peripheral Vascular		
9	DVT/Blood Clots or Pulmonary Embolism	√			Disease / Skin Condition		✓
				28	Present infections		✓
10	Are you on the Pill/ HRT/ Tamoxifen	N/A		29	**Allergies**		✓
11	Anaemia or any blood disorders		✓	30	Any Previous Surgery	√	
12	Are you taking Aspirin/ Dipyridamole/ Clopidogrel/ Warfarin?	√		31	Have you been diagnosed with CJD or a related condition?		✓
				32	Does any close blood relative have CJD?		✓
13	Stroke / TIA	√					
14	Epilepsy		✓	33	Have you ever received growth hormone treatment?		✓
15	Neurological Disease		✓				
16	Muscle Disease		✓	34	Have you had a skin graft donated from another person?		✓
17	Arthritis	√					
18	Connective Tissue Disease		✓	35	Do you have any disabilities	√	
19	Jaundice / Liver Disease / Hepatitis		✓	36	Mental health issues		✓
				37	Other		
20	Indigestion / Heartburn / Stomach problems	√					

Figure 21.4
Examples of variance list expanding on health conditions and leading to actions

Variation _____ Time _____

Code	Variation & reason for it occurring	Action taken & outcome
1	BP meds taken for 10+ yrs. No recent changes	ECG obtained.
2	Angina - feels its controlled Uses GTN x3 x1 every 3/52. Angiogram 2006- by Dr Bloomer, discharged as no new treatment required.	→ Result in notes.
5	Coronary Heart Disease. Uses statin for ↑ cholesterol Echo in notes from 2002	→ in notes.
6	SOB - occasionally when dressing or when walking up incline. ?due to weight Pt States	PtD

Signature of pre-assessment nurse_____

Code	Variation & reason for it occurring	Action taken & outcome
	Exercise tolerance limited by painful knee – can walk steadily for 1+ mile on flat surface.	Peak flow: 350/450/450 predicted: 546
9	DVT – 1954/9 – none since.	To be aware
12	Aspirin taken daily	None
13	??? TIA – 20 yrs ago. No re-occurance	To be aware
17	OA – Shoulders / neck – uses Gel for pain relief. Pain in toes + knee	Neck flexion OK satisfactory Extension restricted but managed to lift Chin well.
20	Gastritis – 2006, noted on Gastroscope. No continuing symptoms	To be aware
25	Hypothyroidism – takes 275mcg daily since Sept 06.	TFT'S checked
30	See Surgery list on page 2	
38	Confused after Hartmanns in 1996 for 2/7. Was OK when had reversal. Anxious re: reoccurance.	Please be aware.
35	Wears glasses. Has Glaucoma. Has twitch in left eye.	To be aware.
N4/4	ECG abnormal	(A) to see on wardly
N5	Urine to test	on wardly
N8	BMI 41	(A) to see ICP Ref to Dietician ✓

Signature of pre-assessment nurse_____

CONCLUSION

While guidelines are now a common part of everyday life, they are absolutely crucial in a complex area such as POA. Guidelines should be made using the best evidence available, be applicable to local circumstance and be subject to regular review. However, unless the use of guidance is embedded in practice, compliance may be low. In the wider world, this problem is often solved by development of rigid processes, designed to increase productivity and efficacy and in some industries improve quality. In healthcare, the use of integrated care pathways can help improve the quality of care by promoting compliance with guidelines and by facilitating audit of the process, while still leaving scope for clinical judgement.

REFERENCES

1. R. Scott (1996). Report of the enquiry into the Export of Defence Equipment and Dual-use goods to Iraq and Related Prosecutions. London: HMSO. In P.J. Schwartz, G. Breithardt, A.J. Howard, D.G. Julian and N. Rehnqvist Ahlberg (1999). The legal implications of medical guidelines – a Task Force of the European Society of Cardiology. *European Heart Journal* **20**: 1152–7.

2. *American Heritage Dictionary* (2007). http://www.Answers.com/topic/protocol (accessed 22.3.2007).

3. European Medicines Agency (2002). Guideline for Good Clinical Practice. http://www.emea.eu.int/pdfs/human/ich/013595en.pdf (accessed 10.04.07).

4. NHS Working in Partnership Programme (2006). Using Clinical Protocols, Standards, Policies and Guidelines to Enhance Confidence and Career Development. http://www.wipp.nhs.uk/uploads/GPN%20tools/Tool5.8-UsingProtocols.pdf (accessed 12.04.2007).

5. R. Broughton and B. Rathbone (2001). What makes a good clinical guideline? Evidence Based Medicine 1(11). www.evidence-based-medicine.co.uk (accessed 12.04.2007).

6. J. Hewitt-Taylor (2006). *Clinical Guidelines and Care Protocols*. Chichester: John Wiley.

7. NHS Modernisation Agency and NICE (2004). What is Protocol-based Care? http://www.modern.nhs.uk/protocolbasedcare/whatis_leaflet.pdf (accessed 14.04.07).

8. NHS Modernisation Agency (2005). *Protocol Redesign – Some Case Studies and Examples*. London: Department of Health. http://www.wise.nhs.uk/PBCIP/br_role-redesign.pdf (accessed 14.04.07).

9. AskOxford.com (2007). On line dictionary. http://www.askoxford.com (accessed 17.04.07).

10. M.J. Field and K.N. Lohr (1992). *Guidelines for Clinical Practice: From Development to Use*. Institute of Medicine, Washington, DC: National Academy Press.

11. National Institute for Health and Clinical Excellence (NICE) (2005). *A Guide to NICE*. London: NICE. http://www.nice.org.uk/page.aspx?o=guidetonice (accessed 17.04.07).

12. National Institute for Health and Clinical Excellence (NICE) (2007). *A Guidelines Manual*. London: NICE. http://www.nice.org.uk/page.aspx?o=guidelinesmanual (accessed 25.04.07).

13. Appraisal of Guidelines Research and Evaluation (AGREE) Research Trust (2004). The AGREE Instrument. http://www.agreetrust.org/docs/AGREE_Instrument_English.pdf (accessed 28.04.07).

14. Guidelines International Network (G-I-N) (2007). http://www.g-i-n.net/index.cfm?fuseaction=about (accessed 28.04.07).

15. The Scottish Intercollegiate Guidelines Network (SIGN) (2007). http://www.sign.ac.uk/about/introduction.html (accessed 28.04.07).

16. NHS Executive (1996). Clinical guidelines: using clinical guidelines to improve patient care within the NHS. Leeds: NHS Executive. Cited in Health Management Specialist Library (2007). Clinical guidelines: A brief introduction. NHS National Library for Health. http://www.library.nhs.uk/healthmanagement (accessed 22.03.07).

17. National Institute of Clinical Excellence (NICE) (2003). *Preoperative Tests: The Use of Routine Preoperative Tests for Elective Surgery*. London: NICE. http://guidance.nice.org.uk/CG3 (accessed 26.04.07).

18. NHS Modernisation Agency Operating Theatre and Pre-operative Assessment Programme (2003). *National Good Practice Guidance on Preoperative Assessment for Inpatient Surgery*. London: Department of Health.

19. NHS Modernisation Agency Operating Theatre and Pre-operative Assessment Programme (2001). *National Good Practice Guidance on Preoperative Assessment for Day Surgery*. London: Department of Health.

20. B. Hurwitz (1998). *Clinical Guidelines and the Law – Negligence, Discretion and Judgment*. Oxford: Radcliffe Medical Press.

21. B. Hurwitz (2004). How does evidence based guidance influence determinations of medical negligence? *British Journal of Medicine* **329**: 1024–8.

22. B. Hurwitz (2000). Clinical practice guidelines: legal, political and emotional considerations. In M. Eccles and J. Grimshaw (eds) *Clinical Guidelines from Conception to Use*. Oxford: Radcliffe Medical Press.

23. J. Tingle 1997). Clinical guidelines and the law. In J. Wilson (ed.) *Integrated Care Management the Path to Success?* Oxford: Butterworth-Heinemann.

24. The Information Centre (2006). Data on Written Complaints in the NHS 2005-06 http://www.ic.nhs.uk/webfiles/publications/nhscomplaints/WrittenComplaintsNHS151106_XLS.xls (accessed 6.05.07).

25. Department of Health (2003). Written complaints about hospital and community services by service area, England, 2002-03 http://www.performance.doh.gov.uk/hospitalactivity/data_requests/download/nhs_complaints/complaint_03_summary.xls (accessed 14.05.07).

26. Royal College of Nursing (2005). Perioperative fasting in adults and children 2005. http://www.rcn.org.uk/publications/pdf/guidelines/PerioperativeFastingAdultsandChildren (accessed 12.06.07).

27. T. Greenhalgh (1997). How to read a paper: Papers that summarise other papers (systematic reviews and meta-analyses) *British Medical Journal* **315**: 672–5.

28. R. Harbour and J. Miller (2001). A new system for grading recommendations in evidence based guidelines. *British Medical Journal* **323**: 334–6.

29. National Institute for Health and Clinical Excellence (2006). Hypertension: management of hypertension in adults in primary care 2006 http://guidance.nice.org.uk/CG34 (accessed 12.06.07).

30. South Devon Healthcare NHS Trust (2005). Perioperative guideline for patients on Warfarin 2005.

31. Heart of England NHS Trust (2006). Peri-op Warfarin guideline.

32. Calderdale and Huddersfield NHS Trust (2007). Guideline for the perioperative management of anticoagulation in Warfarinised Patients 2007.

33. Wikipedia. 'Industrial engineering.' http://en.wikipedia.org/wiki/Industrial_engineering (accessed 12.05.07).

34. Wikipedia. 'Frank Gilbreth.' http://en.wikipedia.org/wiki/Frank_Gilbreth (accessed 12.05.07).

35. National Library for Health. Protocols and care pathways. http://healthguides.mapofmedicine.com/choices/map/index.html (accessed 9.10.10).

Appendix

Accompanying notes for Preoperative Assessment ICP

Proposed Surgery
If patient having surgery listed in surgical criteria refer to Anaesthesia clinic.

- ⇨ Surgical Criteria:
  - Major GI surgery
  - Arterial surgery (Aortic only e.g. AAA or Aortic Bi-Fem)
  - Bi-lateral Hip Replacements (or knees)

- ⇨ For Nephro-ureterectomy, Radical Nephrectomy notes and ICP for review by anaesthetist in HRI.

- ⇨ If Basket Procedure, consider suitability for Day Case Procedure.

Section 1
Language: Assess need for Interpreter for telephone assessment and on admission, ensure relatives who speak English attend anaesthesia clinic.

Religion: If patient is a Jehovah's Witness and is listed for surgery that requires 'group and save' or 'cross match', ensure FBC reviewed in anaesthetic clinic in conjunction with ICP and steps taken to optimise Hb. Anaesthetist in clinic may need to clarify a discussion of risks with the patient, possibly in clinic or possibly by telephone. **Send ICP and medical notes to anaesthetic clinic.**

Add consent form (titled Treatment by patients who refuse to have blood transfusion) to admission pack.

Medicines: If supplements taken then refer to BADS supplement information sheet for advice.

Section 2
Document referrals in designated portion

Social Services referrals: If patient has TCI date then send to Social Services.
If no TCI then file in ICP, to be sent after successful telephone assessment (unless patient needs urgent Social Services assessment).

Occupational Therapy Referrals:
If patient struggling at home and you assess need for pre-op adaptions, refer to OT.

Section 3

Investigations: sign/initial for all advanced arrangements (e.g. G+S, X-match arranged for 10 days pre-op).

Updates: add a fresh observations sheet to the photocopy of the ICP, and date when observations to be recorded.

Oxygen Saturations: if less than 95% then re-check on another finger.
If less than 95%, send ICP and medical notes to anaesthetic clinic.

Abnormal bloods: CRH – seen by consultant anaesthetist in anaesthesia clinic.
HRI – surgical team to review

1) **Hypertension**
   Obtain ECG. See N4
   Have their medications been changed within the last 2 months?

   > **If Yes and patient has TCI within next 2 months then discuss with Anaesthetist**

   ⇨ BP above 140/90 – check their BP 2 more times, **obtain ECG and Electrolytes and send standard letter to GP to let them know that BP is high but not too high for surgery**.
   ⇨ BP above 180/110 – check BP 2 more times, **obtain ECG and Electrolytes and send standard letter to GP to let them know that BP is too high for surgery and operation postponed**. ICP to High BP drawer for monitoring unless operation very urgent.

2) **Chest pain/Angina**
   How often do they get chest pain? Do they get it at rest/night?

   What is their exercise tolerance? Is exercise limited by chest pain, or by lower limb pain/arthritis?

   Can they climb a flight of stairs at a reasonable pace?

   How far can they walk on the flat?

   Has the patient had investigations e.g. Exercise ECG/Angiogram?

   > **If results abnormal then send ICP and medical notes to anaesthetic clinic**.

   Are they under the care of a Cardiologist? What was said at their last clinic OPD?

⇨ **If chest pain more frequent than once a month send ICP and medical notes to anaesthetic clinic.**

⇨ **If chest pain on walking < 200 metres on the flat or upstairs refer to anaesthetic clinic.**

⇨ **Obtain ECG. See N4. Obtain U&E.**

3) **Palpitations/Syncope/Fainting**

What happens? Have they been investigated? Any syncope/fainting?
If recurrent syncope occurs, have they had a 24-hour ECG?
> **If not, then arrange via Anaesthetist.**
⇨ **Obtain ECG. See N4. Obtain U&E.**

4) **MI**

How long ago? How many MIs?

⇨ **Discuss with anaesthetist in clinic for decision re: suitability for day surgery.**

⇨ **Send notes and ICP to anaesthetic clinic if MI within the last 3 months.**

⇨ **Obtain ECG. See N4. Obtain U&E.**

5) **Heart Disease**

What sort of heart disease?
Do they have high Cholesterol?
> If patient taking Statins, obtain ECG.

Have they had Rheumatic Fever as a child?
> **Send ICP and notes to anaesthetic clinic.**

Ask about chest pain/breathlessness/ankle swelling/exercise tolerance.
Do they have a murmur? Have they had an echo?
> **Send ICP and medical notes to anaesthetic clinic.**

Has patient had heart surgery?

> **If CABG or Stenting within last 3 months, notes and ICP to anaesthesia clinic.**
⇨ **Does patient have abnormal heart rhythm? Is it controlled? > If not refer to anaesthesia clinic (unless heart rate over 120 bpm, then refer to Consultant anaesthetist or medical registrar).**
⇨ **Obtain ECG. See N4. Obtain U&E.**
⇨ **If patient has a Pacemaker, send referral letter to Cardiology ASAP to plan for pre-op check prior to surgery.**

6)   Breathlessness

What is their exercise tolerance? Is exercise limited by chest pain, or by lower limb pain/arthritis?

Can they climb a flight of stairs at a reasonable pace? How far can they walk on the flat?

Do they wake up short of breath at night?

Do they get SOB when lying flat?

How many pillows do they sleep on? If more than 2, is it for comfort only?

⇨   **If SOB on lying flat, or use more than 2 pillows due to breathlessness, refer to anaesthetic clinic.**

⇨   **If SOB climbing stairs or on walking less than 200 metres refer to anaesthetic clinic.**

⇨   **Obtain ECG. See N4. Obtain U&E.**

If referred to anaesthesia clinic then measure Peak Flow rate prior to appointment.

7)   Chest Diseases (Asthma, COPD, Bronchitis, Emphysema)

Ask about breathlessness etc. as above

Measure Peak Flow (best of 3, stood up) and compare with value predicted by age, sex and height.

> **If Peak Flow is less than half the predicted rate then send ICP and medical notes to anaesthetic clinic.**

Does patient use inhalers and/or tablets as prescribed?

How often do they use Salbutamol?

If Salbutamol used more than 3 times a day for symptom relief not optimally controlled

> **Send ICP and medical notes to anaesthetic clinic.**

When did they last need to have a course of Steroids?

> **If they have had a course in the last 6 weeks send ICP and medical notes to anaesthetic clinic.**

Have they been an inpatient due to chest condition in the past year? > **If yes send ICP and medical notes to anaesthetic clinic.**

Have they ever been ventilated in ICU? > **If yes, refer to anaesthetic clinic.**

⇨   **If patient has chronic chest condition, refer to Respiratory nurse for Spirometry > Send results, ICP and medical notes to anaesthetic clinic for review.**

Does patient have productive cough? What is colour of sputum?

8) **Snoring/Sleep Apnoea/excessive sleepiness**

Do they ever stop breathing at night?

Do they feel refreshed after sleep?

Do they 'drop off' during the day? Do they find that sleepiness stops your normal ADL's?

Calculate Epworth Score, if ABOVE 12

> **> Send notes and ICP to anaesthetic clinic if TCI is more than 2 weeks, consider oximetry if not had already and wants investigation.**

> **> If TCI is less then 2 weeks then refer patient to Anaesthesia Clinic.**

9) **DVT/ PE?**

When was DVT or PE and under what circumstances? E.g. spontaneous or post-operatively?

If so, were they on Warfarin? When did they stop taking it?

If recurrent DVTs arrange thrombophilia screen if not on Warfarin.

⇨ **If still taking Warfarin, send ICP and medical notes to anaesthetic clinic asking for information about safety of stopping Warfarin pre-operatively.**

10) **Is patient taking the contraceptive pill, HRT or Tamoxifen?**

⇨ Intra-abdominal surgery > stop Pill/HRT one month pre-operatively and advise patient to discuss alternative contraception with source of pill.

⇨ Gynae surgery > to stop HRT 1 month pre-operatively.

⇨ Hip or Knee patients or Major Backs > to stop HRT/The Pill 1 month pre-operatively.

11) **Anaemia/Blood disorders**

What sort of blood disorder? What treatment has been given? Is it still a problem?

⇨ **Obtain FBC and B12, folate, Ferritin and Iron studies.**

⇨ **If the patient has been anaemic in the last 3 months, repeat FBC, B12 folate, Ferritin and Iron studies.**

⇨ **If last FBC abnormal repeat FBC, B12 folate, Ferritin and Iron studies.**

Does the patient bleed excessively after cuts to the skin? > **If so, obtain Coagulation screen.**

12) **Aspirin, Clopidogrel, Warfarin or Dipyridamole taken?**

Why is patient taking Warfarin? What indication? E.g. DVT/PE, AF, Prosthetic valves.

Patients taking Warfarin for mechanical heart valve > **send notes to clinic**.

If needs Enoxoparin pre-operatively, will need District Nurse arranging.

⇨　Patients taking Warfarin for AF only then stop Warfarin 5 days pre-operatively and arrange check INR 1 day pre-operatively.

⇨　If patient has controlled AF together with other cardiac conditions > send ICP and medical notes to anaesthetic clinic.

⇨　If Aspirin, Clopidogrel, Dipyridamole or NSAIDS taken, refer to Consultant surgeon's preference list (June 04). If surgery below the Diaphragm then stop Clopidogrel 1 weeks pre op.

Awaiting Warfarin guidelines clarification with surgical team – Temporary guidelines in place for General surgery and Orthopaedics April 07. Discuss queries with Dr [name].

13) **Stroke/TIA**

When was the stroke/TIA? If less than 12 months ago, have Carotid Dopplers been done?

If any continuing disability then

⇨　**Notes and ICP to anaesthetic clinic if within last 6 months**.

⇨　TIAs: Have they been investigated? Have Carotid Dopplers been performed? What is the result? > **If less than 12 months ago, send ICP and medical notes to anaesthetic clinic**.

14) **Epilepsy**

Are they under the care of a neurologist? How often do they fit?

When was the last fit? If frequent fits or worsening epilepsy > **send ICP and medical notes to anaesthetic clinic**.

If fitted in the last year, patient not suitable for Day surgery.

15) **Neurological Disease**

What is the diagnosis?

How are they affected?

⇨　**Send ICP and medical notes to anaesthetic clinic**.

16) Muscle Disease

What is the diagnosis?

How are they affected?

⇨ **send ICP and medical notes to anaesthetic clinic.**

17) Arthritis

Does patient have pins and needles in arms associated with neck movement?

If yes, > **send for C-spine AP and lateral x-ray and send ICP and medical notes to anaesthetic clinic.**

Severe limitation to neck movement or neck involvement?

If yes, > **refer to anaesthetic clinic.**

Does the patient take steroids? When did they last need to have a course of steroids?

If neck involvement and Rheumatoid Arthritis, > **arrange flexion/extension C-Spine X-rays looking for atlanto axial subluxation via Anaesthesia clinic.**

18) Connective Tissue Disease

What is the diagnosis? How are they affected? Is the patient under the care of the Rheumatology team? If not then

⇨ **discuss with anaesthetist in anaesthesia clinic.**

19) Jaundice/Liver disease/Hepatitis

When? What was the cause?

If Jaundice ever, **obtain LFTs**

⇨ **If Hepatitis B or C make note in ICP to inform anaesthetist & theatre on day of admission. Also note on Waiting list card and 'jobs list' if awaiting telephone assessment.**

⇨ **Arrange LFT s & clotting.**

20) Indigestion/ Heartburn

Symptoms with food or symptoms on an empty stomach?

Do they get heartburn at night?

What do they take for it?

⇨ If heartburn on empty stomach or at night > **advise patient to see GP ASAP.**
Have they had tests for helicobacter pylori? If positive, did they have effective treatment?

⇨ If classic signs of Dyspepsia, **advise patient to see GP.**

21) Kidney/Urinary problems

Expand on nature of the problem, any frequency, urgency, burning, pain, haematuria or nocturia?
⇨ Discuss referral to continence nurse adviser, if appropriate.
⇨ May need to be catheterised pre-op, note in ICP.
⇨ Obtain Electrolytes.

22) Bowel problems

Expand on nature of the problem.
Discuss referral to continence nurse adviser, if appropriate.

23) Is it possible the female patient is pregnant?

If a possibility, counsel re pregnancy test and take test with consent.
⇨ If positive inform secretary, surgery to be postponed
(unless TOP or VERY urgent surgery).

24) Diabetes

What are their normal blood sugars? Advise regarding stopping oral hypo-glycaemics pre-operatively.

⇨ Obtain HbA1C, U&E and ECG.

25) Thyroid problems

What sort of problems?
Is there a goitre? If so > **send ICP and medical notes to anaesthetic clinic.**
Is the thyroid function checked frequently?
⇨ **If not checked in last 6 months or recent dose change, check TFTs.**
⇨ **If goitre present or abnormal TFTs send ICP to clinic.**

26) Unintentional weight loss

If 10% of usual weight has been lost in last 3 months.
⇨ **Calculate nutritional score and refer to Dietician.**
⇨ **If no obvious cause, > send ICP and medical notes to anaesthetic clinic.**

27) Leg ulcers/Peripheral Vascular Disease/Skin condition

Does affected area appear inflamed or infected?

⇨ **Refer to surgeon if significant to planned surgery.**

⇨ **Refer to Tissue Viability or District Nurses if necessary.**

28) Infections

Is the patient taking any antibiotics?

Have they had cough, cold, chest or urine infection in last 4 weeks?

⇨ **If related to chest and productive coloured sputum noted discuss with anaesthetist doing the list, otherwise clinic anaesthetist.**

⇨ **If related to urine or skin, refer to surgeon.**

29) Allergies

Allergies to medicines, foods, metal, rubber or eggs?

⇨ Latex allergy: **> if patient has TBA then place reminder in ICP that will inform Theatre and Ward prior to admission (add reminder on W/L card and job list) > if patient has a TCI then inform Theatre and Ward.**

⇨ **Indicate the nature of allergic reaction the patient has. Ensure red allergy band completed and placed in notes (with patient name on). Document that same completed in the ICP.**

⇨ **If Anaphylactic shock or patient has Scoline Apneoa, send ICP and notes to Anaesthesia clinic.**

⇨ **If any relatives with Scoline Apneoa > send ICP and medical notes to anaesthetic clinic.**

31–34) If patient answers yes to any of these questions, please advise Infection control team and document same in ICP.

31) Have you been diagnosed with CJD or a related condition?

32) Does any close relative have CJD?

33) Have you ever received growth hormone treatment?

31) Have you had a skin graft donated from another person?

35) Disabilities

Please document if glasses/contact lenses/ hearing aid worn, deafness or any other disabilities.

36) Mental Health Issues

Please document if anti-depressants taken or any other mental health problems noted.

37) Anaesthetic/Surgical problems in past?

Document them and discuss with Anaesthetist in Clinic if significant.
Any family history?

⇨ **If any relatives with Scoline Apneoa > send ICP and medical notes to anaesthetic clinic.**

38) Smoking Habit

What does the patient smoke? How many daily?

Offer brief intervention. Document as variance if same declined.

Discuss risks of smoking. Offer smoking cessation advice/support/referral. Supply 'Stop before you Op' booklet.

39) Alcohol consumption

If over 40 units per week, obtain LFTs, clotting studies, Gamma GT.

⇨   **send ICP and medical notes to anaesthetic clinic.**

40) Recreational Drugs

Document what, when and last time used. If history of sustained cocaine or amphetamines use then

⇨ **Obtain ECG. If abnormal then send with ICP and medical notes to anaesthesia clinic.**

41) Family History

Document cardiac, medical history of immediate relatives.

42) Investigations

Does the patient need Group and Save or a Cross Match? (If patient doesn't have TCI the sign for investigation in advance)

⇨ **Refer to maximum blood order protocol.**

⇨ **If Cross Match/Group and Save required then place completed and SIGNED request form and ID bracelet in filing cabinet reception in P/A Unit and also** request FBC and Electrolytes. This ensures that the tests are performed at the same time a few days before admission. Patient will be reminded during pre-op phone call.

⇨ If taking Lithium patient needs Lithium levels and Electrolytes.

⇨ If patients are taking Statins, obtain repeat ECG and Electrolytes prior to admission (if 6 months since pre-op assessment).

N4) Abnormal ECG

Send ICP and medical notes to anaesthetic clinic unless report shows one of the following abnormalities alone:

Sinus bradycardia rate but rate >50.

Sinus arrhythmia

Atrial fibrillation with rate <90 in known AF.

⇨ If alerted by Cardiology Staff that changes are acute then discuss with Consultant anaesthetist or on call medical registrar ASAP.

N5) Abnormal Urinalysis

⇨ If showing signs of infection – obtain C+S, refer to surgeon.

⇨ If showing any other abnormalities, ICP and notes to anaesthetist in clinic.

⇨ If Glucose in urine, obtain Blood sugar finger prick test and HbA1C. If glucose and Blood sugar elevated then postpone surgery and send letter to GP.

N6) BP outside normal limits

Obtain ECG and Electrolytes.

Refer to Hypertension notes above (No 1).

N7) Abnormal temperature, pulse or respirations

If heart rate raised (more than 100bpm) then > recheck manually.

⇨ If still above 90 bpm > check TFTs and obtain ECG.

⇨ Discuss with Anaesthetist in anaesthesia clinic.

N8) BMI outside normal values

If BMI 40 or above, obtain ECG and Electrolytes. Ensure patient is aware of anaesthetic risks. Offer advice regarding diet and refer to Dietician, if patient in agreement and is a TBA. Document as a variance.

⇨ **Send ICP and notes to anaesthetist in clinic**.

If BMI 35 or above, patient not suitable for day case procedure.
If patient having day case Laparoscopic surgery BMI must be 32 or below.

N14) Discharge Planning Problems

If patient needs social services referral and is TBA then complete documentation and place in ICP to be forwarded following successful telephone assessment. If patient has a TCI, send referral to Social Services ASAP, document in ICP under 'referrals' in section 2.

Pre-operative assessment team
Calderdale Royal Hospital

index